CLINICAL
GASTROENTEROLOGY

A practical problem-based approach

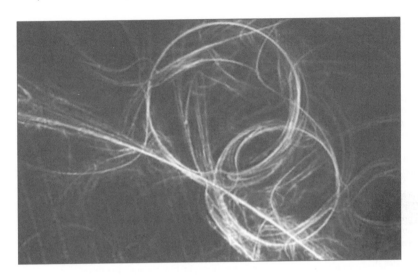

EDITORS

Professor NJ Talley
MD, PhD, FRACP, FRCP (London), FRCP (Edin), FAFPHM, FACP, FACG

Professor of Medicine, Mayo Clinic, Rochester, Minnesota, Consultant Physician, Visiting Professor of Medicine, University of Sydney, Sydney, Australia

Professor CJ Martin
MSc, FRACS

Professor of Surgery, The University of Sydney and Head, Division of Surgery, Nepean Hospital, Sydney, Australia

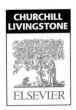

CHURCHILL
LIVINGSTONE

ELSEVIER

Sydney Edinburgh London New York Philadelphia St Louis Toronto

ELSEVIER

Churchill Livingstone
is an imprint of Elsevier

Elsevier Australia
(a division of Reed International Books Australia Pty Ltd)
30–52 Smidmore Street, Marrickville, NSW 2204
ACN 001 002 357

This edition © 2006 Elsevier Australia
First edition © 1996. Reprinted 2004

National Library of Australia Cataloguing-in-Publication Data

---

Talley, Nicholas Joseph.
    Clinical gastroenterology : a practical problem-based
    approach.

    2nd ed.
    Bibliography.
    Includes index.
    For tertiary students.
    ISBN-13: 978-0-7295-3774-2.
    ISBN-10:   0-7295-3774-9.

    1. Gastrointestinal system — Diseases. 2. Gastroenterology.
    3. Digestive organs — Diseases. 4. Gastrointestinal
    system — Diseases — Diagnosis. I. Martin, Christopher J.
    (Christopher John). II. Title.

    616.33

Publisher: Debbie Lee
Publishing Editor: Sophie Kaliniecki
Publishing Services Manager: Helena Klijn
Edited and project managed by Deborah McRitchie
Designed and typeset by DiZign Pty Ltd
Proofread by Tim Learner
Indexed by Max McMaster
Printed by Southwood Press Pty Ltd

FOREWORD

Johann Wolfgang von Goethe (1749–1832) posed the question, 'What is the most difficult of all?', and provided as answer, 'That what you consider the easiest: to see with the eyes what lies before the eyes...'. Clinical practice relies on careful observation and integration of the information—patients usually present with problems, not disease labels. Learning medicine in a problem-based fashion is, therefore, important, and with the second edition of *Clinical Gastroenterology: a practical problem-based approach*, Nicholas Talley and Christopher Martin have produced a teaching gem.

While there is the trend for super-specialisation in modern medicine, a growing need for a straightforward multidisciplinary approach to patients with gastroenterological disorders is recognised. This book represents the current state of the art in the fields of gastroenterology and gastrointestinal surgery and reflects the rapid developments that these two disciplines have made in recent decades. Both disciplines jointly address disorders of the digestive tract, and the specific skills and techniques complement each other. This book reflects best practice in these disciplines.

Applying a clear systematic approach, Talley and Martin provide effective and rational guidance through the clinical presentation, diagnostic work-up and treatment of various symptom categories. Accurate recognition of symptom categories and identification of the most appropriate diagnostic measures and treatment are key issues in this book.

A book devoted to clinical gastroenterology with an emphasis on a practical problem-based approach will never be out of fashion. This new edition provides very valuable information for doctors caring for patients with gastrointestinal disorders and students who wish to obtain a focussed, but sufficiently detailed, overview of the field.

I hope you enjoy studying the fascinating field of gastrointestinal medicine and surgery.

Professor Gerald Holtmann, MD, FRACP, FRCP
Royal Adelaide Hospital
May 2006

FOREWORD

Professors Talley and Martin have drawn on their wide collective experience and encyclopaedic knowledge of the subject matter to produce this very useful and up-to-date text. It is written with characteristic clarity for a wide audience. It will appeal to those who are heading down the road as specialists in gastroenterology or gastrointestinal surgery, its problem-oriented strategy will make it valuable for more generalist doctors such as those in family practice, and it will also be a marvellous reference text for medical students.

To build the book around the symptoms and events that lead a patient to come to a doctor is an intensely practical approach. This is, after all, the starting point of the diagnostic process. This approach will, I suspect, also make the book a valuable text for other health professionals, such as nurses, and I can imagine some patients and their relatives tracking it down and fossicking through it too. But Talley and Martin have not just written a book to help the readers in the art of diagnosis; they take them into basic mechanisms of pathophysiology in a way that is easy to follow and remember, and guide them in evidence-based management as well.

This is a very readable and useful book, which will find its way onto many library shelves and office desks.

Professor ND Yeomans, MD, FRACP, FACG
Dean of Medicine
The University of Western Sydney, Sydney, Australia

PREFACE

It is a great privilege to present the second edition of *Clinical Gastroenterology: A practical problem-based approach*. It is now 10 years since the first edition was published, following the introduction of problem-based learning in universities around Australia and the world. The original goal of this short, integrated textbook of gastroenterology, hepatology and gastrointestinal surgery remains the same: to provide a modern, systematic yet very practical account of the field. This textbook differs substantially from most other textbooks in the field. In order to achieve our goal, we have focused on common and uncommon patient problems as they typically present in clinical practice. A symptom, sign, laboratory test or X-ray finding represents the starting point of each chapter. After a summary of terms and definitions, how to optimally interpret the history and physical examination is reviewed followed by how to logically approach investigations and treatment, ensuring an integration of medical and surgical issues. Finally, each chapter reviews major diseases, including their pathophysiology, natural history and principles of management. Summary tables, management algorithms and illustrations have been incorporated to enhance comprehension. References for further reading based on major review articles and systematic reviews are included. The editors have strived to ensure the chapters provide a uniform approach and are cross-referenced where necessary. Every chapter has been updated to ensure the latest information has been included.

We were very pleased with the positive response to the first edition among medical students and general practitioners, and hope that this new edition will continue to fulfill their needs in this area. We are very grateful to all the contributors who are recognised experts in the field who have provided superb material that is current and easy to read.

We hope that you will find this second edition of *Clinical Gastroenterology* useful in your learning. We also hope that it will provide guidance when you encounter a particular gastrointestinal problem in terms of the best possible management in practice.

NJ Talley and CJ Martin
July 2006

CONTRIBUTORS

Dr PRH Barnes MD, FRACP
Gastroenterologist, North Shore Private Hospital, St Leonards, Australia

Dr S Chew MBBS, FRACS
Senior Lecturer and Staff Specialist in Colorectal Surgery, Nepean Hospital, Sydney, Australia

Associate Professor B Collins BSc, MD, MRCP, FRACP
Staff Specialist in Gastroenterology and Head, Department of Gastroenterology, Royal Perth Hospital, Perth, Australia

Professor IJ Cook MD, FRACP
Professor of Medicine, University of NSW and Director, Department of Gastroenterology, St George Hospital, Sydney, Australia

Dr M Cox MS, FRACS
Senior Lecturer and Staff Specialist in Surgery, Nepean Hospital, Sydney, Australia

Dr V Duncombe MD, MSc, FRACP
Staff Specialist in Gastroenterology, Prince of Wales Hospital, Sydney, Australia

Dr A Keegan BSc (Med), PhD, FRACP
Consultant Hepatologist, Nepean Hospital, Sydney, Australia

Associate Professor JE Kellow MD, FRACP
Associate Professor of Medicine, The University of Sydney, Royal North Shore Hospital, Sydney, Australia

Professor P Kerlin BA, MD, FRACP
Consultant Gastroenterologist/Clinical Professor of Medicine, Princess Alexandra Hospital, Queensland, Australia

Associate Professor D Lubowski FRACS
Associate Professor of Medicine, St George Private Medical Centre, Sydney, Australia

Professor CJ Martin MSc, FRACS
Professor of Surgery, The University of Sydney and Head, Division of Surgery, Nepean Hospital, Sydney, Australia

Dr N Tait
Senior Lecturer in Surgery, The University of Sydney, Westmead Hospital, Sydney, Australia

Professor NJ Talley MD, PhD, FRACP, FRCP (London), FRCP (Edin), FAFPHM, FACP, FACG
Professor of Medicine, Mayo Clinic, Rochester, Minnesota; Consultant Physician, Visiting Professor of Medicine, University of Sydney, Sydney, Australia

Professor G Whelan MD, MSc, FRACP, FAFPHM
Professor/Director of Drug and Alcohol Studies, Physician and Gastroenterologist, Honorary Physician, Department of Gastroenterology, St Vincent's Hospital, Melbourne, Australia

CONTENTS

chapter 1

HEARTBURN, REGURGITATION AND NONCARDIAC CHEST PAIN

HISTORY

Indigestion

Many patients complain of indigestion. What they mean needs to be carefully elucidated as they may be referring to heartburn, acid regurgitation, belching, bloating, abdominal pain, halitosis or even flatus. The exact features of what they mean by 'indigestion' can be elucidated by careful history-taking. Often a combination of symptoms will be elicited.

Heartburn, regurgitation and, to a lesser extent, noncardiac chest pain are symptoms which imply oesophageal disease. The type of oesophageal disease responsible for these symptoms can often be anticipated on the basis of history alone. Physical examination rarely contributes positive findings to support the diagnosis. Heartburn and regurgitation will be discussed together as they often co-exist in patients with gastro-oesophageal reflux disease. Noncardiac chest pain does not imply a particular disease process, but rather a group of disorders and will be discussed separately.

In this chapter, features that help the clinician decide whether symptoms are best described as heartburn and regurgitation will be outlined and associated symptoms supporting the diagnosis of gastro-oesophageal reflux disease and its complications will be discussed. Thereafter, a practical guide to the use of investigations to confirm the clinical diagnosis will be presented as well as an outline of the principles of clinical management. Similarly, a practical algorithm for the diagnosis and management of noncardiac chest pain will be developed.

Heartburn

Heartburn is a term used to describe a specific symptom. Heartburn is a pain or discomfort typically described as burning in nature. Its primary position is usually lower retrosternal, deep to the xiphisternum. Heartburn commonly radiates upwards, retrosternally, occasionally as far as the neck. There may be associated epigastric pain.

The timing of heartburn is characteristic. It occurs intermittently, either postprandially or when the patient bends forward or lies flat in bed, when the gastric contents are level with, or above, the lower end of the oesophagus. When it occurs postprandially, it is most commonly in the early postprandial period, 5 to 30 minutes after a meal. The postural changes that initiate heartburn do so by raising the level of the gastric contents above the level of the gastro-oesophageal junction. The duration of an individual attack, when untreated, rarely exceeds an hour.

The particular factors that precipitate an attack vary considerably from patient to patient. For some, the size of the meal is important, such that it will occur with large meals but not small meals. For others, particular foodstuffs will precipitate an attack. Foodstuffs more commonly incriminated include curries, garlic, red wine, fatty foods, chocolate and citrus juice. The combination of a meal and lying down can be additive in effect. Some patients will describe waking from sleep with severe heartburn a few hours after retiring to bed following dietary indiscretions. Attacks can be precipitated by certain postures but not other apparently equivalent postures. Thus attacks may occur when the patient lies on the right side but not on the left side or supine. Exercise, either isometric, including straining, or isotonic, such as brisk walking or running, can trigger heartburn. Retrosternal burning pain that is triggered by exercise needs to be closely scrutinised to ensure that symptoms of coronary ischaemia are not being overlooked.

Response to medication is often a good sign of whether the patient's complaints are secondary to gastro-oesophageal disease and, therefore, qualify as heartburn. Retrosternal burning pain that is not at least partially relieved by appropriate medication should not be called heartburn, unless there is some other strong evidence supporting gastro-oesophageal reflux disease as the cause of the symptom. Heartburn is usually relieved within several minutes by antacids. Discomfort relieved within much shorter periods or after much longer periods is less likely to be secondary to gastro-oesophageal reflux. Similarly, heartburn usually improves with agents that diminish gastric secretion of acid.

The length of history and frequency of heartburn will vary considerably from patient to patient. Some patients have symptoms dating back over many years, some describe symptoms as occasional only, while others are inconvenienced many times a day. For the individual patient, the temporal pattern of symptoms will be relatively consistent, with little tendency to periodicity, which is more characteristic in 'ulcer patients'.

Heartburn is reported by one-third of the population at least once a month; 10% have daily heartburn. Only a minority of those with reflux symptoms present for medical care.

Regurgitation

Patients with heartburn commonly also complain of acid regurgitation. Although the two symptoms can be closely linked temporally, heartburn tends to be more frequent and, thus, occurs without acid regurgitation on many occasions.

Acid regurgitation describes the intermittent, sudden, and often spontaneous appearance of bitter tasting fluid in the mouth. For some patients, the volume regurgitated is so small that it is not registered as a bolus, but rather a bitter taste. For others, the regurgitated bolus is recognisable as a bolus. Individual patients tend to regurgitate about the same volume of bolus each time. The usual precipitants of heartburn for a particular patient are also the precipitants of acid regurgitation. They include meals (especially big meals), assumption of a horizontal posture, rises in intra-abdominal pressure, and belching. The sensation can usually be cleared by washing out the mouth.

Food regurgitation is described as the predominant form of regurgitation by some patients. This will obviously occur mostly after eating.

Waterbrash is a term used to describe the sudden appearance of a volume of salty tasting or tasteless fluid in the mouth. It is the result of salivary gland stimulation in response to gastro-oesophageal reflux or peptic ulcer disease, but does not have diagnostic value.

Complications of acid regurgitation

Severe acid regurgitation can be associated with other problematic symptoms including choking attacks, a dry cough, asthma, hoarseness of voice, a foul taste in the mouth in the morning, bad breath, a sore tongue, dental caries and nasal aspiration. Some patients complain of waking up episodically with a sensation of choking such that they will cough vigorously, but rarely produce sputum, get up out of bed and even go to an open window to catch their breath. These symptoms subside fairly rapidly. At the onset of such attacks the patient is often described by witnesses as blue in the face. For others, the history suggesting episodic tracheal aspiration will be less dramatic. They may just describe a chronic dry cough perhaps worse in the morning but without sudden exacerbations. When that is the case, other causes of a dry cough will need to be considered and excluded as part of a respiratory work-up. Asthma usually has an allergic basis but, occasionally, it can be precipitated by gastro-oesophageal reflux. Such patients may present later in life without any obvious cause for obstructive airways disease. In these patients, the symptoms of gastro-oesophageal reflux are commonly not severe. Acid regurgitation can result in a chemical laryngitis and cause hoarseness of voice. Usually the regurgitation occurs at night so hoarseness is most evident in the morning, and gradually settles as the day passes. Similarly, waking up with a foul taste in the mouth or bad breath can be attributed to nocturnal gastro-oesophageal reflux. Nasal aspiration is a particularly unpleasant consequence of regurgitation, again usually occurring at night.

Problems with swallowing

Odynophagia

Gastro-oesophageal reflux disease is one of the causes of odynophagia (pain on swallowing). It is usually reported in response to hot or cold foodstuffs (see Chapter 2).

Dysphagia

The sensation of obstructed swallowing is unusual in patients with heartburn and regurgitation and is worthy of special clinical attention. The pathological explanation that should first come to mind when dysphagia is reported is distal oesophageal stenosis secondary to severe, long-standing erosive peptic oesophagitis. In the back of your mind should remain the possibility of an undiagnosed oesophageal carcinoma. It is the implied severity of the reflux disease and the possibility of malignancy that makes investigation by barium swallow and upper gastrointestinal endoscopy mandatory in these patients. The features of dysphagia usually associated with a benign stenosis secondary to peptic oesophagitis are:

- exclusively for solids (not liquids);
- experienced at the lower end of the sternum;

- little variation in severity from day to day given the same sized bolus;
- slow progression in severity over months to years; and
- minimal to no weight loss.

There are some patients with symptoms of dysphagia and reflux for whom an organic cause will not be found by endoscopy or barium swallow; dysphagia in these cases is caused by a motor disorder of the oesophageal body. This abnormality is best evaluated by oesophageal manometry. The symptoms of dysphagia associated with a motility disorder are usually less compelling than those associated with oesophageal stenosis. They are commonly felt higher in the chest and usually vary significantly in degree from day to day.

Belching

Excessive belching is a common complaint of patients with heartburn (see Chapter 7). In some, heartburn may be precipitated by belching.

PHYSICAL EXAMINATION

A typical history of heartburn or acid regurgitation is usually sufficient to diagnose gastro-oesophageal reflux disease. There are no specific signs on physical examination that support the clinical diagnosis. Deep epigastric tenderness may be present, but is not specific and is not of any particular clinical significance.

PATHOPHYSIOLOGY OF GASTRO-OESOPHAGEAL REFLUX DISEASE

The oesophagus and the stomach are separated by a high pressure zone produced by tonic contraction of specialised smooth muscle of the lower oesophageal sphincter. In normal individuals, this functional barrier is maintained except to allow antegrade flow with swallowing and retrograde flow with belching and vomiting. Flow across the lower oesophageal sphincter only occurs when the lower oesophageal sphincter tone is very low (< 3 mmHg). Acid gastro-oesophageal reflux occurs occasionally postprandially in normal individuals during inappropriate relaxations of the lower oesophageal sphincter, or in association with belching.

Acid gastro-oesophageal reflux in patients with gastro-oesophageal reflux occurs by three different mechanisms: 1) spontaneous reflux during inappropriate lower oesophageal sphincter relaxations of increased frequency; 2) retrograde flow prior to recovery of lower oesophageal sphincter tone after swallowing; and 3) increases in intra-abdominal pressure overcoming the weak barrier of a chronically hypotensive lower oesophageal sphincter. Hiatus herniation predisposes to reflux as a result of inadequate clearance of gastric contents away from the lower oesophageal sphincter. Elevation of the head of the bed reduces the chance of retrograde flow of gastric contents other than air in the event of a failure of the lower oesophageal sphincter.

Most of the fluid volume of refluxate is promptly cleared from the oesophagus by one or more swallows. Small amounts of residual acid are neutralised by weakly alkaline saliva with subsequent swallows. Clearance is delayed during sleep when swallowing is less reliably triggered by reflux. Smoking exacerbates the effects of reflux by inhibiting salivation, thereby delaying acid clearance.

Repeated and prolonged exposure to gastric secretions can result in a chemical burn and superficial ulceration of the oesophageal mucosa. The occurrence of injury, expressed as erosive oesophagitis, is dependent on three factors: 1) duration of exposure; 2) the chemical composition of the refluxate; and 3) the natural resistance of the individual. Thereby, we can explain several well-known clinical observations. Firstly, the severity of oesophagitis tends to be worse when oesophageal acidification is prolonged, and reducing gastric acid secretion promotes healing of peptic oesophagitis. Secondly, two patients with similar levels of reflux, as measured by pH monitoring, may have marked differences in mucosal appearance at endoscopy. One may have severe erosive oesophagitis while the other, a normal looking mucosa. The role of bile and pancreatic juice in producing oesophagitis in most patients is limited, but they are responsible for oesophagitis after total gastrectomy.

Heartburn, on the other hand, is dependent primarily on mucosal sensitivity, not mucosal ulceration. Thus, some patients with symptomatically severe heartburn may have no peptic oesophagitis, while others with no heartburn can present with a peptic stricture secondary to long-standing peptic oesophagitis. Therefore, the severity of heartburn is a poor predictor of oesophagitis.

INVESTIGATION OF HEARTBURN AND ACID REGURGITATION

Upper gastrointestinal endoscopy

Gastro-oesophageal reflux results in peptic oesophagitis, but only in a minority of cases. The finding of peptic oesophagitis at endoscopy confirms the clinical suggestion that symptoms of heartburn and regurgitation are due to gastro-oesophageal reflux disease. On clinical grounds, however, many patients with heartburn and acid regurgitation do not need to have their presumed diagnosis of gastro-oesophageal reflux disease confirmed by upper endoscopy. Thus, patients with typical symptoms that occur occasionally and that are completely controlled by simple measures, such as attention to lifestyle (see below) or antacids, do not need upper endoscopy. On the other hand, patients with reflux symptoms and alarm features (such as vomiting, bleeding, weight loss or dysphagia) should always be investigated.

The characteristic endoscopic signs of reflux oesophagitis are shown in Table 1.1 and Figure 1.1. As mentioned above, there is only a weak correlation between the severity of oesophageal acidification and the degree of peptic oesophagitis.

The diagnostic endoscopic examination is always carried as far as the first part of the duodenum looking for incidental pathology. The finding of a chronic duodenal ulcer is significant as, uncommonly, this may be the underlying cause of gastro-oesophageal reflux symptoms; it should be treated medically (see Chapter 5).

Oesophageal biopsy at upper gastrointestinal endoscopy

In some patients, characteristic histological features can be detected in random biopsies of endoscopically normal looking lower oesophageal mucosa. These are:

- relative increase in the papillary height;
- relative increase in thickness of the basal layer of the epithelium; and

- the presence of intra-epithelial neutrophils and eosinophils.

These microscopic findings can be relatively difficult to quantify on routine biopsy specimens. Moreover, the diagnostic value of these findings continues to be disputed, so biopsy is not recommended routinely.

These microscopic signs of 'minimal oesophagitis' should be distinguished from the superficial mucosal ulceration and underlying inflammatory reaction associated with linear erosive peptic oesophagitis.

Upper gastrointestinal endoscopy is usually the only investigation required to assess the cause of heartburn and regurgitation, if any investigation is indicated.

TABLE 1.1: Classification of reflux at endoscopy (Los Angeles—LA—System)

Grade A	At least one mucosal break (erosion) each ≤ 5 mm
Grade B	At least 1 mucosal break > 5 mm but *not* continuous between the tops of 2 mucosal folds
Grade C	At least 1 mucosal break that is continuous between the tops of 2 mucosal folds, but which is *not* circumferential (< 75%)
Grade D	Circumferential mucosal break (≥ 75%)

Upper gastrointestinal radiology

Before the establishment of flexible upper gastrointestinal endoscopy, upper gastrointestinal contrast radiology with barium was the initial investigation for dyspepsia and reflux symptoms. It has been downgraded to a second-line investigation, mainly because it is not a very sensitive detector of the hallmark sign of gastro-oesophageal reflux disease, linear erosive peptic oesophagitis. It does, however, offer

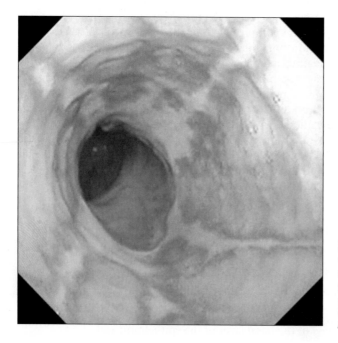

FIGURE 1.1: Endoscopic view of linear erosive peptic oesophagitis (Grade C) of the distal oesophagus.
(From plate 20-4 of the online edition of the Merck Manual, with permission from Dr D Martin.)

complementary information which is sometimes useful. Its main advantages over endoscopy are:

- the diagnosis of a minor degree of oesophageal stenosis secondary to peptic oesophagitis resulting in dysphagia that can be hard to define endoscopically; and

- the more precise definition of the features of an associated hiatus hernia.

Both of these features are relevant if surgery for reflux is contemplated. The radiologist may also detect the occurrence of gastro-oesophageal reflux during the course of the investigation. This finding is only really significant if the reflux occurs freely without stress manoeuvres.

All other investigations of symptoms of gastro-oesophageal reflux have limited roles.

pH monitoring

Episodes of gastro-oesophageal reflux result in oesophageal acidification of the distal oesophagus. Neutral pH is restored by oesophageal peristalsis. These episodes can be monitored and recorded by placement of a pH microelectrode in the distal oesophagus. In the past this test required prolonged nasal intubation, which is unpleasant. That discomfort can now be avoided by attaching the pH electrode to the lower oesophageal mucosa endoscopically. The pH recording occurs by telemetry. The pH electrode subsequently detaches and passes spontaneously. Summation of the duration of episodes over an extended period, usually 24 hours, gives a measure of the underlying pathophysiological process, which can be used to score the severity of the disease. Further, a correlation between symptoms and episodes of oesophageal acidification can be established (see Figure 1.2). The test is not required for diagnosis in the majority of patients with typical symptoms of reflux in whom the diagnosis can be made either endoscopically or, if there is no oesophagitis, on the basis of a successful therapeutic trial with a course of antisecretory treatment. The major indications for pH monitoring are:

- typical symptoms, without endoscopic signs of peptic oesophagitis, not responding to a course of proton pump inhibitors; or

- atypical symptoms, such as cough, asthma, hoarseness or chest pain in patients without endoscopic signs of peptic oesophagitis which do not respond to a course of antisecretory treatment.

Bernstein testing

This is a test of mucosal sensitivity. It involves transnasal oesophageal intubation and perfusion of the distal oesophageal mucosa with dilute (0.1 M) HCl. It is performed in less than one hour. It can be useful if the patient's usual undiagnosed symptoms are reproduced by oesophageal acidification. It can be complementary to pH monitoring in patients whose atypical symptoms are infrequent and do not occur during a pH-monitoring study.

Oesophageal manometry

This test usually has no diagnostic role in the evaluation of symptoms of gastro-oesophageal reflux disease unless anti-reflux surgery is being considered. It may sometimes be useful in the evaluation of patients with symptoms of dysphagia in addition to those of heartburn and regurgitation, where a barium swallow and endoscopy have been normal and the dysphagia remains unexplained (see Chapter 2).

TREATMENT

Clinical management of heartburn and regurgitation

The range of intensity of reflux symptoms extends from a very mild, very occasional discomfort, for which the patient may want little more than some antacid and reassurance, to a regular, incapacitating pain that prevents normal daily activity. Management needs to be commensurate with the magnitude of the clinical problem. Unlike duodenal ulceration, gastro-oesophageal reflux disease is a persistent condition without exacerbations and remissions. Drug therapy has a hierarchy (see Table 1.2). Oesophagitis indicates a need for therapy to heal the mucosa and maintain healing; virtually all patients with severe oesophagitis (LA grade C and D oesophagitis see Table 1.1) will relapse if medical therapy is stopped, as will most (80%) with milder oesophagitis. A review of the clinical management principles for patients with gastro-oesophageal reflux is presented in Table 1.3.

TABLE 1.2: Effectiveness of drugs for gastro-oesophageal reflux

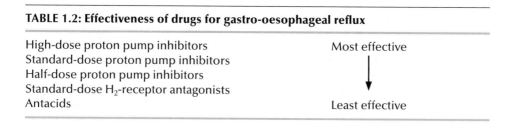

High-dose proton pump inhibitors	Most effective
Standard-dose proton pump inhibitors	
Half-dose proton pump inhibitors	
Standard-dose H$_2$-receptor antagonists	
Antacids	Least effective

Low-level treatment

For most of the population who have occasional and mild symptoms of reflux, low-level treatment is all that is required. Such treatment involves lifestyle changes including:

- weight loss, if overweight;
- avoidance of large meals, particularly before retiring to bed at night;
- postural advice including elevation of the head of the bed by insertion of 20 cm blocks under the bedhead and avoidance of bending; and
- avoiding drugs, cigarettes, alcohol and foodstuffs that might precipitate reflux.

A foodstuff checklist includes: spicy foods, alcohol, fatty foods, chocolates, nuts, tomatoes, as well as many others. Rather than prohibit 'everything' and risk losing patient compliance, it is wiser to establish with the patient which foodstuffs they recognise as triggers, ask them to avoid these, go through the checklist to identify triggers that the patient might not have previously considered and recognised, and then ask the patient to establish relationships between symptoms and triggers so that they might be avoided in the future.

Of these various lifestyle changes, only weight reduction has the potential to change the natural history of the disease. Thus, some patients can clearly identify a critical

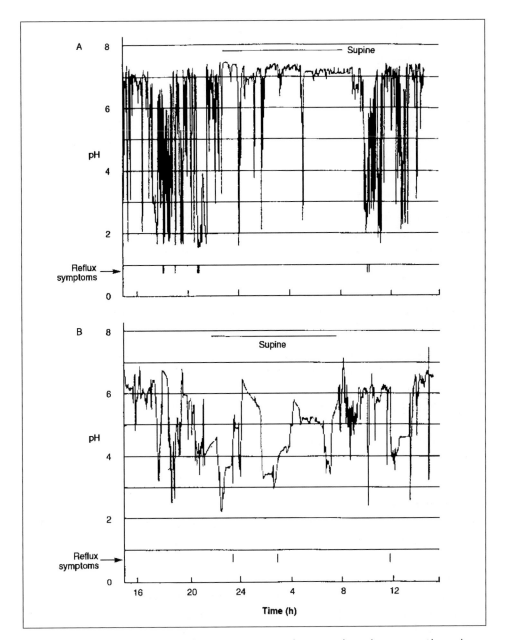

FIGURE 1.2: 24-hour oesophageal pH testing (pH probe 5 cm above lower oesophageal sphincter) **A:** Pathological upright reflux. The lines indicate the times at which the patient had reflux symptoms. These events all coincide with a decrease in pH to below pH 4. The symptoms of this patient are clearly caused by reflux.
B: Pathological reflux during sleep. During sleep, in particular, the oesophageal pH persists longer at a low value due to disordered oesophageal clearance.

A symptom index > 50% ([no. symptoms with pH < 4 ÷ total no. symptoms] x 100%) is considered significant. The symptom-associated probability (SAP) is a more optimal method to estimate if acid reflux episodes are linked to symptoms. The 24-hour recording is divided into 2-min periods, and the 2-min periods before onset of symptoms identified for evidence of reflux (pH < 4.0). The probability (P) that events are unrelated is calculated (using Fisher's exact test). SAP = (1.0 – P) x 100%.
(From AJPM Smout & LMA Akkermans, Normal and disturbed motility of the gastrointestinal tract, *with permission.)*

TABLE 1.3: Features of clinical management of gastro-oesophageal reflux

Low-level treatment

Weight loss, if overweight
Avoidance of large meals
Postural advice such as elevation of bedhead at night
Avoidance of foodstuffs that precipitate reflux
On-demand antacids or H_2-receptor antagonists for breakthrough symptoms

Mid-level treatment

Lifestyle measures of low-level treatment
Regular or on-demand full-dose H_2-receptor antagonist or proton pump inhibitor

High-level treatment

Lifestyle measures of low-level treatment
Regular (or high-dose) proton pump blocker *or* laparoscopic anti-reflux surgery

---

weight above which they experience symptoms and below which they are free of symptoms. It makes good sense to encourage these patients to stay below their critical weight.

Additionally, patients on low-level treatment may benefit from intermittent medication for symptoms. The medication could be antacids if short-term (about 30 minutes) relief is required, or an H_2-receptor antagonist or proton pump inhibitor, if relief for several hours is required.

All of the above lifestyle measures should be presented as part of mid- and high-level treatment. However, there is limited evidence that these lifestyle changes are effective.

Mid-level treatment

Patients requiring the long-term administration of acid suppressants should have the diagnosis confirmed by one of the investigations listed above at some stage. There is very little to choose between the various H_2-receptor antagonists currently available. The end-point of therapy should be complete or near-complete resolution of symptoms. There is no evidence that double-dose H_2-receptor antagonists are more efficacious than standard doses. The onset of action is rapid, but rate of symptom relief is about 50%. Proton (acid) pump inhibitors provide a higher rate of symptom relief (60–80%) and endoscopic healing (80–90%); the onset of action is days. Once symptom relief is achieved, the dose should be stepped down or medication taken as needed (on demand). Patients with no oesophagitis often relapse if medical therapy is stopped, but many do well taking therapy on demand.

High-level treatment

Patients who fail to achieve the end-points of complete or near-complete resolution of symptoms within a reasonable period of 3–6 months should proceed to high-level treatment. The therapeutic options at this level are:

- inhibition of gastric acid secretion by a proton pump inhibitor in standard or, if needed, higher dose; and
- laparoscopic anti-reflux surgery.

TABLE 1.4: Failure of proton pump inhibitor (PPI) therapy to control gastro-oesophageal reflux symptoms: management approach

Mechanism to consider	Management
Misdiagnosis	Review history and investigations
Not taken before meals	Advise taking 30 minutes prior to a meal
Inadequate dosing	Trial of twice-daily therapy
Nocturnal acid breakthrough	Twice-daily PPI; if that fails, H_2-receptor antagonist before bed as needed; consider surgery
Acid hypersecretion	Exclude Zollinger-Ellison syndrome
Drug resistance	Very rare; switch to H_2-receptor antagonist or consider surgery
Oesophageal hypersensitivity	Add a low-dose tricyclic antidepressant

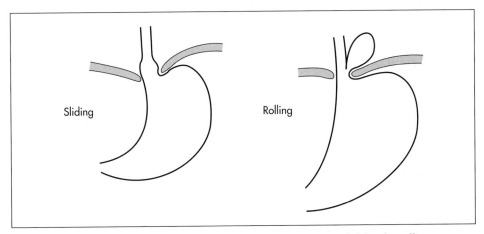

FIGURE 1.3A: Schematic representation of a sliding hiatus hernia (left) and a rolling (paraoesophageal) hernia (right).

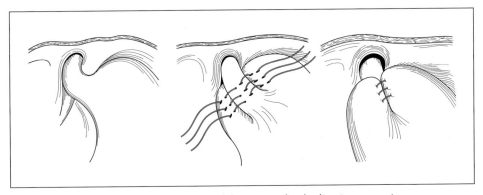

FIGURE 1.3B: Schematic representation of the Nissen fundoplication operation.
(Based on AJPM Smout & LMA Akkermans, Normal and disturbed motility of the gastrointestinal tract, *with permission.)*

There are some patients for whom the end-points of complete or near-complete resolution of symptoms and healing of ulcerative oesophagitis cannot be achieved with proton pump blockade (Table 1.4). Some of these will require higher than conventional doses. An additional nocturnal dose of H_2-receptor antagonists may be of assistance, but benefits often wear off if given continuously. Long-term therapy with these agents is now thought to be safe. Omeprazole, esomeprazole, lansoprazole, pantoprazole and rabeprazole block most acid secretion over a 24-hour period, leading to rises in serum gastrin which exceed normal limits in 20% of patients: in 10% the elevation is pronounced. Hypergastrinaemia leads to enterochromaffin hyperplasia and, in animals, gastric carcinoid tumours. This consequence has not been a problem in humans. Accelerated progression of *Helicobacter pylori* gastritis to atrophy has also been observed with potent acid suppression.

Patients for whom medical therapy results in incomplete resolution of symptoms (e.g., aspiration) can achieve that end-point with anti-reflux surgery. Nevertheless, the majority of patients presenting for surgery present because they are keen to achieve long-term cure, without need for continuing medical therapy and follow-up. Most report the loss of all reflux symptoms without need to take medication from the day of surgery. There is complete control in up to 90% of patients with typical symptoms responding to acid suppression in the hands of an experienced surgeon. However, in some studies up to 50% of cases eventually will have reintroduction of acid suppression therapy over the long term. The risk of postoperative sequelae (see Table 1.5) has limited the more widespread utilisation of anti-reflux surgery. The more troublesome of these are painful abdominal distension (gas bloat) and persistent dysphagia.

The surgical approach for most will be laparoscopic. This conveys the advantages of less postoperative wound pain and early return to full activity. The procedure involves an initial restoration of normal anatomical relationships by reduction of the commonly associated sliding hiatus hernia (see Figure 1.3A) and then wrapping of the lower oesophageal sphincter region with the gastric fundus (see Figure 1.3B). There is still debate as to whether the fundoplication should be complete as shown in Figure 1.3B, or whether the wrap should be incomplete—surrounding less than the 360° circumference of the lower oesophageal sphincter. Current data suggests that patients having the so-called incomplete fundoplication are more satisfied with the outcome because of an apparent reduction in sequelae, even though the long-term control of reflux might not be quite as good as with complete fundoplication. Endoscopic therapies to treat gastro-oesophageal reflux have been developed, including radiofrequency therapy, injection of biopolymer and endoscopic sewing around the lower oesophageal sphincter. These therapies may improve symptoms, but abnormal oesophageal pH often does not resolve. The long-term efficacy is also unknown.

Clinical management of heartburn and regurgitation associated with dysphagia

In the first instance, it needs to be established whether the symptoms are related to:

- a benign distal oesophageal stricture secondary to gastro-oesophageal reflux disease;
- a benign distal oesophageal stricture secondary to gastro-oesophageal reflux disease associated with scleroderma;

TABLE 1.5: Complications of anti-reflux surgery

Complication	Incidence	Impact
Early satiety	Common	Usually minor
Flatulence	Common	Usually not problematic
Gas bloat	5–10% (variable intensity)	Occasionally major
Abdominal distension	Common (usually minor)	Occasionally major
Early dysphagia	Common	Minor or transient
Persistent dysphagia	2%	Occasionally major
Recurrent reflux	5–10%	Rarely uncontrollable with medication
Recurrent hiatus hernia	2–5%	Often asymptomatic

- a functional motor disorder associated with gastro-oesophageal reflux disease; or
- a malignant stricture in a patient with gastro-oesophageal reflux disease.

The presence and site of stenosis can be first defined radiologically. Then the presence or absence of an oesophageal malignancy must be established or disproved by upper gastrointestinal endoscopy and biopsy of the stenosis and any mucosal irregularity. Once malignancy is excluded, oesophageal dilatation should be performed to relieve dysphagia. The dilatation may need to be staged if the stenosis is rigid. Thereafter, the patient should start taking a proton pump inhibitor to achieve mucosal healing, as assessed endoscopically. With this therapy, re-stenosis is uncommon. Anti-reflux surgery should be considered for those who require repeated dilatations or have poor control of heartburn and regurgitation. These patients are sometimes unsuitable for a laparoscopic operation, as oesophageal fibrosis may render the oesophagus short as well as narrow. The established method of surgery for this situation is a Collis gastroplasty, a so-called oesophageal lengthening procedure combined with a Nissen fundoplication.

Patients with oesophageal involvement from scleroderma are usually readily identifiable by the characteristic appearance of their hands and face. These patients have a hypomotile oesophageal body in addition to a failure of the lower oesophageal sphincter. Aggressive high-level medical therapy is to be preferred over surgical therapy. Unfortunately the motility disorder is only poorly responsive to prokinetic agents.

Patients with symptoms of reflux associated with dysphagia but without radiological evidence of stenosis are said to have a functional oesophageal disorder. Usually no specific disorder is identified by oesophageal manometry. Medical therapy may include prokinetic agents.

There are two other issues related to heartburn and regurgitation that should also be considered: hiatus herniation and Barrett's oesophagus.

Hiatus hernia

A hiatus hernia is a protrusion of intra-abdominal contents through the oesophageal hiatus in the diaphragm. Two major types of hiatus hernia are recognised radiologically (see Figure 1.3A).

Sliding hiatus hernia

This type of hernia is extremely common (10–15% of the population) and often asymptomatic. Its prevalence increases with age. It occurs as a result of circumferential telescoping of the segment of stomach which lies just distal to the lower oesophageal sphincter through the oesophageal hiatus. This type of hernia is not prone to obstruction or strangulation, so specific surgical treatment of the hernia is not required; when it is found incidentally in association with gastro-oesophageal reflux disease, attention should be directed at treatment of the reflux disease.

Rolling hiatus hernia

This type of hernia is uncommon. It can range enormously in size from just a small knuckle of fundus protruding alongside the non-displaced lower oesophageal sphincter to the whole stomach twisted and rotated within the posterior mediastinum. With larger rolling hiatus herniae, there is a tendency for the lower oesophageal sphincter to be displaced proximally with the stomach. Such herniae should not be thought of as mixed herniae as the major component is always the rolling component and the symptoms are those of a rolling hernia. These herniae can cause retrosternal pain due to ischaemia of the entrapped portion of stomach. There may be associated vomiting, which is reflex because of visceral ischaemia. Intra-thoracic rotation of the stomach can also result in a different type of vomiting due to gastric outlet obstruction. Early satiety and weight loss form part of a milder obstructive syndrome. Large herniae can cause dyspnoea by occupying part of the thoracic cavity, which would otherwise be available for expansion of the lungs. The only effective treatment is surgical repair of the hernia, which is recommended to prevent further complications.

Barrett's oesophagus

One of the consequences of gastro-oesophageal reflux is a metaplastic transformation of the stratified squamous epithelium of the distal oesophagus to a columnar type of epithelium. The affected oesophagus is called a Barrett's or columnar lined oesophagus. The significance of Barrett's oesophagus is its predisposition to malignant change. The requirement is to identify and treat such patients before they present clinically with an adenocarcinoma of the distal oesophagus (Figure 1.4), when the outlook is likely to be poor (Chapter 15). Identification at a premalignant stage is difficult. There are no clinical signs, and the symptoms, if any, are those of heartburn and regurgitation. The reflux symptoms are often minor so that an endoscopy is not likely to be performed on clinical grounds. As a consequence, many patients remain unaware that they carry this malignant predisposition.

The columnar lining of Barrett's oesophagus is salmon pink in colour and has a matt surface texture, distinguishing it from stratified squamous epithelium, which is pearly pink in colour and shiny in texture. Histological confirmation is necessary. Specialised intestinal metaplasia in the oesophagus is the hallmark finding.

Development of adenocarcinoma in a Barrett's oesophagus is a staged process that probably occurs over several years. The precursors of invasive carcinoma, low-grade and high-grade dysplasia, can only be detected reliably by histological examination of multiple samples of the columnar epithelium. There are no reliable serological markers or even endoscopic appearances. There is no evidence that control of continuing reflux, after the metaplastic epithelial change has occurred, stops progression down the dysplastic pathway, even though this is appropriate for control of reflux symptoms.

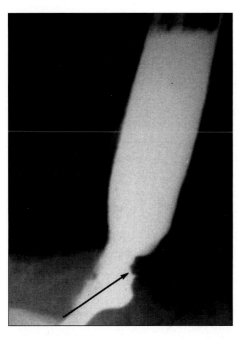

FIGURE 1.4: Adenocarcinoma of the distal oesophagus (arising in Barrett's mucosa) on barium swallow.

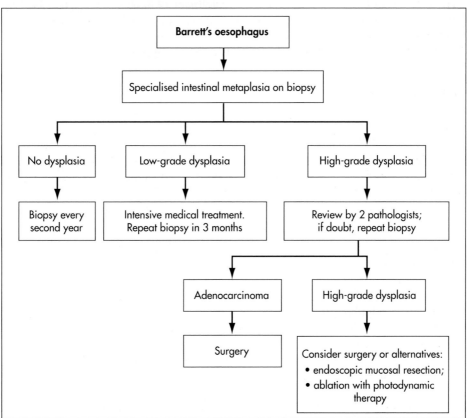

FIGURE 1.5: Recommended surveillance for Barrett's oesophagus.

The aim of the management strategy of patients with Barrett's oesophagus is to identify patients with high-grade dysplasia. These patients are very likely to proceed in the near future to invasive adenocarcinoma (Figure 1.5). It is recommended that second-yearly endoscopic surveillance be conducted, with biopsies (in each quadrant at 2-cm intervals) along the length of the Barrett's mucosa. If high-grade dysphagia is found and confirmed, there is a high risk of underlying adenocarcinoma and removal of the Barrett's epithelium is generally recommended. The current technique involves a surgical resection of the distal oesophagus. The resection is likely to be endoscopic in the future. If low-grade dysplasia is found, repeat endoscopy and biopsy within three months should be considered to determine if high-grade dysplasia has been missed.

NONCARDIAC CHEST PAIN

Noncardiac chest pain is pain not caused by myocardial ischaemia. It is a diagnosis reached by excluding myocardial ischaemia as the cause of the pain by a combination of history-taking, physical examination and one or more investigations.

Historically, cardiac pain due to ischaemia is primarily retrosternal in position. It may radiate to the neck and jaw, and/or down one or both arms. It is pain that is severe in grade, crushing in nature and usually not prolonged in duration. It is commonly precipitated by exercise and causes the patient to stop exercising. Patients with cardiac pain are more likely to have evidence of arterial disease in the lower limbs and cerebral arteries, and cardiac risk factors such as hypertension, diabetes mellitus, obesity, hypercholesterolaemia and tobacco use. Severe retrosternal chest pain that radiates through to the back should lead to consideration of dissection of a thoracic aortic aneurysm.

Chest pain of oesophageal origin is more likely to be prolonged, to radiate through to the back, to be precipitated by eating, and to be associated with dysphagia, heartburn and regurgitation.

In spite of these differences, chest pain of oesophageal origin cannot be distinguished from cardiac chest pain with any degree of certainty on the basis of history alone. Further, physical examination is rarely of any significant help in separating the two. Signs of heart disease such as cardiac murmurs and cardiac failure, or manifestations of peripheral vascular disease, such as bruits and absent pulses, increase the likelihood that the pain is cardiac in origin.

When there is any doubt, and there usually is, investigation is initially focussed on the heart. All patients should have an ECG and troponins measured if they are examined while they are having pain. Those without pain at the time of interview and normal resting ECG, and that will be the usual situation, should have an exercise stress ECG performed. The extent of further cardiac investigation will depend on clinical judgment. This might include echocardiography, radionuclide studies and coronary angiography. Although coronary angiography remains the gold standard, its performance is usually delayed because of its invasive nature and because of the slight risk of complications. The inconvenience and risk obviously need to be weighed against the likelihood that coronary disease will be uncovered and the likelihood that the findings will change the clinical management. One of the advantages of performing coronary angiography that reveals normal coronary arteries is that both patient and doctor can be reassured that sudden death becomes very much less likely.

Microvascular angina. This is a cause of ischaemic chest pain in the presence of normal coronary arteries; abnormalities may be found on non-invasive cardiac function testing (e.g., radionuclide ventriculography or thallium exercise scintigraphy).

Musculoskeletal conditions. Early in the clinical evaluation, before invasive cardiac investigations are performed, the possibility that the chest pain is musculoskeletal in origin will have to be considered and excluded. A history of chest wall injury might indicate a sternal fracture. Palpation of the anterior chest wall may reveal focal tenderness suggestive of costo-chondritis.

Panic attacks. These can cause chest pain. They result in discrete periods of intense fear that occur abruptly with at least four of the following symptoms: chest pain, palpitations, sweating, trembling, shortness of breath, choking, nausea, dizziness, feelings of unreality or detachment, fear of losing control, fear of dying, paraesthesia and flushes or chills.

Oesophageal conditions. Oesophageal conditions that can cause noncardiac chest pain, in order of importance, include:

- gastro-oesophageal reflux disease (most common);
- non-specific motility disorder or hypertensive lower oesophageal sphincter (uncertain significance);
- nutcracker oesophagus (uncertain significance);
- diffuse oesophageal spasm (rare); and
- achalasia (rare).

These conditions can be diagnosed either by endoscopy and pH monitoring in the case of gastro-oesophageal reflux disease, and by oesophageal manometry in the cases of the remainder. Unfortunately it is often difficult to be sure that the oesophageal condition diagnosed is indeed the cause of the pain, as will be discussed below.

The programme of investigation for patients deemed to have noncardiac chest pain that might be oesophageal in origin will depend on how significant the symptoms are in terms of both their severity and frequency. If the pain is significant, then endoscopy and 24-hour pH monitoring should be performed in an effort to diagnose gastro-oesophageal reflux disease. The finding of erosive oesophagitis, which clinches the diagnosis, is unfortunately uncommon in patients with noncardiac chest pain. The finding of oesophageal acidification at the same time as the occurrence of pain on pH monitoring also clinches the diagnosis, but is unfortunately also uncommon. The finding of high levels of oesophageal acidification supports the diagnosis but does not establish it, because this can occur in normal subjects. Nevertheless, as reflux can be effectively treated with proton pump inhibitors, any evidence supporting gastro-oesophageal reflux disease as the cause of the pain should be followed up with a therapeutic trial of proton pump inhibitors for at least one month. If the treatment is effective, it should obviously continue. If the pain only occurs infrequently, the trial may need to be extended. For patients with only infrequent episodes of pain it may sometimes be helpful to perform a Bernstein test, since reproduction of the pain by oesophageal acidification supports the diagnosis. If there is no evidence to support gastro-oesophageal reflux disease as the cause of the pain then oesophageal manometry is the next step. The manometric characteristics of motor disorders that can cause noncardiac chest pain are shown in Table 1.6. A detailed knowledge of these manometric patterns does not need to be committed to memory. Unfortunately, manometry has significant limitations in this clinical setting as it is performed in a laboratory over a short time frame (which is standard) and the chance that the abnormal manometric findings will be observed, except in the case of achalasia, is low. This likelihood can be increased by using provocative agents, such as edrophonium, or extending the period of observation utilising a portable ambulatory manometry system. Effective therapy for diffuse oesophageal spasm, nutcracker oesophagus, non-specific motility disorder and hypertensive lower oesophageal sphincter is currently not available. Therapeutic trials of nitrates or a calcium channel blocker are worthwhile, but should be discontinued if there is no apparent response.

A group of patients will remain for whom no diagnosis will be achieved after all investigations have been completed and therapeutic trials undertaken. These patients probably have oesophageal visceral hypersensitivity, a variant of irritable bowel syndrome. For the sufferer of chest pain, there is likely to be a significant degree of anxiety because of the fear of possible sudden death. Clearly, these patients need to be reassured sympathetically that it is very unlikely that their condition, although distressing, will be progressive or fatal and that continued observation is quite appropriate. Some of these patients will benefit from antidepressant therapy (e.g., low-dose tricyclic antidepressant).

TABLE 1.6: Manometric features of oesophageal motility disorders which may be associated with noncardiac chest pain

Achalasia *(see Chapter 2)*

- Incomplete relaxation of the lower oesophageal sphincter
- Aperistalsis of the oesophageal body

Diffuse oesophageal spasm

- Simultaneous contractions (> 10%)
- High-amplitude contractions (> 180 mmHg)
- Repetitive synchronous oesophageal body contractions (> 2 peaks)
- Prolonged oesophageal body contractions (> 6 sec)

Nutcracker oesophagus

- High-amplitude peristaltic contractions (> 180 mmHg)
- Prolonged oesophageal body contractions (> 6 sec)

Hypertensive lower oesophageal sphincter

- Elevated lower oesophageal sphincter pressure (> 45 mmHg)

Non-specific motility disorder

One or more of the following:
- Nontransmitted contractions (> 20%)
- Repetitive oesophageal body contractions (> 2 peaks)
- Prolonged oesophageal body contractions (> 6 sec)
- Low-amplitude peristalsis (< 30 mmHg)
- Frequent spontaneous contractions

Further reading

Cremonini F, Wise J, Moayyedi P, Talley NJ. Diagnostic and therapeutic use of proton pump inhibitors in non-cardiac chest pain: a metaanalysis. *Am J Gastroenterol* 2005; 100: 1226–32.

Dent J, El-Serag HB, Wallander MA, Johansson S. Epidemiology of gastro-oesophageal reflux disease: a systematic review. *Gut* 2005; 54: 710–7.

Dent J, Jones R, Kahrilas P, Talley NJ. Management of gastro-oesophageal reflux disease in general practice. *Brit Med J* 2001; 322: 344–7.

DeVault KR, Castell DO; American College of Gastroenterology. Updated guidelines for the diagnosis and treatment of gastroesophageal reflux disease. *Am J Gastroenterol* 2005; 100: 190–200.

Moayyedi P, Talley NJ. Gastro-oesophageal reflux disease: a review. Lancet 2006 (in press).

Piterman L, Nelson M, Dent J. Gastro-oesophageal reflux disease—current concepts in management. *Aust Fam Physician* 2004; 33: 987–91.

Sampliner RE; Practice Parameters Committee of the American College of Gastroenterology. Updated guidelines for the diagnosis, surveillance, and therapy of Barrett's esophagus. *Am J Gastroenterol* 2002; 97: 1888–95.

Sharma P, McQuaid K, Dent J *et al.* A critical review of the diagnosis and management of Barrett's esophagus: the AGA Chicago Workshop. *Gastroenterology* 2004; 127: 310–30.

Talley NJ. Review article: gastro-oesophageal reflux disease—how wide is its span? *Aliment Pharmacol Ther* 2004; 20 Suppl 5: 27–37; discussion 38–9.

chapter 2

DIFFICULTY SWALLOWING AND PAIN ON SWALLOWING

PAIN ON SWALLOWING (ODYNOPHAGIA)

Odynophagia is the symptom of pain on swallowing, generally arising from irritation of an inflamed or ulcerated mucosa by the swallowed bolus during its passage through the oesophagus. It is most commonly caused by gastro-oesophageal reflux and less commonly by viral or fungal infections (Table 2.1).

TABLE 2.1: Causes of odynophagia

Infections

Herpes simplex virus
Cytomegalovirus
Candidiasis

Chemical, inflammatory

Gastro-oesophageal reflux
Drug-induced (Slow-K, tetracyclines, quinidine)
Radiation
Graft versus host disease
Crohn's disease
Dermatological diseases (pemphigus and pemphigoid)

Gastro-oesophageal reflux disease

The most common cause of odynophagia is gastro-oesophageal reflux disease, almost always in the context of oesophagitis. The patient typically describes a sensation of pain or discomfort coincident with passage of the bolus through the oesophagus, sometimes combined with a sense of transient bolus hold-up. The sense of bolus arrest can dominate the symptom complex if the oesophagitis has progressed to stricture formation, but is not infrequently perceived even in the absence of a stricture. The symptom of odynophagia always warrants endoscopic investigation. For a detailed account of investigation and management of reflux disease, refer to Chapter 1.

Oesophageal infections

Oesophageal candidiasis

This infection usually occurs in patients receiving prolonged courses of antibiotics or who are immunosupressed by therapy with corticosteroids or other immunosuppressive drugs. Conditions commonly associated with oesophageal candidiasis include diabetes, AIDS, lymphoma and other malignancies, particularly during chemotherapy when these patients are neutropoenic. The oesophageal infection may be accompanied by oral or pharyngeal candidiasis, particularly in the context of AIDS.

The endoscopic features are white plaques on an erythematous mucosa, which can progress to necrosis and ulceration. Diagnosis is confirmed by brushings and biopsy demonstrating hyphae and tissue invasion by the organism. The features can be similar to those of infections due to herpes simplex virus (HSV) or cytomegalovirus (CMV) and biopsy is necessary to distinguish between these conditions.

Therapy is aimed at treating the underlying disease or conditions that predispose to the infection. Modification of drug therapy, such as corticosteroids or antibiotics, may be relevant or the control of diabetes, if present. Specific antifungal therapy, such as oral nystatin is first-line therapy. Amphotericin lozenges are also useful. For severe or refractory cases parenteral antifungal therapy such as amphotericin, miconazole or ketoconazole is indicated.

Herpes simplex oesophagitis

Malignancy, immunosuppressive drugs and immunodeficiency states are predisposing factors, but herpetic oesophagitis can occur spontaneously in the apparently healthy, immunocompetent individual. The causative agent is the herpes simplex virus type 1. The endoscopic appearances can vary from discrete, punched out ulcers to confluent, extensive ulceration. Whitish plaques can also be a feature making differentiation from *Candida* by endoscopic inspection difficult. Endoscopic biopsy will confirm the diagnosis. Treatment involves suspension of drugs such as corticosteroids or cytotoxic agents, if possible. The antiviral agent aciclovir is active against this virus.

Cytomegalovirus oesophagitis

This oesophageal infection is seen most frequently in patients with AIDS, bone marrow transplantation and other immunodeficiency states. Endoscopic features are of extensive ulceration and characteristic inclusion bodies and giant cells are seen on biopsy.

Drug-induced oesophageal ulceration

A number of medications, if allowed to dwell in the oesophagus, can cause severe local ulceration, pain and stricture. A common factor predisposing to this phenomenon is swallowing tablets without water, particularly if taken immediately before lying down at night. Any condition that delays oesophageal transit, such as dysmotility or extrinsic compression, can result in tablet retention where it can cause oesophageal ulceration. Drugs particularly likely to cause this syndrome include: tetracycline, potassium supplements, ferrous sulfate, and quinidine.

DYSPHAGIA

Dysphagia is the symptom of difficulty with the act of swallowing usually causing a sensation of hold-up of the swallowed bolus, frequently accompanied by pain. It can be caused by structural or neuromuscular diseases of the pharynx or oesophagus.

Physiology and pathophysiology

Prior to the swallow, the food bolus is prepared by mastication in the presence of saliva before the oral delivery phase is initiated voluntarily. The bolus is propelled into the pharynx by the sequential upward motion of the tongue against the hard palate and the nasopharynx closing by elevation of the soft palate. At this time, the glottis elevates and the airway closes. A sequential contraction of the superior, middle and inferior constrictor muscles act in concert with the posterior movement of the base of the tongue, propelling the bolus through the relaxed cricopharyngeus muscle into the oesophagus. Liquids traverse the oesophagus primarily under the influence of gravity while solids are propelled through it by the sequence of oesophageal peristalsis. Relaxation of the lower oesophageal sphincter is necessary to permit entry of the bolus into the stomach. Bolus transit through the oropharynx is rapid occurring in 1–1.2 seconds while complete oesophageal clearance is relatively slow occurring over 15 seconds.

The oral and pharyngeal phases of the swallow are executed by the bulbar muscles. The medullary swallow centre is responsible for the triggering of this response and for the timing and sequencing of the responsible muscular actions. Hence, disorders of the medulla may abolish or delay this motor sequence or render it discoordinate. Disorders of the lower cranial nerves, neuromuscular junction or isolated muscle disease may lead to feeble or absent bulbar muscle activity, thereby causing dysphagia.

Oesophageal transport requires intact lower oesophageal sphincter relaxation while adequate oesophageal clearance relies upon coordinated oesophageal peristalsis. Control mechanisms for proximal and distal oesophagus differ. The proximal oesophagus, being composed of striated muscle, is innervated by branches of the vagus nerve whose nicotinic cholinergic terminals end directly onto muscle motor end plates. In contrast, the distal oesophagus is composed of smooth muscle and its innervation and control are far more complex and less well understood. Vagal efferent fibres terminate in ganglia within the myenteric plexus, while the postganglionic intrinsic neurones are a mixture of excitatory (cholinergic) and inhibitory (non-cholinergic, non-adrenergic) nerves. Normal lower oesophageal sphincter relaxation and oesophageal peristalsis are dependent upon intact extrinsic and intrinsic neuronal function and the correct balance between excitatory and inhibitory neurones. For example, in achalasia there is intrinsic neuronal degeneration within the myenteric plexus. It is the loss of inhibitory nerves in achalasia that causes failure or relaxation of the lower oesophageal sphincter.

Causes of dysphagia

Because the physiological mechanisms controlling the different phases of swallowing differ, it is convenient therefore to consider the aetiology of dysphagia under the categories of oral-pharyngeal and oesophageal causes, and whether the disease is a structural or a motility disorder.

Oral-pharyngeal dysphagia is most commonly related to neuromuscular dysfunction, most commonly stroke (Table 2.2). Head and neck surgery and radiotherapy, for malignant disease, are also very commonly associated with oral-pharyngeal dysphagia. Other structural disorders causing oral-pharyngeal dysphagia include strictures, webs and pharyngeal pouch or diverticulum (Figure 2.1).

Because gastro-oesophageal reflux disease is prevalent, peptic oesophageal strictures are a very common cause of oesophageal dysphagia (Figure 2.2, Figure 2.3, Table 2.3). In these cases, there is frequently a prior history of reflux symptoms. Malignant oesophageal obstruction is usually evident on history by virtue of a short history of rapidly progressive dysphagia and significant weight loss (Figure 2.4).

TABLE 2.2: Causes of oral-pharyngeal dysphagia

Functional disorders

Central nervous system
- Stroke
- Head injury
- Parkinson's disease
- Motor neurone disease
- Multiple sclerosis
- Tumour
- Drugs (e.g., phenothiazines)
- Malformations (e.g., syrinx, Arnold Chiari)

Neural
- Motor neurone disease
- Myasthenia gravis
- Radiotherapy
- Poliomyelitis
- Familial dysautonomia

Muscle
- Autoimmune myopathy (polymyositis, dermatomyositis, systemic lupus erythematosus)
- Thyrotoxic myopathy
- Guillain-Barré motor neuropathy
- Muscular dystrophies

Structural disorders
- Head/neck surgery
- Stricture
- Radiotherapy
- Tumour
- Pharyngeal pouch
- Web
- Extrinsic (e.g., osteophytes)

Miscellaneous
- Xerostomia

TABLE 2.3: Causes of oesophageal dysphagia

Structural disorders

- Stricture (peptic, caustic, pill-induced, radiation-induced)
- Tumour
- Rings and webs
- Eosinophilic oesophagitis
- Extrinsic compression (e.g., enlarged left atrium, aberrant right subclavian artery)

Motor disorders

- Achalasia
- Pseudoachalasia (associated with tumour)
- Diffuse oesophageal spasm
- Scleroderma

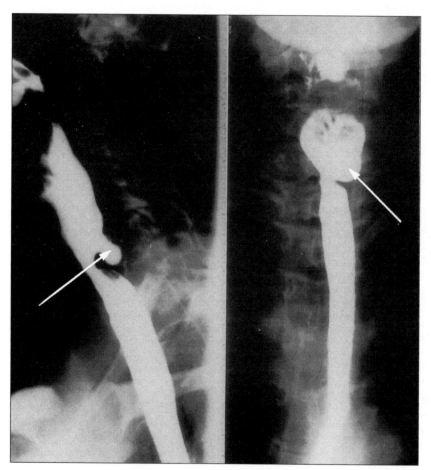

FIGURE 2.1: Lateral (left) and anteroposterior (right) radiographs showing a pharyngeal (Zenker's) diverticulum. This patient described dysphagia with hold-up localised to the neck and regurgitation of food particles, frequently several hours after the meal.

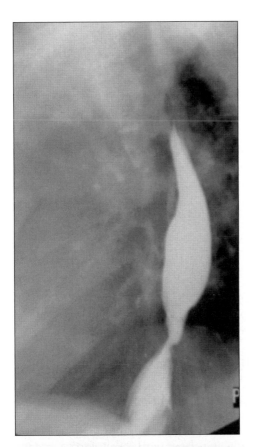

FIGURE 2.2: Barium swallow demonstrating a benign peptic stricture in a patient with gastro-oesophageal reflux disease and dysphagia.

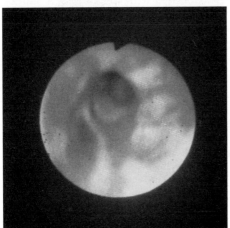

FIGURE 2.3: Endoscopic view of the distal oesophagus in a patient with dysphagia due to gastro-oesophageal reflux disease. Note the extensive ulceration typical of acid reflux and the associated stricture.

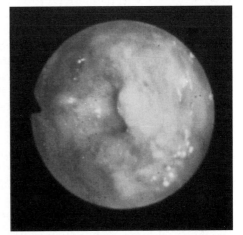

FIGURE 2.4: Endoscopic view of a distal oesophageal carcinoma partially obstructing the lumen causing dysphagia.

Approach to dysphagia

The history and examination of the patient with dysphagia should address four fundamental questions:

1. Does the patient have true dysphagia?
2. Is the dysphagia oral-pharyngeal or oesophageal in origin?
3. Is it due to a structural or motor disorder?
4. Is there an underlying related or causative disease?

An accurate provisional diagnosis can usually be made on the basis of a careful history, thus establishing investigational priorities.

Does the patient describe true dysphagia?

Dysphagia is defined as difficulty with the act of swallowing. The purely sensory symptom of globus can be equated inappropriately with difficulty swallowing by the patient. Globus is a non-painful sensation of a lump or fullness in the throat in which deglutitive food bolus transport is unimpaired. Indeed, globus sensation is usually alleviated by eating and is most noticeable between meals. The patient with globus sensation generally only requires otolaryngological evaluation to exclude local inflammatory or infiltrative disorders followed by explanation and reassurance.

What is the age of onset, duration of dysphagia, how frequent is it and is it progressive?

The duration of symptoms is often an important clue to whether the underlying cause is benign or malignant or whether it is due to a recent, acute event, such as a stroke. Malignant dysphagia usually presents with a short history of progressive dysphagia over weeks or a few months and is frequently associated with weight loss. A sudden onset of dysphagia, often in association with other neurological symptoms or signs, usually indicates a cerebrovascular cause, such as stroke. Frequent dysphagia, that is progressive and predominantly for solids, is more likely to indicate an underlying structural disorder, such as a peptic stricture or tumour.

Intermittent, non-progressive, solid bolus (e.g., steak) obstruction is the hallmark of dysphagia due to a structural lesion such as a Schatzki ring—the so called 'steakhouse oesophagus' syndrome. This is due to a mucosal ring situated at the gastro-oesophageal junction, usually just above a small hiatus hernia. There may be multiple rings, particularly in association with eosinophilic oesophagitis. The multi-ringed oesophagus should be suspected if the patient is male and has had symptoms from an early age.

Intermittent dysphagia, for both liquids and solids, is characteristic of a motility disorder such as achalasia, diffuse oesophageal spasm or scleroderma oesophagus.

Is there dysphagia for solids or liquids?

Dysphagia solely for solids indicates a structural lesion, such as a stricture, ring, web or tumour. Dysphagia for liquids and solids is typical of an oesophageal motility disorder, but this combination is commonly present in pharyngeal dysphagia as well. The patient usually describes other localising symptoms to help differentiate the location of pharyngeal from oesophageal pathology (see below).

Where is the apparent site of bolus hold-up?

The reported site of bolus hold-up can be helpful in localising the location of the underlying cause, but be aware that the patient's perception of the site of hold-up can be misleading. In cases of pharyngeal dysphagia, hold-up is reported in the neck. However, distal oesophageal pathology causing dysphagia can give rise to a sensation of the bolus catching either in the cervical or retrosternal region. Hence, a perception by the patient of apparent bolus hold-up in the neck does not help the clinician distinguish between pharyngeal and oesophageal causes of dysphagia.

Are there associated symptoms indicating the site of the disorder?

Oral-pharyngeal dysphagia can be associated with one or more symptoms relating to disordered bolus delivery to the oesophagus such as: poor bolus control in the mouth; dry mouth; delayed swallow initiation; postnasal regurgitation; coughing or choking during the swallow indicating aspiration; a sense of hold-up immediately following deglutition; and perceived bolus hold-up in the neck. More widespread neuromuscular symptoms, such as weakness, diplopia or movement disorder, are clues to an underlying neurological problem.

Oesophageal dysphagia is usually accompanied by a delayed (15–30 second) sense of hold-up which can be felt either in the cervical or retrosternal region. Patients may attempt to wash the offending bolus down with liquids with varying success. If the oesophagus is totally obstructed by the offending bolus, such attempts can culminate in frank regurgitation and vomiting. Gradually progressive dysphagia for solids on a background of reflux symptoms is suggestive of a peptic stricture. Intermittent dysphagia for liquids and solids suggest a motility disorder, such as achalasia or diffuse oesophageal spasm. Achalasia is often associated with prominent regurgitation and chest pain. Sometimes, regurgitation and vomiting can dominate the symptoms in achalasia. Diffuse oesophageal spasm, a rare oesophageal disorder, is associated with chest pain that commonly occurs during a meal but can also be precipitated by certain foods, such as hot or cold drinks and carbonated beverages. Oesophageal spasm may mimic the features of angina and can also be relieved by sublingual nitrates.

Is there an underlying related or causative disease?

Oral-pharyngeal dysphagia usually has a neurological basis. A prior history of stroke is often obtained. Symptoms of bulbar muscle dysfunction or other brainstem symptoms, such as vertigo, nausea, vomiting, hiccup, tinnitus, diplopia, drop attacks, should be sought. The patient may complain of tremor, ataxia or unsteadiness, which might indicate an underlying movement disorder or may describe muscular weakness suggestive of myopathy (Table 2.2).

Oesophageal dysphagia may present on a background of reflux, hence history of heartburn and antacid use is relevant. Smoking, alcohol and prior caustic ingestion are risk factors for oesophageal carcinoma. Oesophageal dysmotility can be associated with connective tissue disease, particularly scleroderma when Raynaud's phenomenon and typical skin changes may be present. Eosinophilic oesophagitis is frequently associated with a history of atopy and asthma.

Physical examination

Hands and skin. Changes consistent with Raynaud's phenomenon, with or without sclerodactyly, are features commonly found in patients with scleroderma oesophagus. Calcinosis and telangiectasia, if present, complete the features of CREST syndrome, which is always associated with oesophageal dysmotility and reflux. The lilac-coloured (heliotrope) skin changes, typically around the nail beds, bridge of the nose and cheeks and forehead is a feature of dermatomyositis, which can cause severe pharyngeal dysfunction and, to a lesser extent, oesophageal dysfunction as well. Rarely, other skin disorders can cause oesophageal disease and include lichen planus, pemphigus, Behçet's syndrome, acanthosis nigricans and epidermolysis bullosa.

Sweating, tremor and tachycardia of thyrotoxicosis may be present in patients with thyrotoxic myopathy causing pharyngeal dysfunction. The typical features of thyrotoxicosis, however, may not be present in the elderly or individuals taking beta-adrenergic antagonists.

Head and neck. The examiner should palpate the neck for masses, lymph nodes or a goitre. Sometimes a pharyngeal pouch can be felt, nearly always on the left, and may be compressed causing regurgitation of a small amount of food residue into the pharynx with an audible 'gurgle'. Signs of prior surgery, tracheostomy and radiotherapy are obvious and should be noted. The oral cavity including natural dentition or dentures, tongue and oropharynx should be inspected.

Eyes. Thyrotoxic eye signs should be looked for. Ptosis might indicate a myopathy or myasthenia. Unilateral ptosis, if associated with Horner's syndrome (descending sympathetic tract), is typical of lateral medullary infarction causing dysphagia. In addition to dysphagia, the lateral medullary (Wallenberg's) syndrome typically involves hoarseness (10th cranial nerve), vestibular dysfunction (nystagmus, vertigo, vomiting, diplopia and tinnitus), cerebellar limb ataxia, and contralateral loss of pain and temperature sensation over half the body (spinothalamic tract), and hiccup.

Neuromuscular function. Careful examination of cranial nerve function will sometimes detect bulbar muscle dysfunction, but normal palatal motion and an intact gag reflex does not exclude significant bulbar muscle dysfunction in a patient with pharyngeal dysphagia. Tremor and gait disturbances may reflect an extrapyramidal movement disorder, the most common causing dysphagia being Parkinson's disease. Muscle fasciculation, wasting and weakness or fatigability should be sought to detect underlying motor neurone disease, myopathy, or myasthenia.

Watch and listen to the patient swallow. With the index and middle fingers resting lightly on the hyoid and laryngeal cartilages respectively, axial motion of the larynx and hyoid bone should be noted while the patient swallows a mouthful of water. Inadequate laryngeal ascent is frequently seen in neurogenic dysphagia and also impairs airway protection during the swallow and can be associated with aspiration. Aspiration will often (but not invariably) cause coughing or choking during the swallow.

Respiratory and nutritional sequelae. The patient's general nutritional state and body weight are important. The degree of weight loss is a good indicator of the severity of the disease and is most profound in malignant disease. Examination of the chest may reveal signs of respiratory infection suggesting significant aspiration which is common in patients with pharyngeal dysphagia.

Investigation of dysphagia

The initial choice of investigation(s) will depend on the provisional diagnosis determined on the basis of history and, in the first instance, by whether the clinician believes the dysphagia is oral-pharyngeal or oesophageal in location.

Investigation of suspected oral-pharyngeal dysphagia

The initial investigation should be a dynamic, radiographic examination: the videoradiographic swallow study of the oral-pharyngeal phase. This examination should be complemented by static films, but video recordings are mandatory as the motor events of the oral-pharyngeal phase are too complex and too rapid to be resolved by simple observation of fluoroscopy or X-ray films. Static films are only useful in detecting mucosal defects and structural lesions such as strictures, pouches (Figure 2.1) and tumours.

In cases of oral-pharyngeal dysfunction where the cause is not clear, the videoswallow study is a sensitive means of: confirming the site of dysfunction; establishing whether a pharyngeal motor problem exists; defining the mechanisms of dysfunction; and detecting the presence and timing of aspiration. A clear idea of the mechanisms of dysfunction and severity of the disorder is vital in tailoring therapy. In the context of a recent stroke, head/neck surgery or radiotherapy, the underlying cause may be obvious. Nevertheless, in such cases an understanding of the patient's swallow mechanics is vital in deciding on the advisability and safety of oral feeding and the choice of therapy. For example, recognition of timing of aspiration has therapeutic implications. Pre-swallow aspiration results from poor tongue control and premature spill of the bolus over the back of the tongue before laryngeal protective reflexes have been elicited. Intra-swallow aspiration frequently accompanies pharyngeal weakness. Post-swallow aspiration is seen when residual bolus pools in the hypopharynx and spills over into the airway as it reopens following the swallow. Pharyngeal bolus transport abnormalities may be due to defective triggering of the pharyngeal motor response, pharyngeal peristaltic weakness or a combination of both. Pharyngeal muscle weakness may be seen as post-swallow pooling in the pyriform sinuses. If weakness is unilateral, pooling is confined to the paretic side and is associated with pharyngeal bulging on the affected side. In such cases, bolus transport can be facilitated by therapeutic strategies such as head turning towards the paretic side. Diminished upper oesophageal sphincter opening can be due to local stricture, inadequate pharyngeal propulsive forces or incomplete sphincter relaxation. Depending upon the relative contribution of one or more of these features, such patients may benefit from cricopharyngeal dilatation or myotomy.

Laboratory tests are useful in confirming suspected underlying primary diseases that may cause oral-pharyngeal dysphagia. Serum creatinine phosphokinase level, erythrocyte sedimentation rate, antinuclear antibodies, and thyroid function tests will give a clue to most acquired myopathies, but electromyography (EMG) and muscle biopsy may also be necessary as 20% of cases of myositis will have normal biochemistry.

Endoscopy will be required in most patients with pharyngeal dysfunction and certainly all cases in whom it is uncertain whether the problem is oesophageal or pharyngeal. Videoradiography should precede endoscopy, as it may detect a problem that would make endoscopy hazardous or difficult (e.g., pharyngeal pouch, cricopharyngeal stricture, tumour). Furthermore, radiology may detect a structural lesion better appreciated radiologically than it is by the endoscopist and which may be successfully treated endoscopically (e.g., cricopharyngeal stricture, postcricoid web).

If the cause of pharyngeal dysfunction is not apparent after the above investigation, then careful evaluation by an ear, nose and throat (ENT) surgeon is required to exclude pharyngolaryngeal malignancy. Tumours in the region can be readily overlooked by the radiologist and lesions in some locations can be missed by the endoscopist using a standard gastroscope. Features highly suggestive of local malignancy such as recent onset of throat pain on swallowing and hoarseness with dysphagia should prompt early laryngoscopy.

Investigation of suspected oesophageal dysphagia

Endoscopy. With a few exceptions, endoscopy should be the first investigation in cases of suspected oesophageal dysphagia. Endoscopy is more sensitive than radiology in detecting mucosal disease. It also provides an opportunity to obtain biopsies and to combine a diagnostic with therapeutic procedure in cases where dilatation is required. The deficiencies of endoscopy in the assessment of dysphagia are that it cannot diagnose motility disorders and it does not detect all benign structural abnormalities capable of causing dysphagia. This is because an accurate estimation of the narrow-calibre oesophagus is not always possible at endoscopy. Hence, a negative endoscopy does not always exclude a structural cause of dysphagia. If a structural oesophageal abnormality is suspected strongly on history and the oesophagus has a normal macroscopic appearance, then oesophageal biopsy and empiric dilatation is often necessary to rule out conditions such as mucosal rings and eosinophilic oesophagitis.

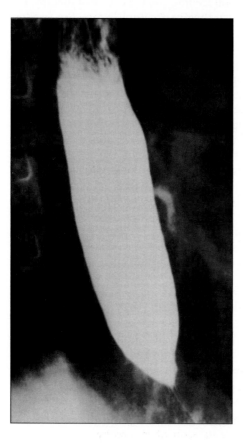

FIGURE 2.5: Radiograph of oesophageal achalasia showing the typical tapered ('bird beaked') appearance at the cardio-oesophageal junction, and retention of food and fluid within a dilated and adynamic oesophagus.

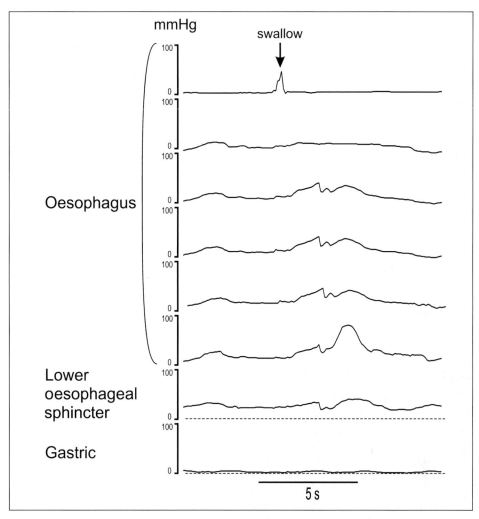

FIGURE 2.6: Manometric tracing from a patient with chest pain, dysphagia and regurgitation showing typical features of achalasia. Note that lower oesophageal sphincter resting pressure is increased. In response to the swallow, the sphincter pressure does not change and does not relax. No peristalsis is seen within the oesophageal body; instead, swallowing induces a low-amplitude, pressure wave, which is identical at all recording sites along the oesophagus.

Radiology. In the investigation of oesophageal dysphagia, there are two situations in which a barium swallow should precede endoscopy: a suspected oesophageal ring and suspected oesophageal dysmotility. Preliminary barium swallow findings in these circumstances may permit definitive treatment of a ring or achalasia at the initial endoscopy or dictate manometry prior to endoscopy if achalasia suspected (Figure 2.5). The patient with a typical history of an oesophageal ring (see above) should have a barium swallow because an oesophageal ring can be easily missed endoscopically. An appropriately tailored barium swallow study, including prone-oblique views and, if necessary, a marshmallow swallow, will usually clearly demonstrate a ring and/or the site of bolus hold-up causing the patient's symptoms. The ring can then be dilated, even if it is not visible to the endoscopist, at the subsequent endoscopy.

Oesophageal manometry. This is usually reserved for cases in whom endoscopy and radiology have failed to achieve a diagnosis. Manometry is the only way to diagnose achalasia with certainty. The manometric features of achalasia are oesophageal aperistalsis, hypertonia and failure of the lower oesophageal sphincter relaxation during swallowing (Figure 2.6). The manometric hallmark of diffuse oesophageal spasm is synchronous oesophageal contractions in at least 20% of water swallows in an oesophagus that can demonstrate peristalsis. Additional features present to a variable extent include: repetitive waves (swallow-induced or spontaneous); high amplitude contractions; and prolonged (> 6 s) contractions. The scleroderma oesophagus demonstrates complete aperistalsis and absent lower oesophageal sphincter tone, both being due to profound smooth muscle degeneration in the distal oesophagus.

Treatment of dysphagia

Specific therapy for dysphagia will be dependent on the cause. Detailed treatment of many problems causing dysphagia is beyond the scope of this chapter and the reader is referred to reviews of these diseases.

Treatment of oesophageal dysphagia

Oesophageal strictures, rings and webs are generally successfully treated by endoscopic dilatation. This is most commonly achieved by passing graduated sizes of silastic (e.g., Savary Gilliard) or steel olive (e.g., Eder Peustow) dilators over an endoscopically placed guide wire. The underlying cause of the stricture must also be treated. Severe reflux disease causing stricture should be treated aggressively with potent acid suppression with a proton pump inhibitor, with the more refractory cases being treated by anti-reflux surgery. Difficult strictures often require repeated dilatations. Oesophageal rings and webs generally respond well to a single dilatation. However, it is now recognised that at least 30% of those with a Schatzki ring will require repeat dilatation over the years. The multi-ringed oesophagus (frequently associated with eosinophilic oesophagitis) requires special caution at the time of dilatation. The rings are often relatively tight and significant post-dilatation tears are not infrequent (Figure 2.7). These patients almost invariably require repeated dilatations over the years. In the presence of confirmed eosinophilic oesophagitis, the frequency of dilatation might be reduced by topical (fluticasone) or systemic steroids, or by the leukotriene inhibitor montelukast although there are as yet no controlled clinical trials to confirm this belief. The management of oesophageal malignancy requires relief of dysphagia and, where appropriate, ablation of the tumour by surgery, chemo-radiotherapy or laser ablation. Due to the advanced nature of the disease at the time of diagnosis, the aim of therapy is palliative in the majority. Relief of dysphagia in difficult circumstances can be achieved by placement of an expanding oesophageal stent. Covered stents are also useful in treating associated oesophago-tracheal fistulae, if they occur.

Oesophageal achalasia is best treated by mechanical disruption of the non-relaxing lower oesophageal sphincter. This can be achieved either by surgical cardiomyotomy or by endoscopic, balloon pneumatic dilatation. The incidence of post-treatment gastro-oesophageal reflux is greater in those treated surgically, hence surgical myotomy is generally now combined with loose fundoplication (e.g., Dor patch). Although smooth muscle relaxants, including the calcium channel blocker nifedipine, do reduce lower oesophageal sphincter pressure, therapeutic results are disappointing. Botulinum toxin is simple and safe to infiltrate into the lower oesophageal sphincter at endoscopy with short-term efficacy approaching that of pneumatic dilatation. However, because botulinum toxin has limited durability requiring repeated injections, it is reserved for

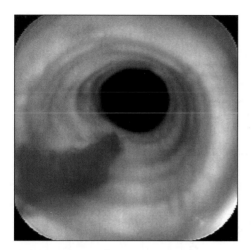
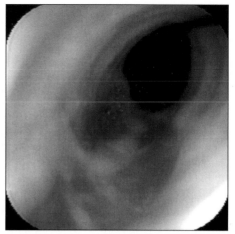

FIGURE 2.7A: Endoscopic appearance in a patient with dysphagia since his teens who has eosinophilic oesophagitis on biopsy. Note the multi-ringed oesophagus and the tear induced by passage of a standard 9 mm endoscope.

FIGURE 2.7B: Note the two significant mucosal tears observed following passage of an 11 mm Savary Gilliard dilator.

the very elderly or those with significant associated co-morbidity, which might put them at high risk for the more invasive therapies.

Diffuse oesophageal spasm is best treated with smooth muscle relaxants such as nitrates and calcium channel blockers. If symptoms are relatively infrequent, sublingual nitrates to abort an episode of chest pain can be useful. Refractory cases with debilitating symptoms can be treated surgically by long oesophageal myotomy, which is effective in 50–70% of cases. The diagnostic and therapeutic steps in the management of oesophageal dysphagia are outlined in Figure 2.8.

Treatment of oral-pharyngeal dysphagia

Identification and treatment of an underlying cause, if present, should be the primary aim. Thyrotoxic myopathy responds well to treatment of the thyroid disorder. Inflammatory myopathies (systemic lupus erythematosus, polymyositis) respond variably to steroids with or without other immunosuppressive agents such as methotrexate or azathioprine. Dysphagia due to myasthenia and, to a lesser extent, Parkinson's disease is also responsive to specific therapy. Avoidance of implicated drugs such as phenothiazines can be helpful, but the effects of these drugs are not always reversible.

Structural disorders such as webs and some strictures can be successfully dilated endoscopically. The dysphagia associated with the posterior pharyngeal pouch is almost invariably successfully treated by surgery (cricopharyngeal myotomy with or without pouch excision or suspension). Head and neck tumours causing dysphagia generally require surgery or radiotherapy.

Pharyngeal dysphagia due to cerebrovascular accident is more difficult to treat. However, substantial spontaneous recovery can also be expected in many cases. Expert treatment of oral-pharyngeal dysphagia requires close cooperation with a speech pathologist and careful assessment of the dynamics of swallowing, as has been outlined. The aims of therapy are to establish a safe means of nutrition by avoiding or minimising aspiration and promote swallowed bolus clearance from the pharynx by

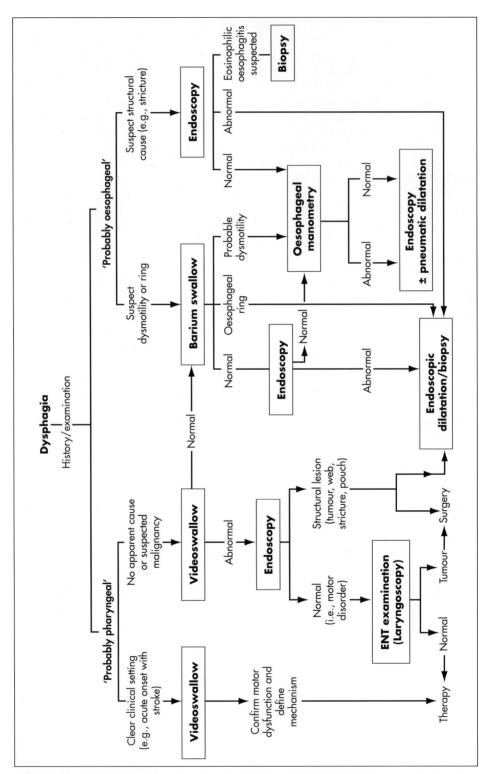

FIGURE 2.8: Algorithm outlining the diagnostic and therapeutic steps in the management of dysphagia.

manipulation of food consistency, swallow technique or the use of prosthetic devices or surgery. The reader is referred to a detailed review of this topic. If aspiration is absent or minimal, oral feeding of modified food consistencies can continue safely. However enteral feeding by alternative means (nasogastric tube; percutaneous gastrostomy) may be necessary to optimise nutrition if feeding via the oral route is considered unsafe. Compensatory strategies minimise the symptoms of aspiration and dysphagia by manipulating the manner in which the food bolus flows through the oral and pharyngeal regions. These techniques involve manipulation of the position of the head and/or body, or altering the characteristics of administered food boluses including volume, rate and viscosity. Direct therapeutic strategies, such as oral sensory stimulation and voluntary modifications to swallow techniques, are designed to alter the mechanics of the swallow and airway protection. For example, the so-called 'supraglottic swallow' is a useful technique to prevent aspiration. The patient is trained to inhale and hold their breath prior to swallowing (thus ensuring early voluntary closure of the true vocal cords), then to swallow and finally cough and exhale following the swallow to clear residual bolus in the region of the laryngeal vestibule.

Intra-oral prosthetic devices can be useful in patients with disordered oral delivery as a result of cancer surgery. They improve oral clearance of boluses by improving tongue and palatal contact or improving velopharyngeal closure. A palatal obturator is useful when part of the palate has been resected.

Disorders of upper oesophageal sphincter opening may be most amenable to cricopharyngeal myotomy, which disrupts the upper oesophageal sphincter and permits it to open more widely. The results from myotomy have been variable, however, and there is no current consensus on who should be selected for myotomy. A range of surgical techniques has been used to alleviate aspiration including laryngeal suspension, partial or complete glottic closure, epiglottopexy, and laryngoplasty. The diagnostic and therapeutic steps in the management of pharyngeal dysphagia are outlined in Figure 2.8.

Further reading

Achem SR, Devault KR. Dysphagia in aging. *J Clin Gasterenterol* 2005; 39: 357–71.

Arora AS, Yamazaki K. Eosinophilic esophagitis: asthma of the esophagus? *Clin Gastro Hepatol* 2004; 2: 523–30.

Castell DO, Richter J (eds). *The Esophagus*, 4th edn. Philadelphia: Lippincott Williams and Wilkins, 2004; 196–220.

Cook IJ, Kahrilas PJ. American Gastroenterological Association clinical practice guidelines: management of oropharyngeal dysphagia. *Gastroenterology* 1999; 116(2): 455–78.

Pandolfino JE, Kaharilas PJ. American Gastroenterological Association medical position statement: clinical use of esophageal manometry. *Gastroenterology* 2005; 128: 207–8.

Spechler SJ, Castell DO. Classification of oesophageal motor abnormalities. *Gut* 2001; 49: 145–51.

chapter 3

HICCUPS, SORE MOUTH, AND BAD BREATH

HICCUPS (SINGULTUS)

Introduction

Hiccup is a common reflex characterised by the act of inspiration against a closed glottis. Almost all individuals experience hiccups. It occurs in utero late in fetal development; in the newborn, and becomes less frequent as the infant matures. Hiccup usually responds rapidly to simple therapeutic measures, however, it can become protracted and is classified as intractable if it persists for longer than 24 hours. Protracted hiccups may be indicative of serious underlying disease and may also have significant deleterious effects such as postoperative wound dehiscence, fatigue, dehydration, weight loss and even death.

Pathophysiology

Electromyographic studies show the reflex involves a transient burst of intense inspiratory activity, involving excitation of the diaphragm and inspiratory intercostal muscles, with reciprocal inhibition of the expiratory intercostal muscles. The discharge burst lasts for approximately 500 ms but the duration of the inspiratory air flow is very much shorter than this because inspiration is halted abruptly, in the presence of continued powerful inspiratory muscle contraction, by glottal closure 35 ms after the onset of inspiration. This phenomenon generates the noxious sensation and the characteristic sound of hiccup. Glottal closure persists for one second or more until the mechanical effect of the hiccup has subsided. Hiccup is most likely to occur during inspiration suggesting the rate of change of lung volume may be a co-stimulus for the reflex.

The reflex is mediated by afferent fibres primarily in the phrenic and vagus nerves as well as dorsal sympathetic fibres. These fibres synapse within the dorsolateral region of the medulla. The main efferent limb of the reflex causing spasm of the diaphragm is then mediated by motor fibres of the phrenic nerve but also via fibres in the vagus, cervical and thoracic nerves. Hence, hiccup can result from direct stimulation or irritation of the afferent or efferent vagal or phrenic pathways; from lesions in the medulla or it can be secondary to metabolic disturbances.

A range of gastrointestinal stimuli can cause reflex excitation of visceral afferent vagal fibres. Vagal afferent receptors in the oesophagus can trigger the responsible medullary centres. This is the proposed mechanism for hiccup occurring during swallowed bolus impaction at the site of a benign stricture or ring or in response to oesophageal distension by retained food and fluid in oesophageal achalasia, or in the context of pill-induced oesophageal ulceration or stricture. Similar vagal afferent stimuli might originate in cases of hiatus hernia or gastro-oesophageal reflux disease, but the evidence implicating reflux as a cause of hiccup remains inconclusive.

Although an association between hiccups and reflux has been well described, whether there is a cause and effect relationship remains controversial. The association may be fortuitous; reflux may cause hiccups or hiccups may cause reflux. Hiccups transiently create a pressure gradient which favours reflux of gastric content into the oesophagus. Hiccups acutely reduce intra-oesophageal pressure by 20–40 mmHg and simultaneously reduce lower oesophageal sphincter pressure. Patients have been described in whom oesophageal acid infusion provoked hiccups, and in whom treatment of reflux cured the hiccups. However, other investigators could not induce hiccups by acid infusion. Furthermore, there are numerous studies reporting failure of fundoplication to cure hiccups even in the context of demonstrable acid reflux, which argues against a causal relationship between reflux and hiccups.

Is hiccup associated with oesophageal dysmotility? An achalasia-like picture during the symptomatic phase of intractable hiccups has been reported. This pattern reverted partially to normal with resolution of the hiccups. Achalasia, presumably secondary to oesophageal distension, can present with hiccups usually during consumption of a meal—a symptom that is alleviated following pneumatic dilatation. A range of non-specific oesophageal motor abnormalities can co-exist during the symptomatic phase. Oesophageal peristaltic abnormalities have been reported by some to be present during hiccups. Several manometric studies have demonstrated oesophageal aperistalsis in response to swallows while patients were symptomatic and a return to normal motility thereafter in the absence of hiccups. However, at least one study reported normal oesophageal peristalsis during hiccups. A non-specific oesophageal motor disorder, with some features consistent with spasm, was reported in one case.

Aetiology of hiccups

The relatively common self-limiting bout of hiccups is frequently induced by gastric distension, emotion, alcohol ingestion or sudden change in temperature. However, most frequently the cause of transient hiccups is unknown. The cause of intractable hiccups can be classified into five groups (Table 3.1):

1. Central irritation of medullary centres;

2. Irritating lesions along the neuronal pathway;

3. Metabolic/endocrine;

4. Psychogenic; or

5. Idiopathic.

Structural or functional disturbances of the dorsolateral medulla, in the region of the vagal nuclei and the nucleus tractus solitarius, can cause hiccups. Medullary lesions causing hiccup include infarction in the territory of the posterior inferior cerebellar artery, tumour, abscess, syrinx, haemangioma, haematoma, aneurysm and demyelination. Central nervous system infections including viral encephalitis, syphilis and HIV encephalopathy are less common central causes for hiccup. Neurogenic hiccup due to brainstem disease is frequently accompanied by localising neurological signs.

Stimulation of visceral afferent vagal fibres originating in the gastrointestinal tract will cause hiccup. Gastro-oesophageal reflux, achalasia, gastric distension, oesophageal or small bowel obstruction and even pancreatic biliary disease can provide the stimulus in these cases. Vagal afferent stimulation of the auricular branch of the vagus nerve supplying the external auditory canal has reportedly caused hiccup—in one instance the stimulus arising from an insect trapped in the auditory canal. Mediastinal disease (e.g., tumour, thoracic aortic aneurysm or diaphragmatic irritation caused by subphrenic and hepatic disease, pleural or pericardial effusion, or myocardial infarction) can similarly result in hiccup by stimulation of vagal or phrenic nerve fibres within the mediastinum or by direct irritation of the diaphragm.

Systemic and metabolic disorders including diabetes, uraemia, hypocalcaemia, hyponatraemia and Addison's disease can cause hiccup. Drugs can cause hiccup, most commonly alcohol and general anaesthetic agents, but others include corticosteroids, benzodiazepines, barbiturates, and etoposide. Psychogenic hiccup has been described although this is speculative as the reflex is truly involuntary.

Approach to the patient with intractable hiccups

A careful history should enquire about neurological symptoms particularly headache and brainstem symptoms such as diplopia, vertigo, nausea, vomiting, hoarseness, ataxia or clumsiness and disordered pain sensation. Chest pain, fever or cough are clues to cardiac, respiratory or mediastinal disease. Gastrointestinal causes may be suspected if reflux, regurgitation, chest pain, dysphagia, vomiting or abdominal pain are reported. A history of metabolic disorders and drug enquiry are also important (Table 3.2).

Physical examination should include examination of cranial nerve, long tract and cerebellar signs. Disordered cognitive function may relate to metabolic derangements or to central causes such as encephalitis. Cardiorespiratory examination should look for signs of pleural or pericardial disease and postural hypotension, which is present in Addison's disease. Examine the external auditory canals for foreign bodies. Abdominal examination should specifically look for signs of gastric stasis (e.g., succussion splash), bowel obstruction or tender hepatomegaly, which may indicate hepatic enlargement, or an intrahepatic lesion such as an abscess.

The priorities in respect of investigations will be dictated by the historical and physical findings. Serum electrolytes including sodium, calcium, blood sugar level and liver function tests should be done. A leucocytosis may indicate an underlying infective process. Chest X-ray and electrocardiogram are important to detect pericardial, plural or myocardial disease such as myocardial infarction. Thoracic CT scan can be performed if mediastinal disease is suspected. Imaging of the abdomen is indicated if a subdiaphragmatic abscess is suspected. Endoscopy is indicated if oesophageal disease or gastric stasis are apparent clinically. The approach to intractable hiccups is outlined in Table 3.2.

TABLE 3.1: Causes of intractable hiccups

Supraspinal lesions

Medullary lesions
- Infarction (e.g., posterior inferior cerebellar artery occlusion)
- Haematoma
- Tumour
- Haemangioma
- Demyelination
- Abscess
- Syrinx

Central nervous system infections
- Viral encephalitis
- Meningitis
- HIV encephalopathy
- Encephalitis lethargica
- Syphilis

Phrenic or vagus nerve irritation

Visceral vagal afferent stimulation
- Oesophageal obstruction (tumour, stricture, ring, pill-induced)
- Achalasia
- Gastro-oesophageal reflux
- Gastric distension
- Small bowel obstruction
- Pancreatic/biliary disease
- Foreign body in external auditory meatus (auricular branch of the vagus nerve)

Irritation of thoracic path of phrenic or vagal nerves
- Mediastinal lesions (tumour, aortic aneurysm)
- Pleural/pericardial effusion
- Pneumonia
- Myocardial infarction
- Diaphragmatic irritation (tumour, subphrenic and hepatic lesions)

Metabolic
- Uraemia
- Hyponatraemia
- Hypocalcaemia
- Addison's disease
- General anaesthesia
- Drugs (alcohol, short-acting barbiturates, methyldopa, steroids)

Idiopathic

Psychogenic?

TABLE 3.2: Approach to intractable hiccups

History

- Neurological enquiry (headache, brainstem symptoms such as vertigo, ataxia, diplopia, hoarseness, dysphagia, pain/temperature sensory loss)
- Cardiorespiratory (chest pain, cough, fever, dyspnoea)
- Gastrointestinal symptoms (reflux, regurgitation, vomiting, chest pain, dysphagia, abdominal pain)
- Known metabolic diseases (renal, diabetes, calcium)
- Drugs (methyldopa, barbituates, alcohol, steroids)

Physical examination

- Cranial nerve and cerebellar function, long tract signs, pain/temperature sensation
- Cognitive function (?encephalopathic features)
- Fever
- Cardiorespiratory signs of pleural or pericardial disease; postural hypotension
- Aural examination for foreign body
- Abdominal examination (gastric splash, signs of bowel obstruction, hepatomegaly)

Investigations *(priority and extent dictated by above findings)*

- Metabolic screen (urea, creatinine, electrolytes, calcium, glucose, liver function tests, ?synacthen stimulation test)
- Blood leucocyte count
- Chest X-ray
- Electrocardiograph
- CT thorax (if suspect mediastinal lesion)
- CT abdomen (if suspect liver or subdiaphragmatic lesion)
- Gastroscopy (if suspect oesophageal or gastric pathology)
- Oesophageal motility studies

Treatment

Treatments for intractable hiccup are many and varied and, due to the nature of the condition, virtually none have been subjected to randomised controlled therapeutic trial. There are at least one hundred physical and pharmacological therapies described. Many of these cures are purely anecdotal and have included prayers to St Jude, the Patron Saint of Hopeless Causes; anger; sexual intercourse; pressing a finger firmly into each external auditory canal (to stimulate the auricular branch of vagus nerve); pharyngal stimulation by swallowing coarse grain sugar; and laryngotracheal stimulation induced by a burst of coughing. Physical measures such as breath holding have been attributed to Hippocrates. There is some physiological basis for this as increasing the partial pressure of CO_2 by rebreathing does reduce hiccup frequency. Other noxious afferent stimuli include strong traction on the tongue or phrenic nerve stimulation.

Primary therapy of any identified underlying cause is appropriate and, in most instances, will lead to rapid resolution of the hiccups. In refractory or idiopathic cases, there are no established guidelines regarding drug therapy for hiccup. A very extensive list of drugs has been described with variable success in hiccup. Notwithstanding, there are numerous reported failures in response to a number of agents and therapy is largely a matter of trial and error. Efficacy studies are largely single case reports and uncontrolled. There is only one randomised, controlled therapeutic trial in hiccup.

This study found the $GABA_B$ receptor agonist, baclofen, to be effective in four patients. There is little objective evidence suggesting that one pharmacological agent is superior to another. Substantial numbers of favourable case reports support the efficacy of dopaminergic antagonists, such as chlorpromazine, haloperidol and metoclopramide in intractable hiccup. Other drugs most frequently reported to be effective include anticonvulsants (phenytoin, sodium valproate, carbamazepine); benzodiazepines (clonazepam); calcium channel blockers (nifedipine, nimodipine), anaesthetic agents (ketamine, lignocaine), and amitriptyline (Table 3.3).

Finally, if pharmacotherapy is unsuccessful, disruption of phrenic nerve traffic by transcutaneous electrical stimulation of cervical phrenic nerve, or left phrenic nerve block may be necessary in severe, refractory cases.

TABLE 3.3: Treatment of intractable hiccups

Physical modalities

Raise pCO_2 by rebreathing

Modification of vagal afferent stimulation
- External auditory canal pressure
- Pharyngeal stimulation by nasogastric tube
- Valsalva manoeuvre

Modification of phrenic efferent traffic
- Transcutaneous electrical stimulation of cervical phrenic nerve
- Phrenic nerve crush

Glossopharyngeal nerve block

Pharmacological modalities
- $GABA_B$ agonist: baclofen
- Dopaminergic antagonists (chlorpromazine, haloperidol, metoclopramide, apomorphine)
- Anticonvulsants (carbamazepine, phenytoin, sodium valproate)
- Calcium channel blockers (nifedipine, nimodipine)
- Other (ketamine, lignocaine, nefopam)

Suggested sequential approach to suppression of hiccups

1. Identification and treatment of underlying cause.

2. Vagal afferent stimulation by pressure in both auditory canals; followed by other simple measures aimed at pharyngeal stimulation (coarse grained sugar, passage of naogastric tube) or Valsalva manoeuvre.

3. Parasympathetic stimulation by per rectal massage.

4. Pharmacotherapy
    either:
    baclofen 5–15 mg tds orally,
    if unsuccessful: add nifedipine 5–10 mg tds
    or:
    chlorpromazine 20–50 mg IVI,
    if unsuccessful: add metoclopramide 10 mg IVI.

6. Phrenic nerve modulation (transcutaneous electrical stimulation) or blockade.

SORE MOUTH

The terminology describing oral sensations varies widely because there is no unanimity in relation to the terms used. The range of terms used include glossodynia, glossopyrosis, stomatodynia or oral dysaesthesia. Soreness in the mouth can be due to objective alterations to the oral mucosa due to ulceration or inflammation. Very commonly, however, the symptoms are variable and there is no evidence of mucosal disease nor any underlying pathology to account for symptoms. The latter situation is classified as the burning mouth syndrome. In contrast to conditions causing oral ulceration in which pain is aggravated by eating, the pain of burning mouth syndrome is often alleviated by eating.

Oral ulceration

Oral ulcers are so common as to be almost universally experienced at one time or another. Serious or recurrent and painful oral ulceration can be an indicator of underlying systemic or gastrointestinal disease.

Aphthous ulceration

These usually take the form of multiple, small, painful, punched out shallow ulcers and can affect the lips, buccal mucosa, and tongue. These lesions can also be quite large, in which case they are usually single. Immunological responses seem to contribute to ulcer formation although trauma to the mucosa is also an important precipitant. The lesions are usually relatively minor and heal over a period of a few days up to two weeks. There is little controlled evidence that topical therapy is effective. However, topical steroid preparations, such as triamcinolone acetonide in dental base (Kenalog in Orabase), or hydrocortisone hemisuccinate lozenges are often used with apparent benefit.

Herpes simplex ulcers

These ulcers are located primarily on the hard palate, gingival and alveolar ridges. They begin as small clusters of vesicles, which transform into small punctate ulcers.

Other causes of oral ulceration

Erythema multiforme is preceded by vesicles. Pemphigus and pemphigoid are preceded by bullae. Behçet's syndrome is a rare, multi-system disease in which oral aphthous ulceration occurs in conjunction with ocular and genital ulceration. Skin, joints and the gut can also be affected.

Glossodynia/glossopyrosis (burning mouth syndrome)

Burning mouth syndrome is characterised by the prolonged sensation of unexplained pain or burning inside the oral cavity, often accompanied by other symptoms, such as dryness, paraesthesia, altered sense of taste (cacogeusia, dysgeusia) or smell. It is at least 2–3 times more common in women and is most prevalent among middle-aged women.

TABLE 3.4: Aetiology of glossodynia

Denture-related
- Dentures (ill-fitting, monomer from denture base)
- Dental plaque
- Oral parafunction

Infective/dermatological
- Candidiasis
- Lichen planus

Deficiency states
- Iron, B12, folate, B2 (riboflavin), B6 (pyridoxine), zinc

Endocrine
- Diabetes
- Myxoedema*
- Hormonal changes occurring during menopause*

Neurologically mediated
- Referred from tonsils, teeth
- Lingual nerve neuropathy
- Glossopharyngeal neuralgia
- Oesophageal reflux*

Iatrogenic
- Mouthwash

Xerostomia

Psychogenic

Idiopathic

---

*Unproven associations

Aetiology

Dentures are commonly implicated in glossodynia. Ill-fitting dentures are reported in 50% of patients with this symptom. It has been proposed that pressure is exerted by the dentures on oral tissues or that muscular tension influences sensory innervation and oral sensory perception. Monomers in the denture base material have also been linked to some cases.

Deficiency states cause macroscopic mucosal alterations, but glossodynia can precede these mucosal changes. Glossitis is a characteristic feature of advanced deficiency of vitamins such as folate and B12 (Table 3.4).

Glossodynia in diabetes can be caused by oral candidiasis, however, a form of oral sensory neuropathy is believed to be a factor in some cases in whom *Candida* infection is not a feature.

Several neurogenic causes of glossodynia are described including trauma to the lingual nerve. Glossopharyngeal neuralgia is characterised by paroxysmal pain, not only in the tongue, but also in the entire distribution of the nerve. Glossopharyngeal neuralgia can be elicited by stimulation of trigger zones in the tonsils, pharynx, tongue base and ear.

Gastro-oesophageal reflux is thought in some cases to be associated with glossodynia but there is little objective evidence to suggest that reflux causes it. Furthermore, the observation that reflux is extremely common and glossodynia relatively uncommon argues against a strong association. Anecdotal experience suggests potent anti-reflux therapy is ineffective in the treatment of glossodynia.

Xerostomia can be associated with a burning sensation in the tongue. Salivary secretion tends to fall with age but xerostomia is commonly caused by drugs with anticholinergic effects and is a major problem after head and neck radiotherapy.

Pathogenesis

The cause of this syndrome is unknown. It is possible that burning mouth syndrome is caused by altered oral sensory function because lowered thresholds for sweet and sour taste, and for tongue pain tolerance have been reported in these patients. Behavioural factors may be important. There is a high prevalence of anxiety, depression, somatic reactions to stress suggesting a psychological basis, but a causal link has not been clearly established. Other studies found regional temperature differences in the tongues of sufferers compared with controls as well as differences in blood flow to the tongue, lips and cheeks suggesting that some form of vascular insufficiency might be implicated.

TABLE 3.5: Approach to the patient with sore mouth

History
- Psychological factors, stress
- Symptoms of systemic disease

Examination
- Mouth, tongue, teeth
- Full examination for signs of endocrine, neurological or haematological disorders
- Otolaryngological assessment

Investigations

Haematological
- Full blood count
- Serum iron, B12, folate
- Blood glucose
- Thyroid function tests
- Serum zinc
- Erythrocyte glutathione reductase activity (riboflavin status)*
- Erythrocyte aminotransferase activity (pyridoxine status)*

Bacteriology
- Swabs from tongue for microscopy and culture

Radiology
- Orthopantomogram (for dental pathology)

Dental opinion

---

*Not widely available

Diagnosis

The first step is to exclude an underlying treatable cause although this will only be identified in the minority. History should include an assessment of the patient's behaviour and life stress factors. A careful inspection of the mouth, tongue and teeth is important. A full physical examination may reveal features of systemic disease such as diabetes, thyroid disease, haematological or neurological diseases (Table 3.5). An otolaryngological examination is also important. A dental opinion should probably be sought in most cases, unless an underlying, correctable systemic disease is found.

Treatment

Identification and treatment of any underlying condition is the first step. Longitudinal studies indicate that the prognosis is poor in idiopathic glossodynia, which persists long term in at least half the patients. It is associated with high levels of patient dissatisfaction and continuing consumption of healthcare resources. If psychopathology can be identified, such as a cancer phobia, therapy directed specifically at this aspect may be helpful.

BAD BREATH (HALITOSIS)

Halitosis, a disagreeable odour detectable in exhaled breath, is common in healthy individuals particularly after sleep (morning breath) or after consumption of certain foods. Halitosis is most commonly caused by the action of oral microflora on oral debris located in gingival crevices, within tongue coating and periodontal pockets. Plaque organisms, particularly *Porphyromonas gingivalis*, fusobacteria and other anaerobes, cause putrefaction and subsequent release of volatile chemicals, particularly sulfide compounds. Halitosis may be physiological or pathological. Physiological halitosis is usually transient and an identifying agent, usually a food or drug, is apparent. For example, high sulfur-containing foods such as garlic, onions, broccoli, radishes, leeks, or drugs such as isosorbide dinitrate, disulfiram and dimethyl sulfoxide (DMSO) can cause halitosis, as can dehydration or starvation. Halitosis may also be a manifestation of significant underlying local or systemic disease, a search for which may be necessary if an oral cause cannot be identified.

Patients frequently do not perceive their own oral malodour, which may be apparent to others. The senses of taste and olfaction are subject to the phenomenon of adaptation making the subject insensitive over time to the offensive odour or taste. Also, chemical senses can be affected by many factors, which themselves can be associated with halitosis, such as normal ageing, poor oral hygiene, xerostomia, craniofacial abnormalities, psychiatric disorders and neoplasm.

Pathogenesis

The majority of cases of halitosis arise from oral conditions (see Table 3.6). The odour is a result of sulfur-containing proteins and peptides being hydrolysed by Gram-negative bacteria in the alkaline environment of the mouth. The resulting volatile sulfur-containing end-products include hydrogen sulfide, methyl mercaptan. Surprisingly, the usual compounds associated with putrefaction of biological tissues (ammonia, putrescine, indole, skatole, and cadaverine) are not contributors to oral malodour. Under normal circumstances the odour of the oral cavity is not static and varies throughout the day and as a function of age, gender, hunger state and, perhaps, menstruation. It is affected by multiple factors, many of which are interdependent, including oral flora, salivary flow, pH, oral musculature, and the presence of appropriate substrates. Conditions favouring production of putrid odours include low ambient oxygen concentration, a shift from Gram-positive to Gram-negative bacterial colonisation, reduced carbohydrates available as bacterial substrates, an alkaline oral pH, and reduced salivary flow.

Any oral inflammatory condition, by its association with tissue degeneration and necrosis, will promote bacterial putrefaction. Gingivitis and periodontal disease favour bacterial putrefaction by increasing local growth factors and substrates available from the inflammatory process. These two conditions produce a very potent halitosis and, because of the increased incidence of these two conditions in the ageing population, they may account for the oral malodour ascribed to ageing.

The surface structure of the tongue provides a suitable environment for a biofilm serving as a repository for periodontal and other bacteria including anaerobes. Deep fissures on the tongue dorsum, present in around 25% of the population, has been associated with higher mouth and tongue odour scores although proof of higher bacterial counts in this population is lacking. The degree of tongue coating (containing a mix of desquamated cells, debris and bacteria) has some correlation with tongue bacterial counts and with halitosis.

Approach to the patient

The approach to the patient is detailed in Table 3.7. The first step is to determine whether the patient does actually have halitosis, by wafting the expired air towards the examiner's nose with the palm of the hand. It is important to be aware, however, that halitosis can be intermittent. Therefore, if it is not apparent to the clinician, corroborative evidence should be sought from family members or close contacts. If the problem cannot be substantiated, the patient may have disordered chemoreception or the problem may be psychogenic. Neurosis can lead to compulsive use of mints, mouthwashes and oral deodorants in the absence of objective malodour. In such cases, halitosis is not physically based and counselling or psychiatric help may be needed.

The next step is to determine whether the odour is perceived predominantly during exhalation via the mouth or via the nose. A stronger odour from nasally expired air indicates a lesion or disease of the nose, nasopharynx, sinuses or respiratory tract. Common causes include local tumours, rhinitis, sinusitis, or nasal foreign body (Table 3.6). Bronchiectasis can cause halitosis. Other respiratory disorders, such as asthma requiring systemic or inhaled corticosteroids, can result in oropharyngeal candidiasis causing halitosis. Conditions in which oral candidiasis is common include cancer, immune deficiency states, diabetes, xerostomia.

A more pronounced odour emanating from oral exhalation indicates an oral, oropharyngeal, hypopharyngeal, or oesophagogastric source. Halitosis is rarely caused by gastrointestinal disorders. Gases from the upper gastrointestinal tract do not normally mix with those of the respiratory tract, but they can in the context of eructation, regurgitation or vomiting. Stagnation of food in a pharyngeal pouch or a dilated oesophagus in achalasia can cause regurgitation or eructation of partially fermented food and secretions.

If the expired air is equally offensive whether exhaled by nose or mouth, a systemic or metabolic cause is suspected.

Finally, a number of patients can present with halitosis and/or altered chemoreception for which no underlying cause can be found. Sophisticated breath analysis (gas chromatography, mass spectrometry) in some of these patients have identified higher than normal levels of volatile sulfur compounds. While some of these individuals have enzymatic or transport abnormalities, it is not known whether a subset of the remainder are heterozygous for sulphur-containing amino acidurias.

Treatment

General

Management of non-oral causes of halitosis requires treatment of the underlying cause. Dental and gingival disease will account for the majority and dental referral should be sought in most cases.

Oral care

Oral care will be dictated by dental opinion. Specific treatment of gingival or periodontal disease may be required. Regular brushing and flossing of teeth, dental review and prophylaxis and plaque removal are important. Adequate frequent cleaning of dentures is also important. If head and neck radiotherapy is planned for any reason, prior initiation of good oral hygiene practices and establishing optimal oral health will minimise the development of post-radiation halitosis secondary to xerostomia. If present, oral candidiasis should be treated with antifungal agents such as nystatin and removal of any removable oral prostheses, which can harbour the organism and recolonise the tissues.

Oral mouthwashes

Chemicals, such as chlorhexidine, chlorine dioxide, metal ions, triclosan or formulations containing essential oils and hydrogen peroxide, can reduce oral bacterial content. While some mouth washes are a useful adjunct in the prevention of halitosis, they are not a substitute for good oral hygiene practices and may only mask oral malodour. Their high alcohol content may further dry out the oral mucosa, and in the context of xerostomia, non-alcohol based fluoridated washes are preferable. Mouthwashes containing chlorhexidine appear to be most effective at reducing plaque and gingivitis. Limited uncontrolled data also support the use of chlorhexidine mouthwashes specifically for halitosis. However, there are no controlled efficacy data and the durability of the effect on oral flora is unclear. Mechanical removal of debris coating the tongue may also be useful although objective efficacy data are lacking. In severe, refractory cases, a trial of metronidazole for 10 days may be considered, although high-level evidence for efficacy is lacking for this approach.

Dietary changes

Eating regularly and avoidance of odiferous foods is important. Low-fat diets and diets high in fruit and vegetables can be helpful.

Treat xerostomia

If xerostomia is a problem, a change in medications may be appropriate as drugs are the commonest cause of dry mouth. Saliva substitutes and sialagogues, such as pilocarpine or sugar-free chewing gum, are useful to increase saliva flow, optimise pH and clean the mouth.

TABLE 3.6: Causes of halitosis

Oral/dental

- Poor oral hygiene/failure to clean dentures
- Dental decay
- Periodontal disease
- Gingivitis
- Oral ulceration (aphthous, infective, traumatic)
- Oral candidiasis (corticosteroids, cancer, immune deficiency, diabetes), xerostomia (drugs, dehydration, ageing, anaemia, hypovitaminosis, diabetes, stress, autoimmune disease, mechanical blockage, malignancy, multiple sclerosis, AIDS, irradiation)
- Oral neoplasm

Nasal/nasopharynx

- Neoplasm
- Rhinitis (atrophic, rhinitis medicamentosa)
- Tonsillitis
- Nasal foreign body
- Sinusitis

Laryngo-pharyngeal

- Pharyngeal pouch
- Neoplasm

Oesophagogastric

- Achalasia
- Oesophageal/gastric cancer

Respiratory

- Bronchiectasis
- Bronchitis
- Tuberculosis
- Lung abscess
- Necrotic neoplasm

Systemic/metabolic

- Starvation
- Uraemia
- Hepatic failure
- Diabetic ketoacidosis
- Inborn errors of metabolism (aminoacidurias, e.g., trimethylaminuria)
- Drugs (alcohol, nitrates, chloral hydrate, iodine-containing drugs)

Psychogenic

- Delusional halitosis
- Hallucinatory feature of schizophrenia or temporal lobe epilepsy

Idiopathic

TABLE 3.7: Approach to halitosis

History

- Onset, constant or intermittent, relationship to time of day, diet
- Dental history: oral habits/hygiene
- Symptoms: dysphagia, regurgitation or coughing; symptoms of systemic disease
- Associated taste disorders that might suggest central cause (7th, 9th, 10th cranial nerves, medulla, pons, thalamus, cortical taste centres)
- Drugs: corticosteroids, drugs causing xerostomia or halitosis

Examination

- Confirm presence of halitosis (if neither detectable, nor supported by close contacts, suspect disordered chemoreception[1] or psychogenic)
- Odour predominantly during *oral* expiration = oral disease in majority (oropharyngeal, oesophagogastric also)
  - ? Upper gastrointestinal evaluation (barium swallow, endoscopy)
  - Oral/dental inspection, oral candidiasis
- Odour predominantly during *nasal* expiration = respiratory tract disease
  - Otorhinolaryngological evaluation (nasopharynx, nose, sinuses)
  - Chest X-ray, sputum examination, bronchoscopy
- Expired air equally offensive via nose *and* mouth = metabolic disorder
  - Blood glucose level, electrolytes, urea, creatinine, liver function tests

1. Test olfactory function (e.g., soaps, wintergreen, cloves).

Further reading

Hiccup

Howard RS. Persistent hiccups [Editorial]. *Brit Med J* 1992; 305: 1237–8.
Ramirez FC, Graham DY. Treatment of intractable hiccup with Baclofen: results of a double-blind randomized, controlled, cross-over study. *Am J Gastroenterol* 1992; 87: 1789–91.
Walker P, Watanabe S, Bruera E. Baclofen, a treatment for chronic hiccup. *J Pain Symptom Manage* 1998; 16: 125–32.

Glossodynia

Grushka M, Epstein JB, Gorsky M. Burning mouth syndrome. *Am Fam Physician* 2002; 65: 615–20.
Murty G, Fawcett S. The aetiology and management of glossodynia. *Brit J Clin Pract* 1990; 44(8): 389–92.
Zakrzewska JM, Forssell H, Glenny AM. Interventions for the treatment of burning mouth syndrome. *Cochrane Database Syst Rev* 2005; (1): CD 002779.

Halitosis

Coventry J, Griffiths G, Scully C, Tonetti M. Periodontal disease. *Br Med J* 2000; 321: 36–9.
Morita M, Wang H-L. Association between oral malodor and adult periodontitis: a review. *J Clinical Periodontol* 2001; 28: 813–9.
Quirynen M, Zhao H, van Steenberghe D. Review of the treatment strategies for oral malodour. *Clin Oral Invest* 2002; 6: 1–10.
Roldan S, Herrera D, Saaz M. Biofilms and the tongue: therapeutical approaches for control of halitosis. *Clin Oral Invest* 2003; 7: 189–97.
Scully C, Porter S, Greenman J. What to do about halitosis? *Brit Med J* 1994; 308(22): 217–8.

chapter 4

ACUTE ABDOMINAL PAIN

Acute abdominal pain is a common ailment experienced by most from time to time. Many episodes of acute abdominal pain resolve spontaneously with analgesia and a period of observation. Acute abdominal pain is a source of anxiety as patients know that it may be the first sign of a serious clinical problem, which may be life-threatening, and that surgery may be the only solution.

Acute abdominal pain is defined as recent onset pain of such severity that medical attention is usually sought shortly after its onset. For the purpose of definition, pain persisting for up to three months is classified as acute; pain lasting more than three months is classified as chronic and is considered in Chapters 5 and 6.

MECHANISMS OF ABDOMINAL PAIN

Visceral pain

The abdominal organs are not sensitive to touch; gentle direct palpation during a laparotomy or a herniorrhaphy performed after infiltration of the anterior abdominal wall with local anaesthesia causes no distress. However, distending or stretching the bowel at these operations causes vague abdominal discomfort, which is mediated by splanchnic sympathetic nerves. This visceral pain is poorly localised, usually to the midline. Distension or stretching of the capsule of the liver, as occurs in acute hepatitis, also causes pain.

Peritoneal pain

The parietal peritoneum, but not the visceral peritoneum, is innervated by pain fibres, which pass to the spinal cord along the segmental nerves. Thus, inflammation of the parietal peritoneum causes abdominal pain that is localised to the inflamed area.

Referred pain

Referred pain is pain experienced at a distance from the area of damage. The best known example is pain felt at the tip of the shoulder, when the parietal peritoneum on the inferior surface of the diaphragm is irritated by, for example, blood or gastric juice. This area of peritoneum is innervated by somatic nerves (C4) as is the skin over the tip of the shoulder.

Abdominal guarding occurs due to a reflex contraction of abdominal wall muscles in response to a noxious stimulus to the pain fibres of the same dermatome.

PATHOLOGICAL CAUSES OF ACUTE ABDOMINAL PAIN

There are certain similarities in the pattern and type of pain that occur when a given pathological process affects different organs within the abdominal cavity. An understanding of these various patterns is important, as it provides a basis for interpreting the clinical effects and consequences of many of the conditions that result in acute abdominal pain. Important pathological causes of abdominal pain are acute inflammation, obstruction, ischaemia and increased pressure within a solid organ. Not uncommonly, an organ is affected by more than one pathological process during the evolution of an illness. An example is acute appendicitis, where the initial process is obstructive and the subsequent one is inflammatory.

Acute inflammation

The common processes leading to intra-abdominal inflammation are bacterial invasion, chemical irritation and ischaemia. The features of pain caused by inflammation depend on whether the organ it affects is intraperitoneal or extraperitoneal.

Inflammation of intraperitoneal organs

Acute inflammation of an intraperitoneal organ results in localised peritonitis if the process involves its peritoneal surface. Ensuing pain results from irritation of pain receptors in the parietal (but not visceral) peritoneum. This pain is described as peritoneal in type. *Peritoneal pain* is well localised; the patient can usually indicate its position with the palm of a hand and, on occasions, with the tip of a finger. The pain is typically aggravated by sudden movement, such as coughing, and minimised by avoidance of movement, such as lying still or using the diaphragmatic rather than the abdominal muscles for respiration. As an example, involvement of a segment of bowel with Crohn's disease, a transmural inflammatory process, can result in peritoneal pain. Inflammation restricted to bowel mucosa, as typically occurs in ulcerative colitis, does not result in peritoneal pain (Chapter 13).

A more common example of acute inflammation as the sole process resulting in peritoneal pain is acute salpingitis. The pain caused by acute inflammation usually develops over a period of hours.

Intraperitoneal inflammation may result from an obstructive process. A well known example is acute appendicitis. The early pain of acute appendicitis is periumbilical and due to obstruction of the appendix (a visceral pain). As the inflammation becomes transmural, the pain becomes peritoneal in type and moves to the right iliac fossa over the inflamed organ.

Intraperitoneal inflammation may be a consequence of perforation of a hollow viscus. Leakage of visceral contents causes pain by chemical irritation. The degree of irritation is dependent on the nature of the leaking material. Thus, leaking gastric juice from a perforated peptic ulcer causes marked irritation. By contrast, gas, which may be the major constituent of the material leaking from a perforated sigmoid diverticulum, causes less irritation and less pain. As the inflammation in response to chemical irritation is rapid, the onset of the pain is rapid. Whether the pain is localised or generalised depends on the degree of soilage. Maximum irritation is usually around the site of leakage (e.g., epigastric for a perforated peptic ulcer and in the left iliac fossa for a perforated sigmoid diverticulum). Other causes of perforation include ischaemia which has progressed to infarction (e.g., gangrenous cholecystitis) and malignancy (e.g., perforated gastric cancer).

With ischaemic bowel, the peritoneal component of the pain is usually a relatively minor component of pain. The major component, which is severe, is visceral in type (see below). Peritoneal inflammation only occurs if the ischaemia of the bowel is transmural. The most sensitive component of the bowel wall to ischaemia is the mucosa. On the other hand, the pain resulting from a splenic infarct is predominantly peritoneal in type.

Inflammation of non-intraperitoneal organs

Acute pancreatitis results in chemical inflammation of retroperitoneal tissues and irritation of visceral nerves. The pain is constant, severe, and not aggravated by movement. If the inflammatory process of acute pancreatitis spreads anteriorly, the patient also complains of a peritoneal pain.

Obstruction

If the bowel is obstructed, then the pain is colicky unless there is some further complication such as gangrene, secondary infection or perforation, when the pain becomes continuous. The colicky pain is severe in degree and midline in position; it is usually epigastric if the organ originated from foregut (down to the second part of the duodenum), periumbilical if the organ originated from midgut (down to the splenic flexure of the colon), and hypogastric if the organ originated from hindgut (left colon and rectum). The pain of biliary obstruction (gall bladder and extra-hepatic biliary tree), described as biliary colic, is constant rather than colicky in nature.

The onset of the pain of obstruction is related to the speed of obstruction. If the occlusion is sudden (e.g., gall bladder outlet obstruction due to a stone or a volvulus of the sigmoid colon), the onset of pain is over minutes. If the occlusion is slowly progressive (e.g., obstructing cancer of the sigmoid colon), the onset of the pain is much slower. If the occlusion is intermittent (e.g., gall bladder outlet obstruction due to a stone), the pain is intermittent.

Obstruction of the gastrointestinal tract may be due to a luminal lesion (e.g., bezoar or calculus), a mural lesion (e.g., a benign or malignant tumour or a fibrous stricture), or an extraluminal lesion (e.g., a fibrous band or the neck of a hernia). The obstruction can occur anywhere along the lumen of the gastrointestinal tract. The obstruction results in proximal distension and stasis. If the obstructed bowel is open-ended proximally, the distension progresses proximally. If the lumen is closed proximally, the luminal contents and the organ itself can become infected (e.g., cholecystitis, cholangitis and appendicitis) or progressive distension can lead to venous obstruction followed by arterial obstruction, and then gangrene and perforation (e.g., closed loop obstruction of bowel).

Ischaemia

Inadequate blood flow results in tissue death (infarction). Arterial ischaemia is caused by an arterial embolus to the bowel, thrombosis or a low output state. The pain is of sudden onset, over a few minutes, severe and continuous (*visceral pain*). The process of venous ischaemia is slower in onset. Consequently, the pain is slower in onset. Otherwise, it has the same characteristics as the pain of arterial ischaemia. When the venous occlusion is complete, as occurs to a loop of bowel strangulated by the neck of a hernia, the tissue drained by the occluded vein becomes oedematous and engorged with blood, and arterial obstruction and thrombosis may follow. With larger vein occlusion by a thrombus (e.g., the portal or the superior mesenteric vein, or occasionally with a volvulus of bowel), the occlusion may be incomplete and alternative venous drainage may save the tissue from necrosis. Acute major mesenteric venous obstruction causes transudation of fluid into the peritoneal cavity, which may be evident as ascites.

Tension in a solid organ

Sudden swelling in solid organs results in a pain of visceral type due to stretching of the capsule of the organ. The pain is dull and constant. The severity of the pain depends on the speed and degree of swelling. Examples include haemorrhage into an ovarian cyst, necrosis of a hepatic metastasis and hepatic venous engorgement due to acute right heart failure.

CLINICAL EVALUATION

From the practical point of view, the clinician should have four goals when managing a patient with acute abdominal pain:

1. relief of symptoms;

2. prompt diagnosis and treatment of life-threatening conditions;

3. early diagnosis and treatment of conditions that have complications which can be averted by prompt treatment; and

4. early diagnosis of conditions for which there is specific rather than symptomatic treatment only.

A simple practical approach to diagnosis of acute abdominal pain, shown in Table 4.1, involves stratification according to:

1. Position of pain
Generalised
Localised, eg:
- epigastric
- right upper quadrant
- central (periumbilical)
- right iliac fossa
- left iliac fossa
- lower abdominal (hypogastric)

2. Nature or type of pain:
- constant
- peritoneal
- colicky

TABLE 4.1: Sites and types of abdominal pain related to different organs

Site	Type of pain	Organ[2]	Radiation
Generalised	Peritoneal[1]	Peritoneum	
Epigastric	Constant	Stomach	
	Constant	Duodenum	± to midline back
	Constant	Pancreas	± to midline back
	Constant	Biliary	± to midline back
	Constant	*Aorta*	commonly to midline back
Right upper quadrant	Constant or peritoneal	Liver	
	Constant or peritoneal	Gall bladder	Commonly around to right scapula
	Constant	Duodenum	
Central/periumbilical	Colicky	Small bowel (midgut)	
	Constant	*Aorta*	Commonly to midline back
Right iliac fossa	Peritoneal	Appendix	
	Constant or peritoneal	Small bowel	
	Peritoneal	Caecum	
	Constant or peritoneal	*Ovary*	
	Constant or peritoneal	*Fallopian tube*	
Left iliac fossa	Peritoneal	Sigmoid colon	
	Constant or peritoneal	*Ovary*	
	Constant or peritoneal	*Fallopian tube*	
Lower abdominal/ suprapubic/ hypogastric	Constant or peritoneal	Colon (hindgut)	
	Constant	*Bladder*	
	Constant or colicky	*Uterus*	

1. Peritoneal pain is defined as constant abdominal pain that is aggravated by movement and relieved by rest.
2. Non-gastrointestinal organs are shown in italics.

TABLE 4.2: Causes of abdominal pain seen at a hospital emergency unit

Cause	Percentage
Non-specific abdominal pain	34
Acute appendicitis	28
Acute cholecystitis	10
Small bowel obstruction	4
Acute gynaecological disease	4
Acute pancreatitis	3
Renal colic	3
Perforated peptic ulcer	2
Cancer	2
Diverticular disease	1
Miscellaneous	9

(Based on de Dombal FT, Diagnosis of Acute Abdominal Pain, 2nd edn, Edinburgh: Churchill Livingstone, 1991, with permission.)

Clinical evaluation is performed with the knowledge that many of the patients who present with acute abdominal pain have a short self-limiting illness for which nothing more than symptomatic and supportive treatment is required. Selection bias results in this proportion being small in patients admitted to hospital, larger in patients presenting to emergency units and largest in general practice. A list of causes of non-trauma-related abdominal pain seen in an English hospital are shown in Table 4.2.

GENERALISED ABDOMINAL PAIN

The common causes of generalised acute abdominal pain are listed in Table 4.3. The first issue to address is whether or not the patient has an abdominal catastrophe. On most occasions, differentiation of a patient with an abdominal catastrophe from one with non-specific abdominal pain is relatively straightforward. As indicated in Table 4.3, the patient with an abdominal catastrophe usually has generalised peritonitis, with generalised tenderness, guarding, rebound tenderness and absence of bowel sounds. However, there may be few signs initially to accompany a mesenteric embolus or thrombosis while the bowel is still viable. Further, the abdominal signs associated with acute pancreatitis may be mild.

There are commonly signs of shock if there has been blood loss or dehydration. These include tachycardia, hypotension, oliguria and peripheral vasoconstriction (cool blue peripheral tissues and a thready pulse). Pallor may be indicative of blood loss. Dehydration is suggested by a dry tongue, reduced skin turgor and decreased eye turgor. The signs of Gram-negative shock are slightly different. Rather than the signs of peripheral vasoconstriction there may be peripheral vasodilatation, evidenced by a bounding pulse and a warm periphery as well as clamminess.

The previous history and associated signs that may be of help in distinguishing the various catastrophes are listed in Table 4.4.

TABLE 4.3: Causes and clinical features of conditions producing generalised acute abdominal pain

Cause	Abdominal signs	Associated signs
Non-specific abdominal pain	Nil or mild	Nil
Perforated appendix	"	"
Perforated diverticulum	"	"
Ruptured ectopic pregnancy	Generalised peritonitis	± Shock
Ruptured pathological solid organ	± Mass/organomegaly	"
Ruptured aortic aneurysm	Tender pulsatile mass	Shock
Strangulated bowel	Focal or generalised peritonitis	Bowel obstruction ± sepsis ± shock
Superior mesenteric thrombosis or embolus	Initially few or no signs (pain out of proportion to signs)	Atrial fibrillation or myocardial infarction ± shock
Ischaemic colitis	Often not severe unless there is transmural infarction	Bloody diarrhoea, atrial fibrillation or myocardial infarction
Pancreatitis	May be few signs (pain can be out of proportion to signs)	± Shock

The management of an abdominal catastrophe includes urgent admission to hospital, cardiopulmonary resuscitation, some simple investigations depending on the gravity of the situation and early laparotomy on most occasions. Conditions for which early laparotomy might not be undertaken include ischaemic colitis and acute pancreatitis.

The investigations that are usually performed are listed in Table 4.5. They include tests aimed at establishing the diagnosis and tests to assist resuscitation. Air under the diaphragm suggests a perforated viscus. It is most commonly present with a perforated peptic ulcer (80% of cases), less commonly present with a perforated diverticulum (20%) and rarely present with a perforated appendix. An amylase estimation is essential in all patients with generalised abdominal pain to avoid an inadvertent laparotomy for acute pancreatitis.

TABLE 4.4: Clinical clues to establish the cause of the abdominal catastrophe

Abdominal catastrophe	Previous history	Possible differentiating physical signs
Perforated peptic ulcer	Dyspepsia or proven peptic ulcer	Lack of liver dullness to percussion Signs maximal in the epigastrium
Perforated appendix	Initial history consistent with appendicitis	Signs maximal in the right iliac fossa
Perforated diverticulum	Preceding history of diverticular disease	Lack of liver dullness to percussion Signs maximal in the left iliac fossa
Ruptured aneurysm	Recent backache Other history of vascular disease	Tender pulsatile mid-abdominal mass Vascular disease elsewhere
Ruptured ectopic pregnancy	Missed period	Signs maximal in lower abdomen Tender pelvic mass on per vagina examination
Ruptured pathological organ	Organ specific	Organ specific
Strangulated bowel	Hernia Previous abdominal surgery	Tender hernia Abdominal scars
Mesenteric thrombosis or embolus	Atrial fibrillation Myocardial infarction Other vascular disease	Vascular disease elsewhere
Ischaemic colitis	Other vascular disease Recent period of low cardiac output Irritable bowel syndrome symptoms	Bloody diarrhoea Signs maximal on the left side
Acute pancreatitis	Alcoholic binges Gallstones	Periumbilical or renal angle blood staining of subcutaneous fat

TABLE 4.5: Investigations for patients with acute generalised abdominal pain	
Investigation	**Possible findings**
Routine	
Erect chest X-ray	Gas under the diaphragm Atelectasis
Erect and supine abdominal X-ray	Distended small or large bowel Thickened bowel Gas in bowel wall Calcified aneurysm
Haemoglobin	Anaemia Haemoconcentration
White cell count with differential	Leucocytosis with left shift
Electrolytes	Unexpected hypokalaemia
Urea and creatinine	Unexpected renal failure
Serum amylase Serum lipase	Hyperamylasaemia suggestive of pancreatitis; marginal elevation seen in small bowel obstruction, acute cholecystitis and mesenteric infarction
Under appropriate clinical circumstances	
Limited gastrograffin meal	Confirmation of duodenal perforation if conservative treatment is contemplated
Beta HCG	Elevated in ectopic pregnancy
Abdominal ultrasound	Confirmation of ruptured aneurysm only if diagnosis in doubt and condition is stable Demonstration of intra-abdominal fluid
CT scan	Confirmation of ruptured aneurysm only if diagnosis in doubt and condition is stable Confirmation of pancreatitis if doubt exists
Limited gastrograffin enema	'Thumb printing' due to mucosal oedema

Specific management of conditions causing generalised abdominal pain

Perforated peptic ulcer

This is diagnosed by a sudden history of prostration with generalised severe abdominal pain of peritoneal type. On examination there is generalised tenderness and guarding, usually maximal in the epigastrium, board-like rigidity, loss of bowel sounds and loss of liver dullness to percussion. The diagnosis is supported by demonstration of gas under the diaphragm on an erect chest X-ray examination (Figure 4.1). A CT scan is more sensitive at dectecting extraluminal (free) gas. If still uncertain, the diagnosis can be made with a limited gastrograffin meal or a laparoscopy.

Initial treatment includes fluid resuscitation, nasogastric suction and broad-spectrum antibiotics. Thereafter, the perforation can be closed either laparoscopically or at open laparotomy. The peritoneal cavity is lavaged at the same time. Closure of the perforation

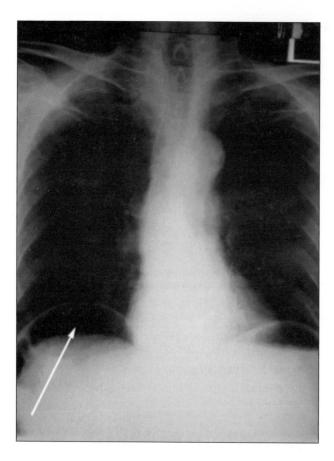

FIGURE 4.1: Gas under the diaphragm from a perforated duodenal ulcer shown on X-ray of erect chest.

is required to prevent continuing contamination of the peritoneal cavity. Laparoscopic closure of the perforation and lavage of the peritoneal cavity to prevent subsequent intra-abdominal abscess formation is the therapy most commonly advocated.

An alternative non-operative approach is possible for selected cases. It is based on the knowledge that in up to three-quarters of cases, the perforation closes spontaneously. Some surgeons give selected patients with perforated duodenal ulcer a trial of non-operative treatment. This involves close clinical observation to detect failure of the peritonitis to resolve, continued fluid resuscitation, and broad-spectrum antibiotics. Non-operative treatment is unsuitable for perforated gastric ulcers and gastric cancers, as the chance of spontaneous closure with these lesions is low. The diagnosis should be established with some certainty before starting a trial of non-operative treatment. A limited gastrograffin meal is required to identify the site of the leaking ulcer.

There is no need to perform a definitive anti-ulcer operation, as the ulcer diathesis can be cured after recovery from the perforation with medication (see Chapter 5).

Perforated appendicitis

The diagnosis might be suspected by a history suggestive of appendicitis (see right iliac fossa pain described below). The patient is toxic with signs of fever, and has tachycardia. The abdominal signs are usually maximal in the right iliac fossa. Air should not be expected under the diaphragm. Appendicectomy is required.

Perforated diverticulum

This may be diagnosed by CT scanning. Preceding pain in the left iliac fossa in a middle-aged to elderly patient is supportive. The abdominal signs may be maximal in the left iliac fossa. There is often a large amount of gas under the diaphragm. The speed of onset is usually slower than with a perforated peptic ulcer.

Resection of the affected segment of bowel is required. In the usual case of a perforated sigmoid diverticulum, a proximal end colostomy is performed and the distal stump oversewn as the bowel has not previously been cleansed of faeces.

Ruptured abdominal aortic aneurysm

The clinical picture is quite different to the conditions above. The patient is usually elderly with risk factors for vascular disease. The pain is central, constant, non-peritoneal in type and often radiates through to the back. Cardiovascular collapse is a prominent feature. A tender, pulsatile epigastric mass is diagnostic. Signs of peritonism are not prominent. If the diagnosis is not made on clinical grounds and the patient is haemodynamically stable, the diagnosis may be made by plain abdominal X-ray examination if the wall of the aneurysm is calcified, or by CT scan, which shows retroperitoneal extravasation of blood as well as the aneurysm. Vascular grafting or stenting of the affected segment is urgently required.

Ruptured ectopic pregnancy

The diagnosis is suspected in a woman of childbearing age who has missed a period. The abdominal symptoms and signs are usually maximal in the lower abdomen. Shock may be a prominent feature. The diagnosis is supported by elevation of beta HCG levels. Local resection is required.

Strangulated bowel

The diagnosis may not be suspected prior to laparotomy, which is performed because of severe pain unrelieved by narcotics in a patient with signs of peritonitis. The site of maximal symptoms and signs is dependent on the position of the strangulated loop of bowel. There may be associated symptoms and signs of small bowel obstruction. On plain radiology of the abdomen, the strangulated loop may be seen as thick walled due to oedema. In addition, there may be radiological features of small bowel obstruction (see Figure 4.2). CT scanning prior to surgery may assist with the diagnosis, and even define the cause of the strangulation.

Local resection is required if the loop of bowel remains non-viable after it is released intra-operatively. Bowel which is pink in colour and exhibits spontaneous peristalsis or peristalsis when stimulated is viable. Further, there should be pulsatile flow of bright red blood through feeding vessels.

A ruptured pathological organ

Presentation and treatment is dependent on the underlying pathology. A delayed splenic rupture, for example, will usually require splenectomy. A ruptured ovarian cyst may require ovarian cystectomy or oophorectomy. A ruptured liver cell adenoma requires a liver resection. Often the underlying problem will only become apparent at laparotomy. A full list of other causes and the appropriate treatment is beyond the scope of this book.

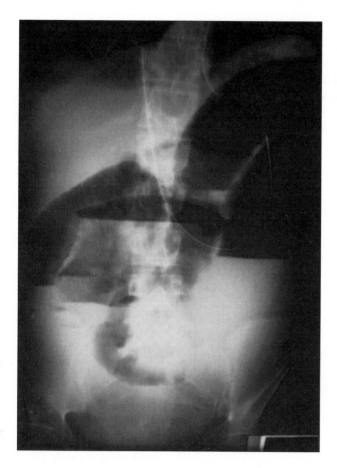

FIGURE 4.2: Plain abdominal X-ray examination of small bowel obstruction showing distended loops of small bowel with multiple fluid levels and absence of colonic gas.

Massive small bowel ischaemia

This is caused by a superior mesenteric artery thrombosis or embolism. It initially presents with severe constant abdominal pain of non-peritoneal type in an elderly patient with risk factors for vascular disease or a patient with risk factors for arterial embolism (e.g., atrial fibrillation or recent myocardial infarction). Early on, when the bowel is still viable, there are minimal abdominal signs. Clinical suspicion in an elderly patient with associated atrial fibrillation, vascular disease elsewhere or a low cardiac output state is the key to early treatment. The diagnosis must be considered in an elderly patient *if the pain is out of proportion to the signs as the abdominal signs are not marked and there are no specific diagnostic signs on plain abdominal radiology*. A triple phase CT scan may be diagnostic and saves valuable time in the lead-up to surgery.

At laparotomy, the bowel is usually non-viable, so that attempted re-perfusion is usually not an option. The extent of bowel ischaemia depends on whether the main trunk of the superior mesenteric artery or a branch is occluded. When the main trunk is occluded, a variable length of proximal jejunum supplied by collaterals from the coeliac artery and a variable amount of the right hemicolon supplied by collaterals from the inferior mesenteric artery remain viable.

There are two initial therapeutic options for massive small bowel infarction:

1. Resection with re-anastomosis of the viable ends.
   Thereafter the patient receives anticoagulation treatment to prevent extension of

the thrombotic process. A 'second-look' laparotomy is usually performed after 24 hours to assess the viability of the remaining bowel.

2. Diagnostic laparotomy only.
   There are some elderly and frail patients who have no realistic chance of returning to an enjoyable lifestyle after massive small bowel resection. For these, a decision against massive resection may be made.

After initial surgical recovery, there is gut adaptation and hypertrophy sufficient to allow maintenance of nutrition by oral means if the residual small bowel length is greater than 45 cm. Patients with shorter residual lengths usually require long-term parenteral nutrition (Chapter 15).

Superior mesenteric venous thrombosis usually results in a more subacute presentation. There can be associated ascites. The demonstration of a venous filling defect on the CT scan confirms the diagnosis. Management is determined by whether the affected bowel is viable or not. If the diagnosis can be made by CT scan and there are no signs of peritonism, the patient can be managed by anticoagulation and observation. After recovery, a predisposing cause is sought. Predisposing causes include the oral contraceptive pill, anti-thrombin III deficiency, protein S and protein C deficiency.

Ischaemic colitis

This is commonly diagnosed without laparotomy because of the associated bloody diarrhoea. The clinical diagnosis is supported by the finding of gross oedema and 'thumb printing' in the left colon on plain abdominal X-ray examination (see Figure 4.3) or CT scan. If there is uncertainty, colonoscopy can be helpful. Ischaemic colitis usually settles with non-operative treatment. If during close observation, however, the abdominal signs become more marked or the patient develops systemic signs of sepsis, laparotomy is required to exclude an occult perforation and resect the ischaemic segment as a Hartmann's procedure. Re-anastomosis is then delayed until after full recovery. Anticoagulation treatment is contraindicated early because of the risk of massive colonic haemorrhage.

Pancreatitis

This is discussed below under *Acute epigastric pain*.

ACUTE ABDOMINAL COLIC

Colicky pain is felt in the midline. It is associated with forceful smooth muscle contraction. It has a characteristic repetitive pattern. There is intense pain for a few minutes, followed by complete relief of pain for a few minutes. It is associated with gastric, small and large intestinal and uterine disorders. Gastric (foregut) colic is experienced in the epigastrium; small bowel and right hemicolon (midgut) colic periumbilically; and left hemicolon (hindgut) and uterine colic suprapubically. So-called 'biliary colic' is a continuous rather than intermittent pain experienced in the epigastrium or the right upper quadrant.

The causes of acute abdominal colic are listed in Table 4.6. The common causes are acute gastroenteritis, food poisoning, constipation and uterine disorders. The life-threatening causes are small and large bowel obstruction.

TABLE 4.6: Causes of acute abdominal colic

- Acute gastroenteritis
- Food poisoning
- Non-specific causes
- Constipation
- Gastric outlet obstruction:
  - Chronic peptic ulceration
  - Gastric cancer
- Small bowel obstruction:

Adhesions:
- Postsurgical
- Inflammatory (e.g., diverticular)
- Radiation
- Meckel's diverticulum
- Metastatic

Hernia:
- Abdominal wall
- Internal

Neoplasm:
- Benign (e.g., leiomyoma)
- Malignant (e.g., carcinoid tumour, adenocarcinoma)

Stricture:
- Ischaemic
- Radiation
- Inflammatory (e.g., Crohn's disease)

Volvulus
Intussusception:
- Tumour (e.g., Peutz-Jegher's syndrome)
Superior mesenteric artery syndrome

Intraluminal bolus
- Gallstone
- Bezoar

- Large bowel obstruction
  - Colon cancer
  - Diverticular disease
  - Volvulus
- Uterine
  - Missed abortion
  - Parturition
  - Period pain

The initial clinical question is: Does this patient have an innocent or a serious cause of abdominal colic? Acute gastroenteritis is usually of viral origin, is associated with diarrhoea and is infectious so that it is likely to have affected others in the household. Food poisoning can usually be related to ingestion of a particular meal. The specific management of the problems that cause abdominal colic with diarrhoea is covered in Chapter 12. Simple analgesics are part of the management.

Constipation of recent origin can often be related to ingestion of drugs (e.g., codeine-containing analgesics) or a change in dietary pattern (Chapter 10). It is managed with simple analgesics, elimination of an identifiable cause and use of a bulking agent.

Uterine causes are associated with vaginal bleeding and menstrual irregularities. Their management is beyond the scope of this book.

Some patients with a non-specific cause may be difficult to distinguish from patients with early bowel obstruction. When there is doubt after the initial clinical evaluation, the patient should have simple investigations, such as plain abdominal radiology, looking for a bowel obstruction. Continued clinical uncertainty may be managed best by close observation in hospital.

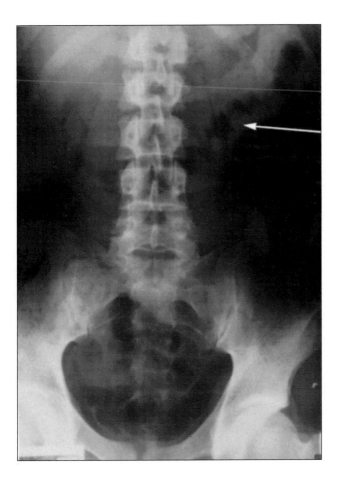

FIGURE 4.3: Plain abdominal X-ray film showing oedematous large bowel and thumb printing due to ischaemic colitis

Bowel obstruction

The four cardinal symptoms of uncomplicated complete bowel obstruction are *colicky abdominal pain, vomiting, abdominal distension* and *absolute constipation*, which includes failure to pass flatus (obstipation) as well as faeces. If the obstruction is incomplete, then one of the cardinal symptoms, constipation, is replaced by diarrhoea. The differential diagnosis of incomplete bowel obstruction is acute gastroenteritis. The degree of abdominal distension is high with colonic obstruction and low with high small bowel obstruction. In contradistinction, the severity of vomiting is less and occurs late with colonic obstruction, and is greater and occurs earlier with proximal small bowel obstruction. The vomitus, although initially bile stained, becomes feculent as the obstruction progresses. If the obstruction continues untreated, a paralytic ileus may supervene and then the hypermotility of the bowel proximal to the obstruction (and the colicky pain) will subside. Alternatively, the unrelieved obstruction may become complicated by strangulation or perforation. These complications are also associated with paralytic ileus. However, rather than the pain settling, it becomes constant and peritoneal in type.

Small bowel obstruction

The most common cause of small bowel obstruction is adhesions from a previous laparotomy. The next commonest cause is hernia, usually inguinal or femoral hernia (Chapter 19). As well as eliciting the symptoms of obstruction, it might be possible to elicit the cause from the history (see Table 4.6).

Physical examination is directed to the demonstration of:

- signs of obstruction (abdominal distension, hyper-resonant abdomen, increased bowel sounds);
- cause of the obstruction (e.g., a previous laparotomy scar raising the possibility of adhesions; an irreducible hernia; an intra-abdominal mass caused by a tumour, intussusception, Crohn's disease, or an appendiceal or diverticular inflammatory phlegmon; or blood mixed with mucus on rectal examination from an intussusception);
- degree of dehydration, so that fluid resuscitation can commence promptly; and
- signs that the obstruction has become complicated (localised peritonism, tenderness in an irreducible hernia), or signs of systemic sepsis (fever and tachycardia).

Specific investigations

- Plain abdominal radiology reveals distended loops of small bowel with fluid levels and absence of colonic gas (see Figure 4.2). Occasionally the cause will be evident, as in Figure 4.4.
- Leucocytosis, particularly if there is a left shift, may indicate ischaemic bowel.
- Abdominal CT scan will show a small bowel obstruction earlier than plain radiology. It will often show the point of obstruction with a transition from dilated bowel to collapsed bowel. The cause may also be evident.

Treatment

After initial fluid resuscitation and gastric decompression with a nasogastric tube, an urgent laparotomy may be required. Factors in favour of early laparotomy include:

- evidence of compromised bowel (constant pain, focal tenderness, unexplained tachycardia (> 100 beats/min), fever (> 37.8°C), and leucocytosis);
- no history of previous surgery that may have caused adhesions; and
- no obvious cause.

An irreducible hernia may be repaired without laparotomy.

If a trial of non-operative treatment is selected, then frequent re-evaluation is imperative lest clinical deterioration be overlooked. If there is no evidence of resolution after 48 hours then laparotomy is required. The duration of the non-operative trial may be extended if the cause is thought to be radiation enteritis, Crohn's disease or involvement of small bowel in a diverticular mass.

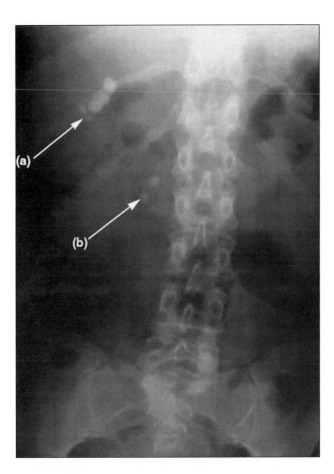

FIGURE 4.4: Radio-opaque stones in the gall bladder (a) and common bile duct (b).

Large bowel obstruction

There are three common causes of large bowel obstruction: colon cancer (75% of cases), diverticular disease (15%), and sigmoid and caecal volvulus (5%).

When managing a patient with an apparent large bowel obstruction on clinical and simple radiological grounds, it is important to be sure that the diagnosis is not simple constipation or acute pseudo-obstruction of the colon, as these conditions are treated non-operatively.

Constipation is associated with a loaded rectum, whereas the rectum should be empty with obstruction. If constipation is the likely diagnosis, bowel washouts from below with enemata should resolve the dilemma. If doubt persists, then a limited gastrograffin enema will be conclusive.

Acute colonic pseudo-obstruction (also called Ogilvie's syndrome) occurs most often in patients in hospital secondary to conditions such as sepsis, acute pancreatitis, electrolyte imbalance, renal failure, spinal cord injury or postoperatively.

If acute pseudo-obstruction is the problem, gastrograffin may produce a return of bowel activity because of its cathartic action. Colonic pseudo-obstruction may mimic organic obstruction. It should be excluded, usually by a limited barium enema. Acute colonic pseudo-obstruction usually resolves within 48 to 96 hours with non-operative treatment. This includes fluid resuscitation, correction of electrolyte abnormalities, withdrawal of medications that might be contributing, such as narcotics and antidepressants, stimulation of colonic motility with neostigmine 2 mg IV under cardiac monitoring, and colonoscopic decompression.

Continued competence of the ileocaecal sphincter prevents retrograde decompression of obstructed large bowel into the small bowel in more than 50% of patients, effectively producing a closed loop. Colonic distension proximal to the site of obstruction is greatest in the caecum and ascending colon. Perforation is usually heralded by localised overlying tenderness. The other useful marker of imminent perforation is colonic distension greater than 10 cm as assessed by plain abdominal X-ray examination. A sigmoid or caecal volvulus is also a closed loop which may perforate if neglected.

Diagnosis and management of large bowel obstruction

Colon cancer. This subject is discussed in detail in Chapter 20. Presentation with complete obstruction is usually preceded by fluctuating incomplete obstruction for several weeks. The tumour is more commonly in the sigmoid or descending colon. The patient may also have noted rectal bleeding. The level of the obstruction may be evident on plain abdominal radiology (see Figure 4.5). Further management is dependent upon whether the obstruction is left-sided or right-sided, and whether the left-sided obstruction settles sufficiently with conservative treatment of bowel rest and gentle enemata to permit mechanical preparation of the bowel. An obstructing cancer in the right hemicolon can be resected with immediate re-anastomosis. An obstructing left-sided colon cancer as far distal as the pelvic brim can be resected with immediate re-anastomosis if all the proximal colon is resected. If a more limited resection is to be performed in mechanically unprepared bowel, and an anastomosis is performed, then either a covering colostomy or ileostomy, or an intra-operative antegrade colonic washout is required. Another approach is to resect the tumour and exteriorise the proximal end as a colostomy (Hartmann's procedure). If the tumour is associated with distant metastases, then a colonoscopically delivered expanding metal stent may be the definitive treatment.

Diverticular disease. Colonic obstruction with diverticular disease is rarely complete. The patient has usually had previous episodes of diverticulitis (see below) prior to the onset of obstruction. Whether or not the patient has a sigmoid colon cancer which is the cause of the obstruction, as well as diverticular disease, can be resolved with colonoscopy. Local colonic resection is reserved for those with obstruction which fails to settle with antibiotic therapy and bowel rest.

Sigmoid and caecal volvulus. The typical patient with a *sigmoid volvulus is* elderly, has chronic constipation and is institutionalised. The patient usually has gross abdominal distension but little vomiting and abdominal pain. The clinical diagnosis is confirmed with a plain abdominal X-ray examination, which has a typical appearance (see Figure 4.6). The single loop based in the left iliac fossa can extend to the right upper quadrant. The volvulus is decompressed using a rigid sigmoidoscope by gently passing a soft rectal tube under direct vision through the point of the rotation at the level of the brim of the pelvis. The torted colon usually reduces spontaneously over two to five days, after which the rectal tube can be removed. As the condition is commonly recurrent, an elective resection of the redundant colon on its long mesentery is advisable unless contraindicated by other medical problems.

A *caecal volvulus* involves the caecum, the ascending colon and the terminal ileum, which rotate on a long mesentery. Typically it affects younger and fitter patients. Radiologically the volvulus extends from the right iliac fossa towards the splenic flexure. The volvulus cannot be reduced radiologically, but may be reduced using the flexible colonoscope. Operative reduction and caecopexy can then be performed electively.

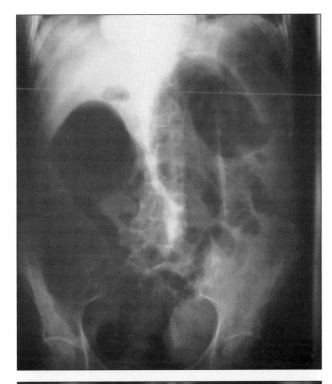

FIGURE 4.5: Plain abdominal X-ray film showing a large bowel obstruction.

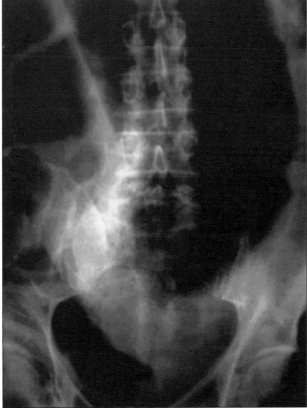

FIGURE 4.6: Plain abdominal X-ray film showing a sigmoid volvulus.

Gastric outlet obstruction

The dominant symptom is profuse vomiting. Pathognomonic features of the vomitus are the presence of foodstuff consumed several days previously, lack of bile staining and a small amount of old blood (coffee grounds). Epigastric pain, particularly colicky postprandial pain, may be a feature. When pain is present, it is relieved by vomiting. Weight loss may be marked.

The major causes of gastric outlet obstruction are distal gastric malignancy and oedema or scarring due to chronic peptic ulceration. In the latter case, there will often be a history of long-standing dyspepsia.

The clinical diagnosis may be supported by demonstrating a gastric splash. This is done by listening to the abdomen whilst shaking the patient from side to side.

Management

Initial management includes intravenous fluid replacement, correction of any electrolyte and acid–base disturbance and nasogastric decompression. There are several points that are salient during resuscitation:

- Gastric fluid losses that need replacement may be as high as 3 L/day;
- Gastric fluid losses may have resulted in a hypokalaemic, hypochloraemic metabolic alkalosis. These are corrected with normal saline and potassium supplements;
- Total parenteral nutrition may be appropriate if weight loss is greater than 10% (Chapter 15); and
- Blood transfusion may be required for severe iron deficiency anaemia.

After gastric decompression the cause should be defined by upper gastrointestinal endoscopy. If active peptic ulceration is found then the gastric outlet obstruction is potentially reversible. Healing the ulcer with parenteral acid suppression may result in resolution of oedema around the ulcer and restitution of luminal patency. Otherwise, the stomach needs to be drained surgically. If the cause is peptic ulceration, this is by vagotomy and distal gastric resection or gastroenterostomy depending on the position of the ulcer. If the cause is gastric malignancy, then this is by distal gastric resection if the tumour is potentially curable, or gastroenterostomy or insertion of an expanding metal stent if it is not curable (see Chapter 15).

ACUTE EPIGASTRIC PAIN

Acute epigastric pain is a common complaint. Often the pain is short-lived and no organic cause is found. A list of causes is shown in Table 4.7. On the basis of an initial clinical evaluation the clinician must decide if:

- the patient requires hospitalisation: and
- further specific investigations, such as upper gastrointestinal endoscopy and/or upper abdominal ultrasound, are needed.

The first of those decisions is difficult and requires clinical experience. It will depend on whether it is considered likely that there is a specific cause and the likely natural history. Factors that assist the clinician to decide include:

- severity, duration of the symptoms and response to the treatment to date;

- associated systemic symptoms and signs; and
- results of initial non-invasive investigations.

There are few features which assist in differentiating specific from non-specific causes. The severity tends to be greater and continuous with organic causes. Radiation of pain to the back is supportive of pancreatitis. Migration to the right upper quadrant suggests cholecystitis. Migration around the side to the scapula or through to the back also suggests gallstones. Associated jaundice may indicate a stone in the common bile duct (Chapter 21).

On many occasions deep epigastric tenderness is the only abdominal sign. If there is focal epigastric peritonism, or more generalised peritonism, a significant cause like a perforated peptic ulcer or acute pancreatitis becomes more likely. The abdominal signs with acute pancreatitis may be unimpressive.

Associated signs of hypovolaemia or Gram-negative sepsis (discussed above under generalised abdominal pain) suggest a perforated peptic ulcer or acute pancreatitis.

Initial investigations

A routine initial screen includes plain radiology of the chest and abdomen, a blood film looking for anaemia and leucocytosis, liver function tests looking for evidence of hepatobiliary disease and a serum amylase test. A marginal elevation of serum amylase (100–400 U/L) is not specific for pancreatitis. Some uncommon but significant radiological signs are listed in Table 4.8. Basal pulmonary consolidation may rarely present with abdominal pain.

Further investigations

The need to proceed with further investigation as either an inpatient or an outpatient depends on the degree of clinical suspicion that an organic cause will be found. For many, symptomatic treatment with antacids or antispasmodics or just simple analgesics is sufficient. The next tier of investigations includes upper gastrointestinal endoscopy and upper abdominal ultrasound. The order in which they are performed depends on the clinical features. The management of abnormalities found on upper gastrointestinal endoscopy is discussed under dyspepsia (see Chapter 5). Hepatobiliary abnormalities found on ultrasound examination are discussed in the next section on right upper quadrant pain and also in Chapter 23.

TABLE 4.7: Causes of acute epigastric pain

- No specific cause found
- Peptic ulceration (uncomplicated)[1]
- Peptic ulceration (perforated)[1]
- Biliary colic[1]
- Acute pancreatitis[1]
- Abdominal aortic aneurysm

---

1. Conditions that also cause right upper quadrant pain.

TABLE 4.8: Specific radiological findings to be looked for in acute epigastric pain	
Sign	**Possible cause**
Gas under the diaphragm	Perforated peptic ulcer
Radio-opaque gallstones	Biliary disease
Colonic cut-off sign	Acute pancreatitis
Sentinel loop	Acute pancreatitis
Pancreatic calcification	Chronic pancreatitis

Acute pancreatitis and its complications

Aetiology

The causes of acute pancreatitis are listed in Table 4.9. The most common causes are passage of gallstones down the common bile duct and alcohol abuse. Pointers towards gallstones as the cause include female gender, older age and abnormal liver function tests.

It is not uncommon for those with alcohol as the cause to deny alcohol abuse, at least initially. If no cause is apparent, serum triglycerides and calcium levels should be measured during convalescence.

Diagnosis

Detection of an elevated serum amylase level is the usual means of diagnosis. The level rises within 12 hours of onset of pain and gradually returns to normal over the next week. This test has a number of false positive and false negative results. False positive results include perforation of stomach or small bowel, small bowel obstruction, mesenteric ischaemia, acute cholecystitis or common bile duct obstruction, morphine, chronic pancreatitis, pancreatic carcinoma, end stage renal failure and chronic alcoholism. Minor elevations can occur with parotitis, tumours, (lung, oesophagus,

TABLE 4.9: Aetiology of acute pancreatitis	
Cause	**Incidence**
Gallstones	50–60%
Alcohol	30–40%
Idiopathic	10%
Post ERCP	2%
Medications, e.g., azathioprine, 6-mercaptopurine, frusemide, hydrochlorothiazide, tetracycline, sulfonamides, oestrogens, sodium valproate, L-asparaginase	Uncommon
Major abdominal trauma, penetrating peptic ulcer	Variable
Mumps	Rare
Hyperlipidaemia	Rare
Hypercalcaemia	Rare
Hereditary (familial)	Rare
Pancreatic tumours	Rare
ERCP = endoscopic retrograde cholangiopancreatography.	

ovarian and breast carcinoma), acute or chronic liver disease, diabetic ketoacidosis and HIV infection. Macroamylasaemia is rare; there are macromolecular aggregates of amylase or IgA and amylase that are not filtered by the kidneys so that the amylase-creatinine clearance is abnormally low.

False negative results may occur in hypercholesterolaemia and recurrent alcoholic pancreatitis. If there is doubt, the diagnosis can be confirmed by CT scan which shows swelling of the pancreas and peripancreatic oedema.

In some centres, serum lipase rather than amylase is used as the biochemical marker of pancreatitis due to its greater specificity. Its rise and fall after acute pancreatitis occur after the same changes in serum amylase.

TABLE 4.10: Poor prognostic factors for acute pancreatitis according to the Glasgow scoring system

Factor	Critical value
AST/ALT	> 200 IU/L
White cell count	> 15 x 10^9/L (15,000/mm^3)
Serum glucose	> 10 mmol/L
Blood oxygen (PaO$_2$)	< 60 mmHg
Serum urea	> 16 mmol/L
Serum albumin	< 32 g/L
Serum calcium	< 2 mmol/L
Serum lactic dehydrogenase	> 600 U/L

ALT = alanine aminotransferase; AST = aspartate aminotransferase.

Assessment of severity

The height of the peak in serum amylase level provides no useful measure of the severity of an attack of pancreatitis. Severity is scored by a combination of predominantly laboratory measurements (see Table 4.10) during the first 48 hours of hospitalisation, and this provides prognostic guidance. Severe pancreatitis is present if there are three or more poor prognostic factors. The mortality rate in cases of mild pancreatitis (less than three poor prognostic factors) is less than 1%, whereas the mortality with severe pancreatitis is greater than 50%.

Initial management

Non-operative management is supportive and directed towards the prevention and treatment of complications. The complications of acute pancreatitis, the time frame of their development and methods for prevention or treatment are listed in Table 4.11.

The important early complications are acute renal failure due to inadequate fluid resuscitation, and respiratory embarrassment due to a combination of inadequate analgesia and physiotherapy, fluid overload and adult respiratory distress syndrome. Some of the causes are at least partly preventable. Patients at risk because of multiple poor prognostic signs, or because of other diseases, fare better in a high dependency or intensive care unit where fluid resuscitation can be managed aggressively with appropriate monitoring. Nasogastric suction to prevent tracheal aspiration, a respiratory complication of paralytic ileus, is required if the patient is vomiting due to ileus.

Severe pancreatitis

The mortality and the morbidity in acute severe gallstone pancreatitis, as graded on prognostic factors (see Table 4.10), can be reduced by urgent endoscopic retrograde cholangiopancreatography (ERCP) and sphincterotomy. Thus an abdominal ultrasound is performed early in the admission to diagnose unsuspected gallstones. If the attack does not settle, then ERCP is performed urgently.

Pancreatic necrosis

The chance of failure of early resolution of pancreatitis, and of developing life-threatening complications, rises if pancreatic necrosis develops. This complication is usually apparent within five days of the onset of the attack if it is going to occur. Pancreatic necrosis is a radiological diagnosis made on a dynamic enhanced CT scan and is evident as unperfused tissue (see Figure 4.7). Its incidence is high in patients who present with three or more poor prognostic signs. It should also be suspected in patients whose pancreatitis fails to settle clinically within a week.

The incidence of the four common major local complications (infected pancreatic necrosis, acute fluid collection, pancreatic pseudocyst and pancreatic abscess) is much higher in patients who have had pancreatic necrosis. These various complications can co-exist.

Infected pancreatic necrosis. The most life-threatening complication of pancreatic necrosis is infection of the necrotic pancreatic and peripancreatic tissue. This complication should be suspected if clinical signs of sepsis develop, usually in the second week after the onset of the illness, or if there is increasing abdominal pain,

TABLE 4.11: Complications of acute pancreatitis			
Organ system	Complication	Time frame	Management (*prevention*[1])
Pancreas	Acute fluid collection	1–6 weeks	Observation, drain if septic
	Pseudocyst	6–12 weeks	Drainage if > 5 cm and persistent
	Necrosis	1–2 weeks	Close observation ± pancreatic culture Antibiotics
	Infected necrosis	2–3 weeks	Operative debridement (often repeated)
	Pancreatic ascites	6–12 weeks	Observation initially, ERCP if persistent
Gastrointestinal	Paralytic ileus	from outset	Nasogastric drainage
	Stress ulceration	1–3 weeks	*Anti-ulcer therapy*
Nutritional	Malnutrition	from outset	*Nutritional support, TPN*
Renal	Acute renal failure	1–3 days	*Adequate fluid resuscitation*, dialysis (if becomes established)
Respiratory	Adult respiratory distress syndrome	2–5 days	ICU/ventilation
	Pneumonia	2–5 days	*Analgesia, antibiotics* and *physiotherapy*
	Pleural effusion	2–20 days	Observation, drain if large

1. Preventative measures are shown in italics.
ERCP = endoscopic retrograde cholangiopancreatography; TPN = total parenteral nutrition.

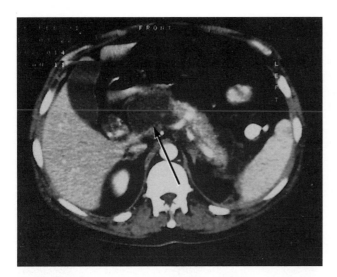

FIGURE 4.7: Dynamic enhanced CT scan showing necrotising pancreatitis (early). Note that the head of the pancreas (arrow) unlike the body and tail does not enhance (unperfused) by IV contrast.

tenderness and swelling, or if unexplained deterioration occurs in another organ system (e.g., cardiac or respiratory). A clinical suspicion of infected pancreatic necrosis can be confirmed by a positive culture from a CT-guided pancreatic fine needle aspirate. The presence of infected necrosis is an indication for pancreatic necrosectomy. As pancreatitis affects the pancreatic and retroperitoneal tissues diffusely, the necrosectomy needs to be repeated every two to three days until the debridement is complete after which the sepsis resolves.

Acute fluid collection. This is a collection of fluid without a fibrous capsule occuring in the lesser sac in the first six weeks after the onset of pancreatitis. It is often asymptomatic, being diagnosed by a CT scan. It may be associated with slow resolution of the symptoms and signs of acute pancreatitis. It may resolve spontaneously or persist to develop a capsule, when it is defined as a pseudocyst. Alternatively, the collection may become infected, or produce gastric outlet obstruction, in which case it should be drained percutaneously under CT or ultrasound guidance. Otherwise, the collection should be monitored by serial CT or ultrasound scans.

Pancreatic pseudocyst. This is an acute fluid collection that has developed a fibrous capsule over six or more weeks. It may be asymptomatic, or be associated with ongoing abdominal pain, nausea and vomiting. It may be complicated by infection or haemorrhage. It may be evident as an abdominal mass (see Chapter 17). If it is asymptomatic, it can be followed by serial scans (Figure 4.8). Smaller pseudocysts (< 5 cm) commonly resolve spontaneously; larger pseudocysts (> 5 cm) tend to persist and eventually need drainage. Drainage is also required for symptomatic pseudocysts (including infected pseudocysts). Drainage needs to be continued until the cavity of the collection shrivels. Drainage can be performed percutaneously through the stomach under CT control, endoscopically through the posterior wall of the stomach, or transgastrically at open operation.

Pancreatic abscess. This is a collection of pus in the peripancreatic tissues. It is not an infected pseudocyst. Clinically, the patient is usually septic and has persistent upper abdominal pain and tenderness. Initial treatment is by percutaneous CT-guided drainage and broad-spectrum antibiotics. Operative drainage is required if the sepsis does not settle after percutaneous drainage.

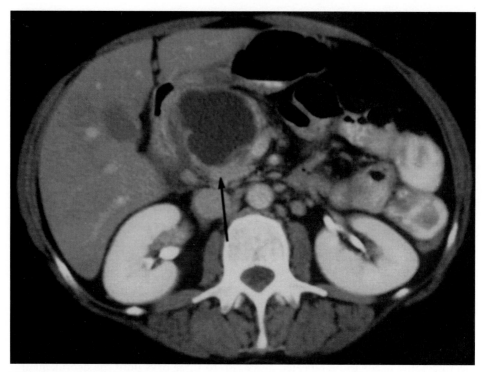

FIGURE 4.8: Dynamic enhanced CT scan showing a pancreatic pseudocyst.

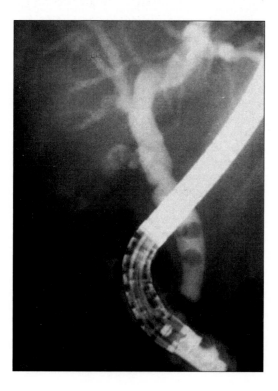

FIGURE 4.9: Endoscopic retrograde cholangiopancreatography showing gallstones in the common bile duct.

Subsequent management

Attention should also be directed towards prevention of further attacks of acute pancreatitis. This involves laparoscopic cholecystectomy and operative cholangiography for patients with gallstones. Only 25% of these cases are found to have persistent stones in the common bile duct (Figure 4.9), which can be removed intraoperatively by exploration of the common bile duct or postoperatively by ERCP. Abstinence from alcohol should be recommended for patients with alcohol abuse.

Acute pancreatitis is only rarely complicated by the development of diabetes mellitus or malabsorption due to pancreatic endocrine and exocrine insufficiency, respectively (Chapter 13). These complications are more common with chronic pancreatitis.

RIGHT UPPER QUADRANT PAIN

Common causes of acute right upper quadrant pain are listed in Table 4.12.

Initial assessment involves making a decision about whether the patient has an immediately life-threatening condition. This view would be supported by finding symptoms and, more particularly, signs of systemic sepsis or shock. Such signs might be attributable to Gram-negative sepsis from cholangitis or cholecystitis, to haemorrhage from a liver cell adenoma or a hepatocellular carcinoma, or one of the life-threatening problems that more commonly causes epigastric pain, such as a perforated peptic ulcer and pancreatitis. Such patients need to be managed in hospital.

Management involves haemodynamic resuscitation and investigation aimed at rapidly identifying the underlying problem. These same investigations are relevant for patients with life-threatening conditions that cause generalised abdominal or epigastric pain as discussed above. They include plain X-ray examinations of the abdomen and chest, a white cell count and a serum amylase test. If there are features of Gram-negative sepsis, blood cultures should be performed and broad-spectrum antibiotics commenced parenterally. The second line of investigation should include an upper abdominal ultrasound looking for cholelithiasis, thickening of the gall bladder wall, dilatation of the biliary tree, air in the wall of the gall bladder or the biliary tree and intra-abdominal fluid. Even though these life-threatening conditions are uncommon, they require prompt, appropriate management.

Most patients who present with acute right upper quadrant pain are not systemically ill. They require analgesia (often narcotic) for the relief of pain. If the pain persists, hospitalisation enables the regular administration of narcotic analgesics.

Gallstones

Gallstones are of two major types: pigment stones and cholesterol-containing stones. Pigment stones occur in patients with excessive haemolysis such as occurs in haemolytic anaemia. Cholesterol and mixed stones occur in patients with bile secreted from the liver that is supersaturated with cholesterol. Cholesterol-supersaturated bile results from either enhanced cholesterol secretion (e.g., obesity, pregnancy, fasting) or decreased bile acid secretion (e.g., small bowel disease). Gall bladder hypomotility (e.g., fasting, pregnancy, hyperalimentation) also predisposes to gallstone formation.

TABLE 4.12: Causes of right upper quadrant pain

- No specific cause found
- Biliary colic[1]
- Acute cholecystitis
- Acute cholangitis
- Gall bladder dysfunction
- Sphincter of Oddi dysfunction
- Metastasis[1]
- Abscess[1]
- Hepatitis
- Primary liver tumour
- Hydatid cyst
- Other causes of acute liver swelling
- Peptic ulceration[1]
- Acute pancreatitis[1]

---

1. Conditions that also cause acute epigastric pain.

Biliary pain (colic)

Biliary colic is severe pain of gradual onset, which reaches a peak that may be sustained for minutes to hours and then resolves slowly. It is more commonly experienced in the right upper quadrant than in the epigastrium. The pain can be severe enough to cause agitation and a secondary tachycardia. It may radiate around the side to the right scapula. It can be associated with nausea and vomiting. If the patient has had the pain previously, gallstones may already have been demonstrated by upper abdominal ultrasound. As well as upper abdominal ultrasound, the following investigations are also performed:

- a white cell count looking for a leucocytosis which suggests the development of cholecystitis;
- a serum amylase test so that pancreatitis is not overlooked; and
- liver function tests looking for evidence of occult choledocholithiasis.

Once the diagnosis of biliary colic is confirmed, initial management depends upon whether the pain is adequately controlled and whether the development of acute cholecystitis has complicated the attack of biliary colic. The complications of gallstones are listed in Table 4.13.

Acute cholecystitis

Obstruction of the outlet of the gall bladder (Hartmann's pouch) by a gallstone initially causes biliary colic. The obstruction eventually results in chemical inflammation of the gall bladder, which may be complicated by secondary bacterial infection. The pathological process takes about 24 hours to develop. The pain of acute cholecystitis is peritoneal in type. There may be associated fever. Abdominal examination reveals right upper quadrant peritonism. Usually the tenderness is too great to allow detection of a gall bladder mass, even if one is present at this stage. As the attack resolves, and the gall bladder swelling settles, the gall bladder with residual inflammation may be evident as a tender area beneath the costal margin during deep inspiration. This sign is called Murphy's sign.

TABLE 4.13: Complications of gallstones

- Persistent biliary colic
- Acute cholecystitis
- Empyema of the gall bladder
- Mucocoele of the gall bladder
- Acute cholangitis
- Obstructive jaundice
- Acute pancreatitis
- Gallstone ileus (cholecystoduodenal fistula)

An attack of acute cholecystitis usually settles within 24–48 hours. Recovery is assisted by the use of broad-spectrum antibiotics administered parenterally. Resolution of the attack is associated with dislodgment of the obstructing gallstone from the gall bladder outlet. The diagnosis of cholecystitis is confirmed, if necessary, by demonstrating a thick-walled gall bladder on ultrasound.

Failure of acute cholecystitis to resolve leads to one of four complications:

1. **Empyema of the gall bladder.** Empyema of the gall bladder is an 'abscess of the gall bladder'. Clinically, the patient remains septic and has continuing right upper quadrant pain of peritoneal type, tachycardia, high spiking fever, marked right upper quadrant peritonism, with an underlying grossly thickened, inflamed gall bladder surrounded by an omental phlegmon. The mass may not be evident on clinical examination because of overlying guarding, but will be quite apparent on ultrasound. Antibiotics alone are not enough to produce resolution; drainage of the intravesical pus is required either percutaneously under ultrasound (or CT) guidance, or by cholecystostomy or cholecystectomy. Clinical neglect may result in perforation of the gall bladder, septicaemia or a right subphrenic or subhepatic abscess.

2. **Gangrenous cholecystitis.** Gangrenous cholecystitis is usually indistinguishable from empyema of the gall bladder on clinical grounds; the pathological diagnosis is made at laparotomy when patchy areas of necrosis are found as the gall bladder is shelled out of its omental phlegmon. The diagnosis may be made radiologically or by ultrasound on the basis of air in the gall bladder wall usually from anaerobic organisms. The treatment is as for empyema. Perforation is more common here than with empyema.

3. **Cholecystoduodenal fistula.** This complication is only recognised after it has occurred. The fistula forms when a gallstone trapped in the neck of the gall bladder slowly erodes through into the second part of the duodenum. This might be recognised after the event by the presence of air in the biliary tree (see Figure 4.4). It may become evident after a large gallstone impacts in the terminal ileum causing small bowel obstruction.

4. **Mucocoele of the gall bladder.** If the gall bladder outlet remains obstructed and the contents do not become infected, a mucocoele of the gall bladder develops over several weeks. The bile is absorbed and the gall bladder distends with mucus secreted by the gall bladder mucosa. Clinically, an avocado-sized, slightly tender mass is evident in the right upper quadrant. The treatment is cholecystectomy.

Acute acalculous cholecystitis

This is a rare form of cholecystitis usually seen in the intensive care unit, where it occurs in debilitated patients, following major trauma, recent major surgery or severe sepsis. Some of these patients are so unwell that they do not complain of right upper quadrant pain. If the patient complains of pain, then diagnosis is by ultrasound. If there are no complaints of pain, as is common in this situation, the diagnosis is made incidentally on a CT scan or during laparotomy performed as a result of unexplained deterioration thought to have an abdominal cause. Cholecystostomy rather than resection may be required because of the patient's poor physical state.

Definitive management of cholelithiasis

The definitive treatment of gallstones is cholecystectomy. If possible, the procedure is performed laparoscopically because this has a lower morbidity and more rapid recovery time than open cholecystectomy. An operative cholangiogram is performed at the same time to ensure that unsuspected stones are not left behind in the common bile duct and that the common bile duct has not been injured during cholecystectomy. The risk of unsuspected choledocholithiasis at cholecystectomy is 3–7%. This possibility becomes more likely if one or more of the risk factors listed in Table 4.14 are present.

The timing of cholecystectomy depends on the severity of the inflammatory process at presentation and the general medical state of the patient. Cholecystectomy might be delayed for six weeks to allow an acute inflammatory process to resolve, since the operation can be completed more often laparoscopically without need to convert to open operation if the inflammation has resolved. Failure of the acute inflammatory process to resolve is suggested on clinical grounds by persistent sepsis, and severe continuing pain and tenderness. Under these circumstances, intervention is required. This may be either percutaneous or surgical drainage, or surgical excision in the acute phase.

Currently, other treatments of cholelithiasis have only a limited use. Extracorporeal lithotripsy, even when combined with dissolution therapy (e.g., ursodeoxycholic acid), fails to completely remove stones from the gall bladder in over 50% of patients with asymptomatic gallstones. This therapy is not recommended for symptomatic stones.

TABLE 4.14: Preoperative risk factors for common bile duct stones

- History of obstructive jaundice
- History of pancreatitis
- Elevated hepatic transaminases
- Elevated alkaline phosphatase
- Elevated bilirubin
- Dilated common bile duct on ultrasound (> 6 mm)

Acute right upper quadrant pain and jaundice

Most patients with both acute right upper quadrant pain and jaundice have acute cholangitis. This diagnosis is supported if fever is also present. This triad of symptoms is known as Charcot's triad (Chapter 21). Initial management involves resuscitation and treatment of associated Gram-negative sepsis. An urgent ultrasound examination should reveal cholelithiasis, a dilated common bile duct and sometimes a stone in the common bile duct. ERCP with sphincterotomy should be performed urgently if the signs of sepsis are severe or they do not settle rapidly with parenteral antibiotics.

If the cholangitis settles promptly with parenteral antibiotics, then the underlying cause of the cholangitis still needs to be treated during that hospital admission. This might be by ERCP (Figure 4.9) and sphincterotomy or cholecystectomy and exploration of the common bile duct, performed either laparoscopically or open. If the clearance is endoscopic, elective cholecystectomy is performed subsequently, unless the patient is elderly or frail.

If the ultrasound examination does not demonstrate gallstones, other causes must be sought. In a small subset of patients, as discussed below, the explanation is apparent on the ultrasound of the liver. As mentioned above, a normal serum amylase level essentially eliminates unsuspected acute pancreatitis. Peptic ulceration is diagnosed by upper gastrointestinal endoscopy. For the remainder, no further investigation is required if the pain resolves without recurrence.

If the pain recurs, the ultrasound examination should be repeated because small stones may be missed in up to 5% of cases. If the cause is still not apparent, a cholecystokinin (CCK)-DIDA test should be performed. This is a test of gall bladder function. Initially, DIDA is taken up by the liver, excreted in the bile and concentrated in the gall bladder. If the gall bladder is non-functional or contains tiny stones, it contracts minimally in response to cholecystokinin. If the cystic duct is obstructed by a small stone, the gall bladder will not be outlined (Chapter 23).

Differential diagnosis of biliary colic

Occasionally, a patient with a clinical picture suggestive of acute biliary colic has an alternative explanation, which is apparent on ultrasound examination. More usually the pain is less severe in degree and more prolonged in duration. On review, there may be other clinical clues, which are summarised in Table 4.15.

Hepatic metastasis

Haemorrhage into a liver metastasis, or necrosis of a metastasis can produce a dull ache in the right upper quadrant. The primary tumour is usually gastrointestinal and, on questioning, has symptoms attributable to it. Occasionally the primary tumour is in the breast or the lung.

On ultrasound examination, usually multiple solid lesions are found throughout the liver. A CT scan is used to confirm the ultrasound findings and to assess the pancreas. Management of metastatic liver disease is covered in Chapter 23.

Hepatic abscess

With a hepatic abscess, the symptoms of sepsis (spiking fevers, night sweats, poor appetite and loss of weight) tend to overshadow the right upper quadrant pain.

Hepatic abscesses are of two types: amoebic and pyogenic. An amoebic abscess is caused by the protozoan *Entamoeba histolytica,* which invades the colonic mucosa, and is carried to the liver via the portal circulation. Infestation is rare in Western societies and usually follows a visit to an endemic area. Confirmation that the abscess is amoebic is usually made serologically. Treatment with metronidazole should result in resolution of the abscess. Percutaneous drainage is indicated if the diagnosis is uncertain, the abscess is likely to rupture or there is no improvement after 48 hours.

TABLE 4.15: Causes of right upper quadrant pain other than gallstones found on ultrasound examination

Diagnosis	Ultrasound findings	Clinical clues
Hepatic metastases	Multiple solid lesions	Previous carcinoma Irregular hepatomegaly
Pyogenic liver abscess	Cystic lesion(s)	Spiking fevers Anorexia Loss of weight Risk factors
Amoebic liver abscess	Cystic lesion(s)	Spiking fevers Anorexia Loss of weight Recent travel to endemic area
Right-sided cardiac failure	Dilated hepatic veins	Pulsatile liver Cardiac symptoms Respiratory disease Peripheral oedema
Hepatic adenoma/ focal nodular hyperplasia	Solitary solid lesion	Young woman Oral contraceptive pill
Hepatocellular carcinoma	Solid lesion Satellite lesions	Risk of hepatitis B or C Known cirrhosis Ascites
Hydatid cyst	Cystic lesion with daughter cysts or calcified wall	Rural exposure
Budd-Chiari syndrome	Caudate lobe hypertrophy Ascites	Ascites

The causes of pyogenic abscesses are listed in Table 4.16. Management of pyogenic abscesses involves elucidation of the cause, drainage of the abscess, usually percutaneously using ultrasound or CT guidance and broad-spectrum antibiotics.

Hepatic adenoma and focal nodular hyperplasia

The benign liver tumours, hepatic adenoma and focal nodular hyperplasia (FNH), can cause right upper quadrant pain by intraperitoneal rupture, by bleeding into the lesion or expansion of the lesion. Their diagnosis is discussed in Chapter 23. Symptomatic and complicated lesions are usually managed by liver resection.

Hepatocellular carcinoma

As with hepatic adenoma and FNH, hepatocellular carcinoma can cause right upper quadrant pain as a result of rupture, haemorrhage or expansion. The lesion usually arises in a cirrhotic liver, so that the patient may also have signs of chronic liver disease, portal hypertension or ascites. The diagnostic features on scanning are discussed in Chapter 23.

Hydatid cyst

This lesion may be asymptomatic or cause a dull ache in the right upper quadrant. It is caused by *Echinococcus granulosus* (rarely *Echinococcus multilocularis*). The appearance of the liver cyst on ultrasound examination are often diagnostic. In a living cyst, usually there are also daughter cysts. Calcification of the wall of the cyst indicates that the contents are no longer viable (Chapter 23). The diagnosis is confirmed serologically, with an enzyme-linked immunosorbent assay (ELISA) and a complement fixation test. Viable cysts need to be removed to prevent complications such as intraperitoneal rupture. Intraperitoneal spillage needs to be avoided during intra-operative clearance of the live cyst contents to avoid the risk of anaphylaxis and intra-abdominal seeding with infective material. Preoperative therapy for several weeks with anthelmintics, such as albendazole, reduces risk of recurrence.

Budd-Chiari syndrome

Hepatic vein thrombosis or Budd-Chiari syndrome that develops acutely is a rare cause of right upper quadrant pain. Ultrasound examination will show ascites and caudate lobe enlargement. The venous drainage of the caudate lobe is directly into the inferior vena cava, so that this segment hypertrophies as it is not affected by the hepatic vein thrombosis. Doppler flow studies are useful but liver biopsy is necessary to confirm the diagnosis. Management is by treatment of the underlying cause (e.g., anticoagulation) and usually a portosystemic venous shunt (Chapter 22).

Right heart failure

Severe or acute right heart failure may cause right upper quadrant pain by venous engorgement of the liver and stretching of the capsule. The symptoms and signs of cardiac failure are gross and dominate the clinical picture. Palpation of the liver may show it to be pulsatile.

Right upper quadrant pain after previous cholecystectomy

Recurrence of pain suggests that the original problem may not have been biliary colic due to gall bladder stones. The cause may be due to a biliary or a non-biliary cause. Possibilities include biliary causes such as a retained or recurrent stone in the common bile duct or sphincter of Oddi dysfunction; non-biliary causes include peptic ulceration, pancreatitis (see Chapter 5) and irritable bowel syndrome.

As discussed above for right upper quadrant pain without prior cholecystectomy, the initial question is whether the patient has an immediately life-threatening illness.

Patients with life-threatening conditions such as acute cholangitis are managed along lines discussed above. Thereafter, investigation is first aimed at exclusion of common duct stones as the cause. The finding of a dilated common bile duct, with or without a stone on ultrasound examination, or abnormal liver function test results supports the diagnosis of choledocholithiasis which needs to be confirmed or excluded by ERCP or magnetic resonance cholangiopancreatography (MRCP). Choledocholithiasis evident after previous cholecystectomy is usually managed by endoscopic techniques.

If choledocholithiasis is not found, the cause may be *sphincter of Oddi dysfunction*. This is a syndrome characterised by biliary-type pain following cholecystectomy. There are two types:

- Type 1: characterised by a demonstrable stricture of the sphincter with a dilated duct on ultrasound examination, abnormal liver function test results during episodes of pain, and relief of symptoms after endoscopic sphincterotomy;

- Type 2: characterised by a non-dilated duct, variable abnormalities in liver function test results during episodes of pain and a less certain response to endoscopic sphincterotomy.

Findings of a normal diameter bile duct with normal liver function test results make a biliary cause for right upper quadrant pain less likely.

TABLE 4.16: Aetiology of pyogenic liver abscesses

Mechanism of infection	Examples
Cholangitis	Biliary obstruction from stone or malignancy Bile duct instrumentation
Portal pyaemia	Acute/subacute diverticular disease Appendiceal abscess
Direct spread	Penetrating duodenal ulcer
Systemic bacteraemia	Intravenous drug abuse Subacute bacterial endocarditis
Secondary infection of primary liver lesion	Traumatic haematoma Necrotic hepatic metastasis Hydatid cyst Amoebic abscess

RIGHT ILIAC FOSSA PAIN

The exact cause of right iliac fossa pain commonly remains undetermined. The pain often resolves spontaneously after a short period and does not recur. Patients, on the other hand, have a different perspective. They commonly believe that they have acute appendicitis and require urgent appendicectomy.

The causes of right iliac fossa pain are listed in Table 4.17. Differentiation between the various causes is not always possible on clinical grounds, and investigations frequently do not help. Acute appendicitis remains largely a clinical diagnosis; CT scanning can occasionally help. Right iliac fossa pain seldom represents an intra-abdominal catastrophe.

The initial aim of the clinician is to determine whether there is sufficient clinical evidence of localised peritonitis to require surgery. A patient with a typical history of periumbilical, usually colicky pain that shifts to the right iliac fossa, together with a low grade temperature, and localised and rebound tenderness maximal over McBurney's point in the right iliac fossa, is likely to have acute appendicitis and should proceed to appendicectomy. Other signs of acute appendicitis are listed in Table 4.18. If the clinical picture is not clearly one of appendicitis, the next priority depends upon the gender of the patient. In women, consideration must be given to possible gynaecological causes of right iliac fossa pain (Table 4.17), some of which require surgical intervention. A history of abnormal or missed periods or a vaginal discharge is sought. A vaginal examination and speculum examination may demonstrate localised tenderness, a mass or a purulent discharge. Relevant investigations include a pregnancy test and pelvic ultrasound. Laparoscopy may be required to confirm a gynaecological diagnosis and/ or deliver definitive treatment.

TABLE 4.17: Differential diagnosis of right iliac fossa pain

Gastrointestinal causes
- Non-specific right iliac fossa pain
- Acute appendicitis
- Mesenteric adenitis
- Terminal ileitis
- Acute inflammation of a Meckel's diverticulum
- Crohn's disease of the terminal ileum
- Caecal carcinoma
- Inflammatory caecal lesion (e.g., diverticulitis in a solitary caecal diverticulum)
- Inflammatory lesion of the terminal ileum (e.g., foreign body perforation)

Non-gastrointestinal causes
- Ruptured ovarian follicle (Mittelschmerz)
- Acute salpingitis (pelvic inflammatory disease)
- Rupture/torsion or haemorrhage of an ovarian cyst
- Endometriosis
- Ectopic pregnancy
- Urinary tract infection

Those patients of the cohort without evidence of localised peritonitis are observed and reviewed. Most are afebrile and have a normal white cell count. If the clinical signs progress and become more suggestive of appendicitis, then surgery is indicated. If the pain resolves spontaneously, no further investigations or follow-up are required.

Other inflammatory conditions of the terminal ileum and caecum may mimic acute appendicitis. Occasionally there are clinical clues that indicate that the localised peritonitis is not due to appendicitis. An elderly patient may have a right iliac fossa mass suggesting a caecal carcinoma or a complication of a diverticulum. If a mass is found, the presence of tumour or pus within it should be ascertained by ultrasound or CT scanning. An appendix abscess, if diagnosed preoperatively, can be drained percutaneously with ultrasound or CT control. A caecal carcinoma is treated by right hemicolectomy. The principles of treatment of diverticulitis of a solitary caecal diverticulum are the same as for left-sided diverticulitis if the diagnosis is known. Often, however, the diagnosis is only established after the affected caecum is removed.

A patient with acute right iliac fossa pain and diarrhoea may have acute terminal ileitis. Recurrent right iliac fossa pain and diarrhoea or previous episodes of perianal sepsis may suggest Crohn's disease.

TABLE 4.18: Other signs of acute appendicitis	
Name	**Sign**
Jump tenderness	Jumping or hopping induces pain. Useful in children
Cough tenderness	Cough produces localised pain over McBurney's point
Psoas sign	Pain on elevating right leg (due to inflammation adjacent to psoas muscle)
Rovsing's sign	Tenderness felt in the right iliac fossa while palpating the left iliac fossa
Rectal tenderness	Tenderness palpable on the right side accentuated by bimanual palpation

Specific management

Acute appendicitis

The treatment for acute appendicitis is appendicectomy. Traditionally this is performed open through a muscle-splitting incision. That approach is still best for children. In adults the operation is commonly performed laparoscopically for several reasons:

- The accuracy of the clinical diagnosis is relatively low in adult women (53–78% of cases); it is higher in men (85–90%). The inaccuracy relates to gynaecological diseases that mimic acute appendicitis;
- If the cause is gynaecological, then laparoscopy is a more accurate diagnostic tool than laparotomy through an incision in the right iliac fossa; and
- Laparoscopic appendicectomy is associated with a more rapid postoperative recovery.

Terminal ileitis

Some patients with a clinical diagnosis of acute appendicitis are found to have terminal ileitis. Diarrhoea will have been a feature of the disease. The usual cause is *Yersinia enterocolitica* (Chapter 12). This should be confirmed by convalescent serology. Occasionally, this illness is the first manifestation of Crohn's disease.

Mesenteric adenitis

Mesenteric adenitis is quite common in children and adolescents. It is presumed to be a viral illness with enlargement of the mesenteric lymph nodes. There is often a preceding history of a viral-like illness. This is a self-limiting condition that resolves without specific therapy.

Meckel's diverticulum

A Meckel's diverticulum is a congenital remnant of the vitelline duct. It is a true diverticulum that occurs on the antimesenteric border of the terminal ileum, 45–60 cm from the ileocaecal sphincter. It occurs in 2% of the population and complications are unusual. If the base of the diverticulum is narrow, the diverticulum can become obstructed and present with an appendicitis-like illness. Other complications include:

- bleeding from peptic ulceration caused by ectopic gastric mucosa[1]; and
- small bowel obstruction due to a congenital adhesion to the umbilicus.

    These complications are managed by local resection of the diverticulum.

Crohn's disease

The management of Crohn's disease diagnosed prior to surgery is covered in Chapter 13. When a segment of Crohn's disease is found at operation for presumed appendicitis, a resection only needs to be performed if there is a local complication (perforation, fistula or obstruction).

Caecal carcinoma

A caecal carcinoma found at laparotomy is treated by right hemicolectomy and primary anastomosis (Chapter 20).

LEFT ILIAC FOSSA PAIN

There are only a limited number of causes of acute left iliac fossa pain. They can be subdivided into gastrointestinal causes (Table 4.19) and the same non-gastrointestinal causes as right iliac fossa pain (Table 4.17).

When approaching the patient with acute left iliac fossa pain, the first decision to be made is whether the patient needs an urgent laparotomy. The decision is made on clinical grounds. If there is shock due to sepsis or hypovolaemia, and marked signs of peritonitis, or radiological evidence of bowel perforation, an urgent laparotomy is required. Such presentations are uncommon so that most patients are managed non-operatively.

Initially, for those managed non-operatively, investigation is the next step. Age and gender are important pointers. Most gynaecological causes affect women in their reproductive years (15–45) whereas diverticular disease and colonic ischaemia affect older patients of both sexes. Gastrointestinal causes are also associated with disturbances of bowel habit. Acute diverticulitis may be associated with constipation or diarrhoea, while ischaemic colitis is invariably associated with bloody diarrhoea.

Diverticular disease

Increasing age is associated with the development of pulsion diverticula of the colon. This process is also associated with consumption of a diet low in roughage. Each diverticulum consists of a mucosal pouch only and is located at the mesenteric attachment of the colon. Diverticula are most commonly present in the sigmoid colon (Figure 4.10). They occur with decreasing frequency from sigmoid colon to caecum. They do not occur in the rectum which has a complete outer longitudinal layer of muscularis propria. There may be hypertrophy of the muscularis propria of the sigmoid colon.

Uncomplicated diverticular disease is usually asymptomatic. Treatment of patients with diverticular disease with long-term high roughage diet reduces the incidence of the complications of diverticular disease; this treatment also reduces the incidence of recurrence of these complications. The infective complications of diverticular disease, acute diverticulitis, abscess, perforation and fistula formation, result when the neck of a diverticulum, which is narrower than the sac, becomes obstructed by faecal material and the contents of the sac become infected.

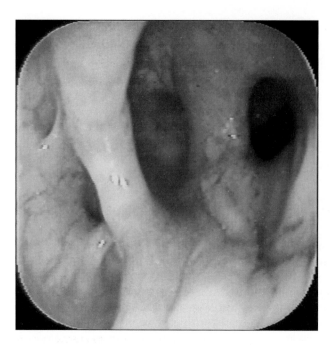

FIGURE 4.10: Diverticulosis on colonoscopy.

Acute diverticulitis

The signs of acute diverticulitis can be remembered as those of 'left-sided appendicitis'. The usual position of the pain is explained by the fact that it is nearly always the sigmoid colon that is most severely affected by diverticular disease and the sigmoid colon lies most often in the left iliac fossa. Unlike acute appendicitis, the peritoneal pain of acute diverticulitis is usually not preceded by colicky midline pain. The presence of a tender mass in the left iliac fossa, often palpable by concurrent abdominal and rectal palpation, is common. A diverticular mass may or may not have a significant amount of pus at its centre. It usually takes several days to decide if the mass is a simple phlegmonous mass or whether there is an underlying diverticular abscess. If there is an underlying abscess, the symptoms and signs are likely to persist in spite of the non-operative treatment with bowel rest and broad-spectrum antibiotics. The differentiation can be made on CT scan if there is doubt.

TABLE 4.19: Gastrointestinal causes of acute left iliac fossa pain

- Non-specific left iliac fossa pain including constipation
- Acute gastroenteritis
- Acute diverticulitis
- Colonic carcinoma
- Colonic ischaemia
- Localised small bowel perforation

Patients with deep tenderness in the left iliac fossa as the only specific sign of flare-up of acute diverticular disease can be treated at home with oral fluids, broad-spectrum oral antibiotics, analgesia and early review. Once the flare-up has settled completely (usually four to six weeks), the diagnosis is confirmed with a barium enema. If there is concern that there is both diverticular disease and a sigmoid colon cancer, then colonoscopy should be performed.

A diverticular abscess needs to be drained if there are continuing signs of severe sepsis and left iliac fossa peritonism after 48–72 hours. The drainage may be percutaneous with ultrasound or CT-guided control or by laparotomy. Surgical drainage often involves a Hartmann's procedure.

Complications of diverticular disease

The complications of diverticular disease include colo-vesical fistula, colo-vaginal fistula, colo-enteric fistula, small bowel obstruction (discussed above under acute abdominal colic), large bowel obstruction (discussed above under acute abdominal colic) and massive gastrointestinal bleeding (see Chapter 9).

The outstanding presenting feature of a colo-vesical fistula is pneumaturia or faecuria. There may be hypogastric pain due to associated urinary bladder inflammation. The fistula is usually the size of a pinhole. It is unusual to be able to demonstrate the fistula with either a barium enema or cystogram.

The outstanding presenting feature of a colo-vaginal fistula is a faeculent vaginal discharge. A previous hysterectomy is common; this allows the segment of sigmoid colon to come into contact with the apex of the vagina.

The outstanding presenting feature of a colo-enteric fistula is profuse diarrhoea. Treatment of all fistulae is resection of the affected segment of colon and oversewing the defect in the bladder or vagina, or resection of the affected segment of small bowel.

Ischaemic colitis

The clinical presentation of ischaemic colitis may be similar to acute diverticulitis. Differentiating features include a history of cardiac disease, arrhythmia or other vascular disease, as well as a history of profuse bloody diarrhoea (Chapter 9).

Ischaemic colitis is managed non-operatively unless there is clinical evidence of sepsis or a progressive deterioration on repeated clinical assessment. The management of ischaemic colitis is discussed in generalised abdominal pain above.

Sigmoid colon cancer

Localised perforation of a sigmoid colon cancer can closely mimic acute diverticulitis.

Constipation

Constipation may be associated with a dull aching pain in the left iliac fossa. The management of constipation is discussed in Chapter 10.

Further reading

Dang C, Aguilera P, Dang A, Salem L. Acute abdominal pain. Four classifications can guide assessment and management. *Geriatrics* 2002; 57: 30–2, 35–6, 41–2.

Korotinski S, Katz A, Malnick SD. Chronic ischaemic bowel diseases in the aged—go with the flow. *Age Ageing* 2005; 34: 10–6.

Mackay S, Dillane P. Biliary pain. *Aust Fam Physician* 2004; 33: 977–81.

Murtagh J. Acute abdominal pain: a diagnostic approach. *Aust Fam Physician* 1994; 23: 364–74.

Renzulli P, Jakob SM, Tauber M *et al.* Severe acute pancreatitis: case-oriented discussion of interdisciplinary management. *Pancreatology* 2005; 5: 145–56.

Sajja SB, Schein M. Early postoperative small bowel obstruction. *Br J Surg* 2004; 91: 683–91.

Trowbridge RL, Rutkowski NK, Shojania KG. Does this patient have acute cholecystitis? *J Am Med Assoc* 2003; 289: 80–6.

Wagner JM, McKinney WP, Carpenter JL. Does this patient have appendicitis? *J Am Med Assoc* 1996; 276: 1589–94.

Werner J, Feuerbach S, Uhl W, Buchler MW. Management of acute pancreatitis: from surgery to interventional intensive care. *Gut* 2005; 54: 426–36.

chapter 5

INDIGESTION (CHRONIC EPIGASTRIC PAIN OR DISCOMFORT)

INDIGESTION AND DYSPEPSIA

The terms indigestion and dyspepsia mean different things to different people. It is therefore important to clarify with a patient what they mean by indigestion. The term is generally used by patients to describe symptoms related to the upper abdomen or chest. Dyspepsia is a term usually only used by medical practitioners. The current internationally accepted definition of dyspepsia is persistent or recurrent pain or discomfort centred in the upper abdomen. However, many also include classical symptoms of gastro-oesophageal reflux, namely heartburn or acid regurgitation, as part of dyspepsia, which has caused confusion (see Chapter 1).

Despite problems with definitions, there is no doubt that dyspepsia is very common in clinical practice. It is also one of the most common gastrointestinal symptoms in the community, occurring in 25% of the adult population, although only a minority seek medical care.

A diverse range of physiological or pathological mechanisms can result in chronic or recurrent epigastric pain. These include: 1) inflammation, not only acute, but also chronic; 2) abnormal motor activity producing distension or excessive contraction of hollow organs; 3) stretching of the capsules of solid viscera, for example, the liver; 4) malignant invasion of nerves; 5) organ-specific responses, such as acid and pepsin acting on nerve fibres in the base of a peptic ulcer. Based on the afferent relays or pathways for pain impulses, activated by these processes, three different types of pain can be appreciated clinically. These types can occur in isolation or together in the one individual. *Visceral* pain arises from nociceptors situated in the walls of the abdominal viscera, *somatic* pain from nociceptors situated in the parietal peritoneum and supporting tissues, and *referred* pain by activation of strong visceral impulses spilling over to the somatic afferent neurones in the same spinal cord segment. Visceral pain tends to be dull, perceived in the midline and poorly localised; it may be described in terms other than 'pain', and may be accompanied by symptoms of autonomic disturbance. Somatic pain, like referred pain, tends to be sharp or aching, sustained, lateralised and yet relatively poorly localised; it may be worse on movement. Referred pain tends to be sharp or aching in character, lateral or bilateral and roughly localised to the somatic dermatome. When patients describe pain as superficial, it may arise from lesions in the abdominal wall or hernial sac, but may occasionally also represent referred pain, from disease in intra-abdominal or thoracic viscera.

CLINICAL ASSESSMENT

Epigastric pain should be distinguished from discomfort; the latter refers to a subjective, negative feeling which does not reach the level of pain. Discomfort can include a number of other symptoms including early satiety or satiation (inability to finish a normal sized meal), postprandial fullness, nausea (Chapter 8) and upper abdominal bloating (Chapter 7).

Determine if epigastric pain or discomfort is the major complaint; it may or may not be related to meals, and may be intermittent (recurrent or cyclical) or continuous. As with any pain, the other specific features need to be ascertained, including site, radiation, mode of onset, intensity, character, and precipitating/relieving factors (see Chapter 6). For the purposes of this discussion, a duration of three months or longer is taken as indicating chronicity, which distinguishes dyspepsia from the acute symptoms present in disorders such as perforated peptic ulcer, acute cholecystitis, and acute pancreatitis (Chapter 4).

Patients with dyspepsia may present with distinct clusters of symptoms. One classification of dyspepsia divides patients into the following subgroups: those patients who have chronic epigastric pain (epigastric pain syndrome or ulcer-like dyspepsia), those who have postprandial symptoms such as postprandial fullness or early satiation (postprandial distress syndrome or dysmotility-like dyspepsia), those with chronic unexplained nausea (chronic idiopathic nausea) or those who have dyspeptic symptoms that do not clearly fall into either grouping (unspecified dyspepsia). However, there is considerable overlap among the subgroups in practice. Also, they appear to correlate poorly with documented disorders such as peptic ulceration, and they do not correlate well with specific pathophysiological disturbances such as delayed gastric emptying or *Helicobacter pylori* gastritis.

Symptoms of gastro-oesophageal reflux disease (GORD) and dyspepsia often overlap. Because of the high specificity of the symptoms of GORD, however, if the patient has predominant symptoms of heartburn or regurgitation, as well as upper abdominal pain/discomfort, the condition should usually be classified as symptomatic GORD, irrespective of the presence or absence of endoscopic oesophagitis (see Chapter 1). Likewise, while retrosternal chest pain, and even dysphagia, may be regarded by the patient as indigestion, they should not be classified as dyspepsia. Both cardiac causes (e.g., ischaemic heart disease) and noncardiac causes (e.g., GORD or oesophageal motility disorders) may be the underlying aetiology in these instances.

Upper abdominal complaints also occur frequently in patients with features compatible with other functional gastrointestinal disorders; irritable bowel syndrome (IBS) is the commonest of these disorders (see Chapter 6). Despite this overlap, approximately two-thirds of patients with dyspepsia and no peptic ulcer or other organic disease report a normal bowel habit, which suggests that they constitute a distinct group from IBS. Aerophagia refers to the repetitive pattern of swallowing air and belching to relieve the sensation of abdominal distension or bloating. It is best regarded as a specific functional gastroduodenal disorder and is considered further in Chapters 6 and 7.

Differential diagnosis of dyspepsia

The differential diagnosis of dyspepsia is extremely wide, including diseases not only of the gastroduodenum, but also all of the other organs situated in the upper abdomen. Therefore, it is crucial to identify the precise symptoms. Leading questions are often required to elicit the complaints that trouble the patient most. Even when a detailed history has been obtained, the exact clinical diagnosis is often difficult—symptoms such as weight loss, nocturnal waking, or relief or aggravation by eating often fail to discriminate between the different diagnoses. Patients with dyspepsia can, however, be subdivided into two main categories, based on the known or proposed underlying pathophysiology (Table 5.1). Thus dyspeptic symptoms may be ascribed to:

1. various organic diseases ('organic' dyspepsia), where there is an identified cause for the symptoms and if the disorder is improved or eliminated, symptoms also improve; or

2. various functional disorders ('functional' or 'non-ulcer' dyspepsia), where there is no definite structural or biochemical explanation for the symptoms but there may be an identifiable pathophysiological or microbiological aberration of uncertain relevance.

TABLE 5.1: Differential diagnosis of epigastric pain or discomfort	
Organic	**Functional dyspepsia**
• Chronic peptic ulcer (gastric ulcer, duodenal ulcer)	• Sensorimotor dysfunction of gastroduodenum:
• Gastro-oesophageal reflux disease (with or without oesophagitis)	- idiopathic gastroparesis/gastric antral hypomotility
• Drugs/medications	- gastric dysrhythmias
• Symptomatic cholelithiasis	- gastric/duodenal hypersensitivity
• Chronic pancreatitis	• *H. pylori* gastritis but no peptic ulcer
• Malignancy (gastric, pancreatic, colonic)	• Psychosocial factors:
• Mesenteric vascular insufficiency	- chronic life stress
• Metabolic causes (e.g., renal failure, hypercalcaemia, diabetes mellitus with gastroparesis)	• Idiopathic
• Abdominal wall pain	

Organic dyspepsia

Usually a targeted history and examination can provide a provisional diagnosis of the disorders in this category. In most instances, physical examination of the dyspeptic patient will not reveal any abnormality except deep tenderness in some cases. Evidence of weight loss, dysphagia, vomiting, bleeding, a family history of gastric or oesophageal cancer, anaemia, lymphadenopathy, or an abdominal mass indicates a greater likelihood of an organic disorder (these are referred to as 'alarm features' or 'red flags').

CHRONIC PEPTIC ULCER

Patients with uncomplicated peptic ulcer classically describe intermittent symptoms of 'burning' or 'gnawing' epigastric pain, which they can locate by finger point; the pain tends to be worse before meals and is relieved by taking food or antacids. Epigastric pain may waken the patient at night, commonly at about 2.00 am, when it is again relieved by food or antacids. The diagnosis is further strengthened if the history is clearly episodic with symptoms present for a few months at a time, followed by periods of remission (periodicity). The intensity and duration of pain vary from recurrence to recurrence, and the symptom-free intervals vary unpredictably. A history of prompt and good symptomatic relief by a course of H_2-receptor antagonists or proton pump inhibitors suggests an acid-related disorder (either peptic ulcer or reflux). There may be associated symptoms of heartburn and occasional vomiting. It is usually not possible to differentiate between gastric and duodenal ulceration by symptoms alone; in gastric ulcer, however, pain relief associated with food may be short-lived and anorexia, nausea and weight loss are more prominent. Unfortunately, classical ulcer-type symptoms also do *not* discriminate peptic ulcer disease from non-ulcer dyspepsia.

Chronic peptic ulcer, in most cases, is caused by *H. pylori* infection or non-steroidal anti-inflammatory drugs (NSAIDs); acid hypersecretory states (e.g., the Zollinger-Ellison syndrome due to a gastrin-producing tumour) are rarely a cause.

Gastric cancer

A short history of dyspepsia occurring in a patient over the age of 55 years should raise the suspicion of gastric cancer (Chapter 15). Symptoms of pain or discomfort on a daily basis, together with early satiety (inability to finish a normal meal), increase the probability. Weight loss, anorexia and vomiting are common symptoms especially when the malignancy is advanced (hence not curable). Dysphagia occurs with tumours arising from the cardia or distal oesophagus.

Chronic pancreatitis and pancreatic cancer

This less common condition presents as deep, boring upper abdominal pain, often radiating through to the back. There may be other symptoms of pancreatic insufficiency, for example steatorrhoea and possibly diabetes mellitus.

Similar symptoms of shorter duration, often with weight loss, may be associated with carcinoma of the pancreas, although this condition can typically present late when the patient is cachectic and jaundiced (Chapter 15).

Cholelithiasis

'Biliary colic' is associated with the sudden onset of severe or very severe epigastric pain which may pass through or around to the back (Chapter 4). Typically there are episodes of pain that occur unpredictably. With inflammation of the gall bladder, the pain may shift to the right upper quadrant and become 'peritoneal' in type. With biliary colic, movement does not aggravate the pain. The pain is usually not 'colicky' but sustained, albeit varying in intensity. Symptoms may be induced by a fatty meal. In the absence of typical biliary pain there appears to be no association between the presence of gallstones in the gall bladder and dyspepsia. If a gallstone enters the common bile duct, there may be associated features of intermittent jaundice, dark urine, pale stools, or episodic fever and rigors (see Chapter 21).

Other causes

Drugs are an important cause of dyspepsia, especially in the elderly. All NSAIDs may be associated with dyspepsia, whether or not there is chronic peptic ulcer. A number of antibiotics, digoxin, theophylline, and potassium or iron tablets can induce upper abdominal discomfort.

Intestinal ischaemia can sometimes cause dyspepsia. **Intestinal or mesenteric angina** causes the classical triad of upper abdominal pain induced by eating, a fear of eating (sitophobia) and weight loss (Chapter 6).

Metabolic causes such as renal failure, hypercalcaemia or thyroid disease can at times present with dyspepsia. Dyspepsia can occur in patients with long-standing diabetes mellitus who have autonomic neuropathy, gastroparesis, or diabetic radiculopathy. Other metabolic causes are discussed in Chapter 6. **Referred pain** from the chest or back may also occasionally cause chronic upper abdominal pain.

Not infrequently, the **abdominal wall** can be the source of unexplained upper abdominal pain or discomfort, arising from nerve entrapment or from a previous abdominal wall surgical scar. On physical examination in the latter condition, there is localised tenderness that is not abolished when the abdominal wall muscles are tensed (Carnett's test).

Functional or non-ulcer dyspepsia

This category represents the most common cause of dyspepsia in both patient and community populations. The term 'functional' implies a true disturbance of function, or an awareness of disturbed function, in the upper abdomen; it is inappropriate to use the term to denote a psychosomatic disorder. At present, patients with a past history of documented chronic peptic ulcer disease or evidence of pathological gastro-oesophageal reflux should not be classified as having functional dyspepsia.

MANAGEMENT OF DYSPEPSIA

A careful history is important to document the symptoms; in particular gastro-oesophageal reflux disease and biliary disease can usually be readily suspected from the history and relevant further investigations and treatment undertaken. Otherwise, if there are no symptoms or signs to indicate a higher probability of organic disease, and the patient is less than 55 years of age and is not taking regular aspirin or other NSAIDs, then immediate investigation may not be warranted (Figure 5.1). Depending on the age of the patient, and the duration and severity of symptoms, reassurance regarding the low probability of serious disease, and a full explanation of the mechanisms currently believed to underlie the symptoms may be associated with an improvement in symptoms. A short-term empiric trial of an H_2-blocker or proton pump inhibitors for 4–8 weeks may be useful but patients must be followed up. An alternative approach is to test for *H. pylori* infection (e.g., a urea breath test) and treat positive cases with specific antibiotic therapy as described below. In late middle-age and elderly patients, the threshold for investigation should be much lower, as organic disorders occur more frequently in this age group.

If symptoms are not fully relieved after 8 weeks following empiric drug treatment, investigation of the upper gastrointestinal tract, preferably by endoscopy, is advisable.

The aim of endoscopy is to definitely exclude peptic ulcer, reflux oesophagitis, and malignancy. Endoscopy is superior to the double-contrast barium meal and is now considered the 'gold standard' because it allows direct visualisation and biopsy of the oesophagus, stomach and duodenum. Ideally, endoscopy should be performed during a symptomatic phase when the patient is not on potent antisecretory drugs, to help ensure an active ulcer is not missed. All gastric ulcers should be biopsied to exclude gastric cancer (unless there is a contraindication, such as active bleeding, use of anticoagulants or known portal hypertension). *H. pylori* can be accurately detected by histological examination of gastric mucosal biopsies, or by subjecting such biopsies to rapid urease testing, as described below.

Screening blood tests, such as full blood count and blood film for anaemia and biochemical testing for glucose intolerance and abnormal liver function are recommended, although these tests generally have a low yield. Urea and electrolyte estimation should be performed in patients with persistent vomiting, as uraemia may present with dyspepsia and vomiting. Hypercalcaemia, usually due to hyperparathyroidism, is an uncommon cause of nausea but may be associated with duodenal ulcer. Serum amylase or lipase levels are usually not helpful in chronic pancreatitis except following an acute exacerbation. Upper abdominal ultrasonography in the absence of symptoms or biochemical test results suggestive of biliary tract or pancreatic disease is not recommended as a routine screening test because outpatient studies have shown that most dyspeptic patients have no detectable abnormality. However, if the latter disorders are suspected, ultrasonography should be performed early in the course of investigations.

Do not forget that gallstones may be incidentally found on ultrasonography; in the absence of typical biliary pain or alarm features, these should be usually ignored. Barium studies can be useful, especially if mechanical obstruction of the proximal small bowel is suspected. Psychological disorders, such as depression, somatoform disorder and eating disorders, should be considered in patients with chronic symptoms.

The benefit of scintigraphic gastric-emptying studies in routine clinical practice is not established. However, in selected cases with certain symptoms (e.g., severe postprandial fullness or recurrent vomiting), and normal endoscopic findings, documentation of the presence and extent of delayed emptying or abnormal handling of solids, especially in regard to the lag phase and rates of emptying, can improve diagnostic precision and indicate lines of further therapy. Gastric manometric and myoelectrical assessments of gastric and proximal small bowel motility are specialised techniques available in some centres and, at the present time, remain indicated for severe or unusual cases only.

If gastroparesis is identified, systemic disorders such as diabetes mellitus, thyroid disease, and connective tissue diseases, as well as drug side effects, should be excluded. The demonstration of gastroparesis also indicates that particular therapies may need to be pursued more vigorously. Small, frequent low-fat meals combined with a prokinetic plus, if nausea is prominent, an antiemetic can be helpful in the setting of gastroparesis. Gastric electrical stimulation may improve symptoms but does not accelerate gastric emptying.

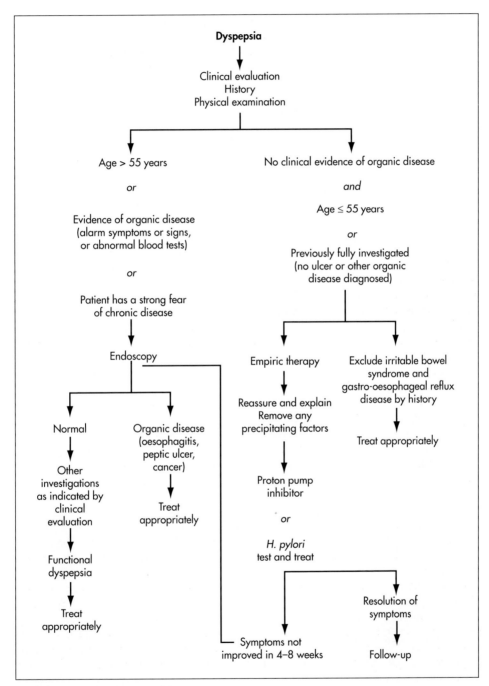

FIGURE 5.1: Management of dyspepsia.

DISEASES ASSOCIATED WITH EPIGASTRIC PAIN OR DISCOMFORT

Chronic peptic ulcer

Aetiology and pathophysiology

Chronic peptic ulcer can be defined as a break in the mucosa of greater than 5 mm with depth (Figure 5.2). An erosion, on the other hand, is smaller, lacks depth and is not associated with symptoms. In the general population, a chronic ulcer can be demonstrated in about 20% of patients with dyspepsia who are investigated; the risk is higher in the elderly.

Gastric acid secretion (from the parietal cells in the body and fundus of the stomach) is controlled by several interrelated factors in health, but the major stimulus is food. The cephalic phase comprises the acid response to the anticipation of food, or the sight, smell or taste of food, and is mediated by the vagus nerve. The gastric phase comprises acid secretion in response to food (primarily amino acids and amines) via gastrin release from the antral G cells. The intestinal phase occurs in response to food (especially protein) reaching the small bowel. Coffee and alcohol also stimulate acid secretion. A negative feedback loop operates when the gastric pH drops below 3, causing gastrin release to be strongly inhibited, probably by release of somatostatin from antral D cells.

The three major causes of chronic ulcer are *H. pylori* gastritis, NSAIDs and gastrinoma (the Zollinger-Ellison syndrome).

Helicobacter pylori. H. pylori is a chronic infection of the stomach that causes chronic histological gastritis. The bacterium is a spiral-shaped Gram-negative rod with flagella at one end. It is probably most often acquired in childhood by close contact in families and, once acquired, persists for life in most cases. The mode of transmission is unclear but both oral and faecal spread has been suggested. In Western countries, approximately 30% of the population is infected, with older persons and those from lower socioeconomic groups being more often infected. The higher prevalence with age reflects higher infection rates in the past; the risk of adult acquisition is low (< 1% per

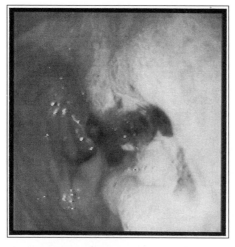

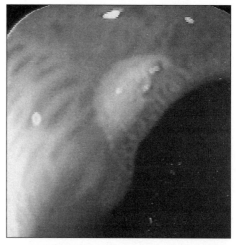

FIGURE 5.2A: Chronic duodenal ulcer (anterior wall) with clot on the base (at endoscopy). This was caused by *H. pylori*.

FIGURE 5.2B: Chronic gastric ulcer with no signs of recent haemorrhage (at endoscopy). This was caused by aspirin.

year. In developing countries (and in migrants from these countries), approximately 80% of adults are currently infected.

H. pylori is uniquely adapted to the gastric mucosal environment; for example, it produces the enzyme urease in very large amounts. It protects itself from gastric acid by breaking down endogenous urea using urease to produce a protective ammonia cloud. The infection induces gastric inflammation characterised by mononuclear and polymorphonuclear cell infiltration of the mucosa. The antrum is predominantly inflamed in Western countries but the gastritis often also involves the gastric body.

Most duodenal ulcer patients (> 90%) and many gastric ulcer patients (80%) have this infection. *H. pylori* causes an elevation in serum gastrin (because D cells in the antrum that produce the inhibitory peptide somatostatin are reduced due to the gastritis, disinhibiting antral G cells). The elevated gastrin increases meal-related acid secretion in those predisposed. These changes in gastrin reverse with cure of the infection. Increased acid secretion probably damages the mucosa in the first part of the duodenum leading to areas of gastric-type epithelium in the duodenum (called gastric metaplasia) that can be infected by *H. pylori* (these bacteria can live only on gastric epithelium). The localised inflammation in the duodenum caused by *H. pylori* (duodenitis) can progress to an ulcer. Duodenal ulcer will heal with acid suppression but usually recurs in *H. pylori*-infected patients (the duodenal ulcer diathesis) (Figure 5.3). The pathogenesis of gastric ulcer is also strongly linked to *H. pylori*. Cure of the infection leads to resolution of the gastritis (but not gastric metaplasia in the duodenum) and eliminates the ulcer diathesis (in both duodenal and gastric ulcer) where the ulcer was caused by the infection. Other factors, such as virulence of *H. pylori* infection (based on the *cag* pathogenicity island), smoking, chronic psychosocial stress and 'genetic' factors, such as blood group status, probably act as disease modulators.

H. pylori infection can be diagnosed at endoscopy by taking gastric biopsies from the antrum and examining them histologically for the bacteria (one of the 'gold standard' tests) (Table 5.2). A screening test, the rapid urease test, has a high sensitivity and specificity (> 95%). It involves placing an antral biopsy in a pH-sensitive medium containing urea. Urease produced by the bacteria splits the urea to ammonia that changes the pH and produces a colour change (Figure 5.4). Culture is insensitive and is reserved for determining antibiotic resistance in selected cases that have been difficult to cure with therapy.

Non-invasive tests are also available that do not require endoscopy and gastric biopsy. The bacteria induce an antibody response (IgG) that can be measured, but this is not useful for distinguishing past from current infection. Breath tests are performed by having patients ingest urea labelled with ^{14}C (requiring a low dose of radiation) or ^{13}C (non-radioactive); urease, if present from *H. pylori*, splits the urea to ammonia, and the resulting CO_2 production is absorbed and expired in the breath where the labelled ^{14}C or ^{13}C can be measured (Figure 5.5). Also, a stool antigen test for *H. pylori* is accurate for diagnosing current infection.

Non-steroidal anti-inflammatory drugs (NSAIDs). Traditional NSAIDs inhibit the enzyme cyclooxygenase and hence reduce the production of prostaglandins such as PGE2 and PGI2, impairing gastrointestinal mucosal defence. NSAIDs (whether given orally, rectally or systemically) induce subepithelial haemorrhage and erosions in the stomach and/or duodenum in about two-thirds of patients. Up to 15–20% of NSAID users develop chronic gastric ulceration, while perhaps 5–10% develop duodenal ulcers. Chronic NSAID users are at a three- to six-times increased risk of serious gastric and duodenal ulcer complications (bleeding, perforation or death) compared with non-users. Unfortunately, complications are the presenting feature rather than dyspepsia in more than half the patients who develop NSAID-related peptic ulceration.

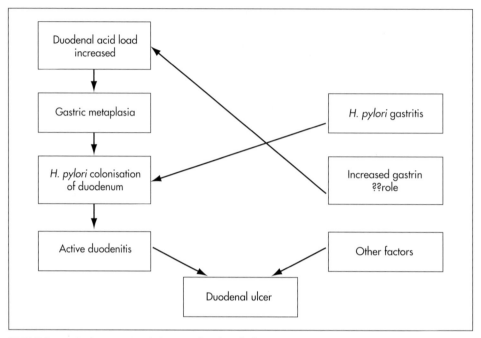

FIGURE 5.3: Pathogenesis of chronic duodenal ulcer.

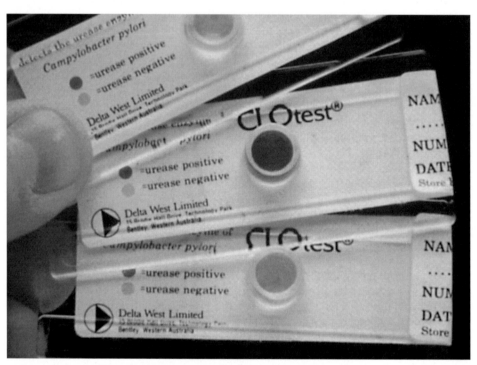

FIGURE 5.4: A rapid urease test—a gastric biopsy is placed in the pH-sensitive medium. Top and bottom tests: no colour change. Middle test: change to magenta within 3 hours, indicating the presence of urease (and hence *H. pylori*).

TABLE 5.2: Diagnostic tests for *H. pylori*—testing should only be performed if treatment is planned

Methods	Advantages	Disadvantages	Usefulness
Non-invasive			
Serology	Non-invasive, relatively cheap	Requires validation in local patient	Initial diagnosis, not follow-up after therapy
^{14}C urea breath test	Rapid, allows distinction between current and past infection	Involves ingestion of radioactivity Reduced sensitivity with acid suppression or antibiotics	Initial diagnosis, follow-up of treatment regimens
^{13}C urea breath test	No radioactivity, as for ^{14}C	Complex equipment, expensive Reduced sensitivity with acid suppression or antibiotics	Initial diagnosis, follow-up of treatment regimens
Stool antigen test	Allows distinction between current and past infection	Reduced sensitivity with proton pump inhibitor	Initial diagnosis, follow-up of treatment regimens
Invasive			
Rapid urease test	Rapid, inexpensive	Invasive Reduced sensitivity in those on acid suppression or with recent or active bleeding	Initial diagnosis
Histology	Allows assessment of mucosa	Invasive, costly	Assess gastritis, metaplasia and atrophy etc, initial diagnosis
Culture	Specificity: 100%	Invasive, costly, slow, less sensitive	Initial diagnosis, antimicrobial sensitivities, strain typing (macrolide resistance 4–12%); metronidazole resistance is common

NSAID ulcers and ulcer complications occur more commonly in the elderly (> 60 years of age), with high doses, in those with a prior history of peptic ulcer or bleeding, with multiple NSAID use or steroids, with concurrent use of anticoagulants, and in the presence of other serious illness. Those with *H. pylori* infection and exposure to NSAIDs may be at higher risk of ulcer than those with just one of these factors, but this is controversial. NSAIDs may also cause small bowel disease (ulceration, perforation) and colonic disease (stricture, colitis). COX-2-selective NSAIDs are associated with significantly less peptic ulceration.

Gastrinoma. The Zollinger-Ellison syndrome refers to a gastrinoma causing gastric acid hypersecretion and, frequently, peptic ulceration. The tumours producing this syndrome may be found in the pancreas (85%) or the duodenal wall. Two-thirds are malignant with metastases. Ulcers in this syndrome may be single or multiple. The increased gastrin may cause gastric hypertrophy with prominent folds. Diarrhoea with or without steatorrhoea occurs in one-third of cases (because the high acid level

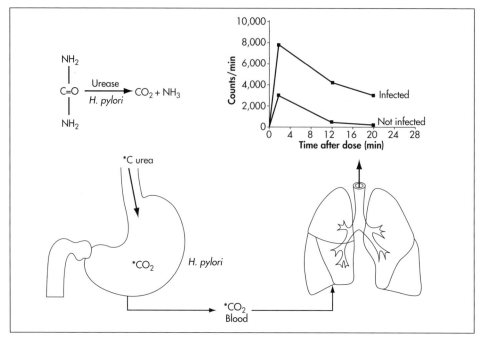

FIGURE 5.5: Schematic representation of the ^{14}C and ^{13}C breath test. After ingestion of labelled urea, urea is metabolised by urease and labelled CO_2 is produced. This is exhaled via the lungs and the concentration of labelled carbon atoms can be determined in the exhaled air. The value at 20 or 30 min may be used to define a positive urea breath test (upper curve). An early peak can occur in both *Helicobacter pylori*-positive and -negative cases from hydrolysis of urea by mouth flora.
(*Based on Holtmann G, Talley NJ,* Infections of the Gastrointestinal Tract, *Raven Press, with permission.*)

damages small bowel mucosa and inactivates pancreatic lipase as well as deconjugating bile salts); in 10% of cases, diarrhoea is the only presenting symptom. The Zollinger-Ellison syndrome can also occur as part of the multiple-endocrine neoplasia (MEN) type I syndrome where there is hyperplasia, adenoma or carcinoma of the pancreatic islets, parathyroid and pituitary. This is an autosomal dominant condition, so there may be a family history of ulcer. In addition to the clinical features found with a gastrinoma, there is usually hypercalcaemia, secondary to parathyroid disease (Chapter 23). Serum gastrin levels should be checked to screen for this diagnosis if patients have multiple or refractory ulcers, enlarged gastric folds or a dilated duodenum, an ulcer plus diarrhoea or steatorrhoea, or hypercalcaemia, associated with ulcer disease. A serum gastrin concentration greater than 1000 pg/mL in patients producing gastric acid (which can be measured by testing the pH of gastric juice at endoscopy or by formal gastric secretory function testing) is virtually diagnostic. Conditions such as pernicious anaemia or post vagotomy surgery can cause a high serum gastrin level, but gastric acid secretion is low. In difficult cases, a secretin test is helpful; gastrinomas cause a paradoxical rise in gastrin in response to a secretin bolus of greater than 100 pg/mL above baseline. Once a diagnosis of Zollinger-Ellison syndrome is made, consideration should be given to whether there is evidence of MEN I (e.g., hyperparathyroidism). Thereafter, evidence of metastatic spread (> 60% are malignant) and tumour localisation is sought by a contrast CT (5 mm sections). Endoscopic ultrasound may identify small tumours. Imaging may still miss up to 30% of tumours in this syndrome. Even if no tumour is found by scanning, it can usually be located by surgery.

Initial regimen	Dose	Duration	Eradication rate
TABLE 5.3: Treatment of *H. pylon*—current regimens			
Proton pump inhibitor (triple therapy)			
Any PPI (e.g., omeprazole, esomeprazole, pantoprazole or lansoprazole)	Full dose bid	1 week	80%
- plus clarithromycin	500 mg bid		
- plus amoxycillin	1 g bid		
- or metronidazole	400 mg or 500 mg bid		
In the event of treatment failure to first-line triple therapy *Quadruple therapy (second line)*			
PPI	Twice daily	2 weeks	75%
- plus Pepto-Bismol (or bismuth subcitrate)	2 tablets qid (or 240 mg)		
- plus tetracycline	500 mg qid		
- plus metronidazole	400 mg or 500 mg qid		
Alternative triple therapy (third line)			
PPI	Twice daily	10 days	> 80%
- plus rifabutin	300 mg once daily		
- or levofloxacin	250 mg bid		
- plus amoxycillin	1 g bid		
PPI = proton pump inhibitor; qid = four times per day; tds = three times per day; bid = two times per day.			

The tumour should be resected where feasible (liver metastases may also be amenable to resection); otherwise, patients are managed with high dose proton (acid) pump inhibitors to control gastric acid. Approximately 50% of patients who cannot be completely resected die from tumour spread in 10 years; newer chemotherapy regimens may reduce disease progression.

Treatment

All cases of chronic peptic ulceration associated with *H. pylori* should be treated with combination antibacterial therapy. A number of combination regimens are now available and appear to be effective. Such regimens include triple therapy with a proton pump inhibitor such as omeprazole 20 mg, esomeprazole 40 mg, lanzoprazole 30 mg or pantoprazole 40 mg twice daily together with two antibiotics (e.g., metronidazole, amoxycillin, tetracycline or clarithromycin) for 1 to 2 weeks (Table 5.3). Antisecretory therapy is usually then continued for a further 4 to 6 weeks to ensure ulcer healing although this may not be absolutely necessary. With this type of therapy, successful cure of the infection in over 80% of patients and resolution of the ulcer can be achieved.

Side effects include, diarrhoea (including, in rare cases, pseudomembranous colitis from the antibiotics), anaphylaxis, nausea or taste disturbances, photosensitivity reaction (tetracycline), peripheral neuropathy (metronidazole) and a disulfiram-like reaction with alcohol ingestion (from metronidazole).

As well as efficacy, the choice of regimen is dependent on other factors, in particular compliance with the drugs and costs of the therapy. It is recommended that cure of infection be checked by a breath test or stool test (or endoscopic biopsy) at least one month after ceasing therapy, although in the future this may not be necessary if a regimen with a high cure rate has been employed, no ulcer complications have occurred in the past and there has been clinical improvement. If initial therapy fails for *H. pylori*, a repeat course with different agents can be tried. Gastric ulcers still need to be followed up by endoscopy to ensure healing and exclude malignancy. If treatment regimens to eradicate *H. pylori* fail, then long-term proton pump inhibitor maintenance therapy can be utilised.

Ulcers associated with NSAID use are ideally treated by stopping the NSAID—at least while ulcer healing therapy is given. In this situation, any conventional ulcer healing regimen can be employed, such as a proton pump inhibitor, as single therapy. If *H. pylori* is present, it should also be treated. Gastric ulcer healing should be assessed 8–12 weeks after initiating therapy to ensure healing, and further gastric biopsies taken to exclude malignancy.

If traditional NSAID therapy is required long term, the lowest dose of a short-acting and less toxic NSAID (e.g., ibuprofen) should be prescribed. Enteric-coated or rectal NSAIDs do not significantly reduce the risk of ulcer. Co-prescription with a prostaglandin analogue such as misoprostol is a reasonable option and is more effective than prophylaxis with H_2-receptor antagonists (which at standard dose reduce duodenal but *not* gastric ulcer recurrence from NSAIDs). Misoprostol has been shown to reduce the occurrence of gastric and duodenal ulcer by more than 60% over the subsequent months as well as ulcer complications. A proton pump inhibitor is an alternative and commonly prescribed option.

Surgery is now rarely indicated for control of peptic ulcer disease as cure is attainable (Figure 5.6). When surgery is required, the surgery is directed at treating the complication (e.g., oversewing the perforation or under-running the bleeding ulcer). Rarely, a gastric resection will be required if a gastric ulcer is resistant to healing and malignancy cannot be confidently excluded. The ulcer diathesis can be treated by conventional therapy (listed above) after the patient has recovered from the operation. However, many patients in the past underwent gastric surgery for this disease. The complications that may arise in these cases are summarised in Table 5.4.

TABLE 5.4: Complications of peptic ulcer surgery

1. Recurrent ulceration
   Consider incomplete vagotomy, gastrinoma, retained antrum

2. Dumping syndrome
   Early—30 min after eating due to hyperosmolar contents entering the small bowel. This results in tachycardia, sweating and collapse
   Late—90–180 min after eating due to hypoglycaemia (reactive)

3. Malabsorption and diarrhoea
   Mild steatorrhoea due to rapid intestinal transit after gastric resection. If the stool fat is unexpectedly high, consider bacterial overgrowth, coeliac disease, gastrojejunocolic fistula or gastroileostomy, and Zollinger-Ellison syndrome

4. Bile reflux gastritis after partial gastrectomy
   This results in early satiety, vomiting and distension

5. Gastric remnant carcinoma
   After partial gastrectomy: risk increases after 15 years

6. Retained antrum after Billroth-II
   This results in gastric hypersecretion

7. Afferent loop syndrome after Billroth-II
   This results in pain relieved by vomiting, in bloating and bacterial overgrowth

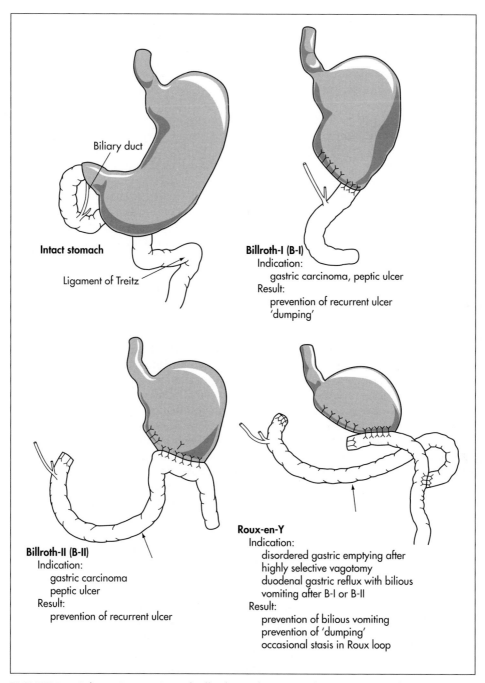

Biliary duct

Intact stomach

Ligament of Treitz

Billroth-I (B-I)
Indication:
gastric carcinoma, peptic ulcer
Result:
prevention of recurrent ulcer
'dumping'

Billroth-II (B-II)
Indication:
gastric carcinoma
peptic ulcer
Result:
prevention of recurrent ulcer

Roux-en-Y
Indication:
disordered gastric emptying after
highly selective vagotomy
duodenal gastric reflux with bilious
vomiting after B-I or B-II
Result:
prevention of bilious vomiting
prevention of 'dumping'
occasional stasis in Roux loop

FIGURE 5.6: Schematic overview of Billroth-I and B-II partial gastrectomy and Roux-en-Y reconstruction with their indications and their consequences for gastric emptying.
(*Based on AJPM Smout and LMA Akkermans,* Normal and disturbed motility of the gastrointestinal tract, *with permission.*)

Functional (non-ulcer) dyspepsia

Pathophysiology

Although the pathogenesis of functional dyspepsia remains unknown, a number of physiological factors appear to be associated with the disorder. Most attention has been directed towards assessment of upper gut sensorimotor function.

In health, the major motor functions of the stomach are to temporarily store ingested food during the process of breakdown of solids, to empty chyme appropriately into the small bowel, and to empty indigestible solids remaining in the stomach after a meal. During ingestion of a meal, vagally-mediated receptive relaxation of the proximal stomach occurs in response to swallowing. This relaxation prepares the proximal stomach to receive oesophageal contents, and is followed by gastric accommodation, whereby the proximal stomach progressively relaxes to accommodate increasing volumes, while maintaining a relatively constant intragastric pressure. Solid emptying is largely controlled by antral and pyloric motor activity. Phasic contractions (the migrating motor complex, or MMC) sweep from the mid-stomach to the pylorus, at a frequency of three per minute, mixing and grinding the food until particles are approximately 1 mm in size. Emptying of liquids is controlled by coordinated motor activity in the fundus, body and antrum. Proximal gastric tone appears to be of particular importance in liquid emptying. The pylorus is an important functional component of the gastroduodenal region and also regulates solid and liquid emptying. The rate of gastric emptying is regulated by additional factors such as the osmolality and fat content of the meal, the amount of gastric acid secreted and duodenal motility. Liquids empty more rapidly than solids; the time taken for half the gastric contents to empty after ingestion of a standard mixed meal is about 90 minutes for the solid phase, and about 30 minutes for the liquid phase.

Gastric stasis. Delayed gastric emptying, predominantly for solids, but also for liquids, is observed in 25% of patients with functional dyspepsia. Abnormalities in intragastric distribution of the meal can also be documented. Postprandial antral hypomotility is accepted as the cause of delayed gastric emptying in most cases, but alterations in duodenal motility may also play a role. The underlying cause of such motility abnormalities is unknown. The presence of gastric stasis, however, correlates poorly with symptoms in individual patients and, thus, its importance in the syndrome of functional dyspepsia is not established.

Impaired fundic relaxation. Failure of the fundus to relax normally after meal ingestion occurs in up to 40% of patients with functional dyspepsia. This can cause the symptom of early satiety in some of these patients. The mechanical accommodation of the stomach to gastric distension (compliance), however, does not appear to be different between patients and control subjects.

Altered gastroduodenal sensitivity. At least some cases of functional dyspepsia appear to be associated with an enhanced gastroduodenal sensitivity to distension (Figure 5.7). The relationship between this phenomenon and the alterations in upper gut motility described above is not clear, but it is likely that in some cases these may be a consequence of altered visceral afferent function. Gastric volumes required to induce feelings of distension and pain have been shown to be significantly lower in patients with functional dyspepsia than in control subjects.

***H. pylori* gastritis.** *H. pylori* gastritis histologically is found in 30% of dyspeptic patients with no evidence of peptic ulcer disease. However, *H. pylori* gastritis is common in totally asymptomatic subjects. The presence of the gastritis does not appear to have an important influence on the prevalence or type of gastric motor dysfunction. Cure of infection results in symptomatic improvement in a minority long term (with a 10% benefit over placebo).

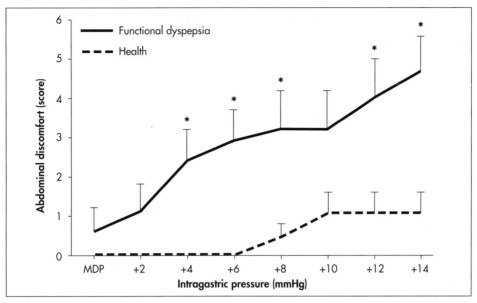

FIGURE 5.7: Heightened gastric sensitivity to balloon distension of the stomach in patients with functional dyspepsia versus control subjects. Note the onset of symptoms at lower pressures in patients with functional dyspepsia.

MDP = minimal distending pressure.

(Based on data from Mearin et al, Gastroenterology *1991; 101: 999–1006, with permission from the American Gastroenterological Society.)*

Psychosocial factors. Although acute stress can alter gastrointestinal function and induce symptoms in healthy subjects, the role of life-event stress in the pathogenesis of chronic functional dyspepsia remains controversial. It appears, however, that life events which are highly threatening or which lead to frustration of goals are associated with functional dyspepsia. It is important to note that no characteristic personality profile is demonstrable in patients with functional dyspepsia. Psychosocial disturbances such as neuroticism, anxiety and depression probably, however, influence the decision to seek health care.

Treatment

The approach to treatment is outlined in Table 5.5. Once a positive diagnosis has been made, management of functional dyspepsia is based on reassurance regarding the absence of serious disease, and an explanation of the possible factors producing symptoms. Patients should be advised to avoid specific foods that aggravate their symptoms such as coffee and alcohol and also to avoid any medications that may be provoking symptoms. A reduced-fat diet may be beneficial, as fat delays gastric motor function more profoundly than other dietary constituents. For postprandial symptoms, a decrease in meal size with more frequent meals should be tried. The presence of anxiety, depression and/or chronic stress should be explored and can be addressed from the outset with simple forms of counselling; untreated anxiety or depression may impair the response to other forms of therapy. An explanation of the ways in which stress can affect upper gut function is often valuable, and is used to emphasise the recurrent or episodic nature of the symptoms. If the dyspeptic symptoms are long standing, a psychological precipitant (e.g., a stressful life event or fear of organic disease)—rather than the specific gastrointestinal symptoms themselves—may account for the current visit. Recognition of this may avoid multiple visits and extensive gastrointestinal investigations.

If symptoms are affecting quality of life significantly, drug therapy should be considered. Medical therapy can usually provide at least partial relief of symptoms; this may be related to the high placebo treatment effect (up to 60% in functional dyspepsia).

All *H. pylori*-positive patients with functional dyspepsia may be offered eradication therapy for dyspeptic symptoms, but many will not benefit. Trials with antisecretory drugs, particularly the proton pump inhibitors, have indicated that these medications are modestly superior to placebo in the therapy of functional dyspepsia; patients with epigastric pain may be more likely to respond. Thus, it is reasonable to suggest that these medications should be first-line medications. If there is no improvement, a prokinetic drug (e.g., domperidone, 10 mg, three times per day) can be tried.

The prokinetic drugs have been shown to be effective in improving symptoms in functional dyspepsia. The original agent in this class was metoclopramide, and although early studies suggested symptomatic improvement when compared with placebo, recent assessments are not available. Moreover, the side-effect profile, especially extra-pyramidal reactions, is more frequent than with newer agents. Domperidone, a dopamine receptor antagonist with fewer side effects than metoclopramide, has been shown to be more effective than placebo in relieving symptoms, although the data in functional dyspepsia are limited. Tegaserod is a serotonin type 4 receptor partial agonist that accelerates gastric emptying and probably relaxes the fundus; however, benefit in functional dyspepsia has been limited.

TABLE 5.5: Key features of functional dyspepsia

Clinical features

- Chronic or recurrent (≥ 3 months) abdominal pain or discomfort centred in the upper abdomen
- May be symptoms of early satiety, postprandial fullness, nausea, retching, vomiting, or upper abdominal bloating
- No clinical, biochemical, endoscopic or ultrasound evidence of organic disease likely to explain symptoms (not all these tests are necessary to make the diagnosis)

Treatment

1. Make a positive clinical diagnosis based on the history and physical examination, and limit tests
2. Minimise invasive investigations and avoid giving 'mixed messages'; do not perform repeated testing without substantial indication
3. Determine the patient's agenda; ask why the patient with chronic symptoms has presented now
4. Provide education and firm reassurance
5. Try dietary modification (e.g., low-fat diet, small more frequent meals)
6. Set realistic treatment goals and centre therapy on adjustment to illness and patient-based responsibility for care
7. Prescribe drugs sparingly targeting the symptom(s) of most concern to the patient; remember the placebo response:
   - short-term trial of a proton pump inhibitor or prokinetic agent or H_2-receptor antagonist
   - consider combination drug therapy or antidepressants in resistant cases
8. Consider behavioural treatments or psychotherapy for moderate to severe cases
9. Organise a continuing care strategy

In general, long-term drug treatment should be avoided in most patients with functional dyspepsia. For those patients with frequent relapses, short intermittent treatment courses (for example 1 to 2 weeks) may be considered when no other management is successful and symptoms are significantly affecting the patient's quality of life. Antidepressants may have a role in difficult cases. Newer medications, such as drugs that modify visceral afferent function, may allow a wider choice of therapeutic agents in the future.

Chronic pancreatitis

The most common cause of chronic pancreatitis is alcohol (Table 5.6). Alcohol leads to hypersecretion of a proteinacious fluid that can precipitate first in the small pancreatic ducts and later in the main pancreatic ducts. These deposits block the ducts and cause dilatation of the ducteals; later, inflammatory infiltrates appear. It is unclear whether or not the normal pancreas secretes a specific protein that inhibits calcium carbonate stone formation (stone-inhibitor protein). Smoking increases the risk of chronic pancreatitis.

TABLE 5.6: Causes of chronic pancreatitis

1. Chronic alcoholism
2. Idiopathic
3. Hypertriglyceridaemia
4. Hypercalcaemia
5. Trauma
6. Hereditary (autosomal dominant)
7. Cystic fibrosis
8. Tropical (nutritional)
9. Haemochromatosis
10. Prolonged parental hyperalimentation
11. Obstruction:
    - benign, e.g., pancreas divisum with obstruction of the accessory ampulla
    - cancer, e.g., of the ampulla or duct (short history)
12. Autoimmune (may be misdiagnosed as pancreatic cancer)

Clinical presentation

While patients with chronic pancreatitis may present with episodes of acute pancreatitis (Chapter 4), the common mode of presentation is intermittent abdominal pain, usually in the epigastric region after eating (15 to 30 minutes) and radiating to the back. It may be made better by sitting upright and leaning forward. The pain may also occur in the right or left upper quadrant. It is typically severe and is unrelieved by eating or antacids. Alcohol and fatty meals may make the pain worse. It tends to become more continuous pain with disease progression. There may be diarrhoea and steatorrhoea as well as weight loss due to pancreatic insufficiency (Chapter 13). Commonly these patients have a history of high analgesic use and abuse. The clinical problem may be very difficult to evaluate if the patient has become narcotic dependent. Thus, it may be hard to be sure which of the symptoms are due to chronic pancreatitis.

On physical examination, there may be signs of wasting and malnutrition. Rarely, jaundice is present because of obstruction of the common bile duct. Patients may also have evidence of diabetes mellitus with advanced disease. Other complications of chronic pancreatitis include the development of pseudocysts, which may become infected (Chapter 4). Pancreatic ascites can also occur (Chapter 18). Clinical evidence of vitamin deficiency is rare (fat soluble vitamins [A, D, E, K] or B12)

Diagnosis

Levels of amylase and lipase are unhelpful. A plain abdominal X-ray examination may show pancreatic calcification (in 30% of cases) which is virtually diagnostic. An abdominal CT scan will detect pancreatic calcification more often. A CT or ultrasound scan may also show a shrunken pancreas with dilatation of the main pancreatic duct that is a pointer to the diagnosis. Endoscopic retrograde cholangiopancreatograhy (ERCP) or magnetic resonance cholangiopancreatograhy (MRCP) is the next test to perform if the diagnosis of chronic pancreatitis is suspected, but other tests have been unhelpful. This provides information on the morphology of the ducts. ERCP complications (2%) include acute pancreatitis, sepsis and cholangitis. Endoscopic ultrasound is an alternative and may be as useful as ERCP.

If patients have diarrhoea or suspected steatorrhoea, a 3-day faecal fat estimation should be obtained. A faecal fat excretion of > 40 g per day is usually only seen with pancreatic steatorrhoea (Chapter 13). Cystic fibrosis needs to be considered in children or young adults in such cases and a sweat electrolyte test should be obtained. It is also important to check serum calcium and triglyceride levels to exclude these rare causes of chronic pancreatitis.

Non-invasive tests of pancreatic function, such as the bentiromide and the pancreolauryl tests are useful in patients with moderate or severe chronic pancreatitis but both false positive and false negative results do occur. Intubation studies, such as the secretin test (which stimulates pancreatic exocrine secretion that is measured by obtaining a duodenal aspirate), is not widely available.

The differential diagnosis must include pancreatic cancer, as well as rare diseases such as autoimmune pancreatitis and pancreatic endocrine tumours.

Treatment

Control of abdominal pain is the major problem in most patients. Narcotic addiction needs to be avoided. Total alcohol absence is essential as this may reduce the pain. Oral pancreatic enzyme preparations reduce pain (because they reduce cholecystokinin secretion leading to a negative feedback on the pancreas, putting it at rest). Large doses are required with meals. Pancreatic steatorrhoea is also treated with pancreatic enzyme replacement. The usual dose is six to eight Viokase or Cotazym tablets, or three capsules of enteric-coated pancreases. One to two tablets should be taken on starting the meal, and during and just after the meal. Prescribe small, low-fat meals. If this fails, antisecretory therapy to reduce gastric acid secretion (acid inactivates the enzymes) can be helpful. Pain control may be achieved with a short course of narcotics plus a low-dose tricyclic antidepressant and an NSAID long term. Hospitalisation keeping the patient nil by mouth may be needed until pain control is achieved. The usefulness of octreotide is uncertain, but may be worth a trial.

In difficult cases, relief of pancreatic duct obstruction with endoscopic removal of stones or extracorporeal lithotripsy may sometimes be helpful. Temporary insertion of a stent into a proximally obstructed pancreatic duct may be of value. If a pseudocyst is present in a patient with pain, it may respond to drainage, which can be done radiologically, endoscopically or occasionally by surgery. Coeliac axis nerve blocks are worth a trial, and bilateral thoracoscopic splanchnectomy has shown promise.

Extracorporeal shock wave lithotripsy for pancreatic stones, if available, may be helpful in selected cases.

Surgery (e.g., a lateral pancreaticojejunostomy [Puestow] procedure) can alleviate pain when the pancreatic duct or system is dilated. Another approach is lateral pancreaticojejunostomy with saucerisation and drainage of the head of the pancreas (Frey's operation). This procedure is also effective in patients without a dilated main pancreatic duct. Focal disease in the head or tail of the pancreas can be treated by a pylorus-preserving pancreaticojejunostomy or distal pancreatectomy. Resection may also be indicated if carcinoma of the pancreas cannot be excluded; this complication occurs in 5–10% of patients with chronic pancreatitis. Surgery has approximately a 70 to 90% rate of success.

Further reading

Camilleri M, Talley NJ. Pathophysiology as a basis for understanding symptom complexes and therapeutic targets. *Neurogastroenterol Motil* 2004; 16: 135–42.

Cremonini F, Delgado-Aros S, Talley NJ. Functional dyspepsia: drugs for new (and old) therapeutic targets. *Best Pract Res Clin Gastroenterol* 2004; 18: 717–33.

DiMagno MJ, DiMagno EP. Chronic pancreatitis. *Curr Opin Gastroenterol* 2005; 21: 544–54.

Duggan A. Management of dyspepsia at the beginning of the twenty-first century. *Intern Med J* 2003; 33: 604–9.

El-Serag HB, Talley NJ. Systemic review: the prevalence and clinical course of functional dyspepsia. *Aliment Pharmacol Ther* 2004; 19: 643–54.

Feinle-Bisset C, Vozzo R, Horowitz M, Talley NJ. Diet, food intake, and disturbed physiology in the pathogenesis of symptoms in functional dyspepsia. *Am J Gastroenterol* 2004; 99: 170–81.

Moayyedi P, Deeks J, Talley NJ *et al*. An update of the Cochrane systematic review of *Helicobacter pylori* eradication therapy in nonulcer dyspepsia: resolving the discrepancy between systematic reviews. *Am J Gastroenterol* 2003; 98: 2621–6.

Moayyedi P, Delaney BC, Vakil N *et al*. The efficacy of proton pump inhibitors in nonulcer dyspepsia: a systematic review and economic analysis. *Gastroenterology* 2004; 127: 1329–37.

Tack J, Bisschops R, Sarnelli G. Pathophysiology and treatment of functional dyspepsia. *Gastroenterology* 2004; 127: 1239–55.

Talley NJ. Dyspepsia. *Gastroenterology* 2003; 125: 1219–26.

Talley NJ. What the physician needs to know for correct management of gastro-oesophageal reflux disease and dyspepsia. *Aliment Pharmacol Ther* 2004; 20 Suppl 2: 23–30.

Talley NJ, Vakil N, Moayyedi P. AGA technical review on the evaluation of dyspepsia. *Gastroenterology* 2005; 129: 1756–80.

chapter 6

CHRONIC LOWER ABDOMINAL PAIN OR DISCOMFORT

INTRODUCTION

Most chronic lower abdominal pain is not due to organic disease, and often represents a source of frustration and confusion to both patient and physician. The commonest cause is irritable bowel syndrome; related functional bowel disorders, such as functional abdominal bloating, together with the separate entity of chronic functional abdominal pain, account for the majority of other cases. These functional gastrointestinal disorders represent a substantial source of morbidity and cost to the community. Because the management of the different causes can be quite different, it is important to make a positive diagnosis of the cause of the abdominal pain.

HISTORY

The key to diagnosing the cause of chronic or recurrent abdominal pain is a precise history. In most cases, a skilled physician can make an accurate diagnosis or at least narrow the range of possible diagnoses even before the physical examination. Even so, chronic abdominal pain is more difficult to diagnose than acute pain, because the characteristics of the pain tend to be less specific and can be difficult for patients to describe. The essential features that need to be elicited are described below.

Perception of pain

The terms used by patients to describe abdominal pain vary greatly. In particular, some refer to pain, and others to discomfort, fullness or even indigestion. Moreover, individual responses to a given painful stimulus also vary: thus, while one patient may describe very severe pain, to another it may be mild in intensity. A number of factors may account for these individual differences, and in this regard it is important to remember that the experience of pain includes: 1) nociception whereby a noxious stimulus conveys an impulse centrally; 2) conscious perception of this sensation; 3) an affective response such as distress; and 4) a behavioural response.

Site, radiation and referral of pain

It is helpful to ask the patient to indicate with his or her hand where the pain is felt; this is best elicited during the physical examination with the patient in the supine position. If the pain is midline, the region on the abdomen can give a clue to the origin, e.g., pain from the small bowel tends to be peri-umbilical, while pain from the colon tends to be perceived in the lower abdomen. The more the painful area can be localised (e.g., to a finger-tip point), the more likely it is that the site reflects the origin of the painful stimulus. Radiation of pain can be characteristic of certain organs. For example, pancreatic pain can be referred to the back, while radiation to the groin occurs in disorders of the ureter and testicle.

However, in functional bowel disorders, such as irritable bowel syndrome, the radiation of pain—from the colon particularly—can be to any of these sites but also to other extra-abdominal areas; it may also shift in location.

Character, intensity and duration of pain

The nature or character of the pain is important to define, as certain disorders are associated with pain of a particular quality. Thus the pain of intestinal obstruction is usually cramping, while pain of inflammatory origin is often continuous in nature. Other descriptions can be suggested to the patient by the examiner, or the patient can be asked to relate the current pain to previous pains he or she may have experienced. The intensity or severity of pain does not always provide reliable information, and it is important to appreciate that the intensity of pain cannot differentiate between 'functional' and 'organic' disorders. Sometimes, however, associated signs and the manner in which the patient describes the pain can give clues to the intensity. Asking the patient to rate the pain on a numerical scale from one to ten can be used to compare the intensity of recurrent episodes of pain. The mode of onset of pain can be helpful; in general, chronic lower abdominal pain has a gradual onset, with a slow increase in intensity, when compared with the sudden onset of pain from mechanical or vascular causes. Some types of recurrent lower abdominal pain, however, can occur in discrete episodes of sudden onset.

The overall duration of pain is often an important indicator of the significance of the disorder causing the pain—thus, continuous pain which has been present for months or years, in a patient not obviously unwell, is usually functional in origin. When pain is recurrent, the timing (frequency and duration, time of day) are important to establish. Pain that wakes the patient from sleep usually indicates an organic disorder, although it can occur in the functional bowel syndromes. It is important to determine whether the patient actually wakes because of pain, or whether other factors initially wake the patient.

Modifying factors

Factors which modify the pain can also be important. Routinely, the relationship of pain to meals, bowel motions, exertion, menstruation and sexual intercourse should be obtained. A diary of the timing of pain in relation to meals and other activities can help both the patient and the doctor to determine provoking or relieving factors. Patients often state that eating exacerbates the abdominal pain, and in some instances this can provide discrimination, such as mesenteric ischaemia with 'intestinal angina'. In general, however, the timing of pain in relation to food intake is not of great help in diagnosing disorders causing chronic lower abdominal pain. Similarly, consumption of particular foods is usually not of great relevance, as food allergy or intolerance is an uncommon disorder (Chapter 16). Excessive ingestion of sugars (such as lactose present in milk products, and fructose and sorbitol present in fruits, some soft drinks and confectionery) may provoke bloating, abdominal discomfort, flatulence and diarrhoea.

Relief of pain by bowel movements or by passing flatus is suggestive of a colonic origin for the pain: such relief is usually perceived rapidly, but can be short-lived. Colonic pain can be experienced in a variety of abdominal regions, and is often associated with a disordered bowel habit.

Musculoskeletal causes of pain can be exacerbated by different postures or exercise and relieved by rest, although once again this distinction cannot be relied upon. The patient can be asked to demonstrate the postures that can bring on the pain. Pain originating in the anterior abdominal wall is aggravated when the abdominal wall is tensed by, for example, raising the lower limbs in the supine position. Episodes of pain related to menstruation raise the possibility of pelvic inflammatory disease or endometriosis; it should be remembered, however, that abdominal discomfort from a wide variety of causes can be aggravated premenstrually, and alterations in stool pattern are also common at this time.

DIFFERENTIAL DIAGNOSIS OF CHRONIC LOWER ABDOMINAL PAIN OR DISCOMFORT

As for indigestion, the differential diagnosis of chronic lower abdominal pain is wide, and the same principles apply (see Chapter 5). The two main categories that need to be considered are various 'organic' disorders and various 'functional' bowel disorders (Table 6.1). In the case of organic disorders, the cause can be identified and, if improved or eliminated, symptoms improve. In the case of functional disorders, there is no structural or biochemical explanation for the symptoms, although in some there may be an identifiable pathophysiological dysfunction present. Indeed, as further research is conducted, it is likely that the distinction between 'organic' and 'functional' disorders will become increasingly blurred.

'Organic' bowel disorders

Uncomplicated *diverticular disease of the colon* is not normally associated with symptoms. A proportion of individuals, however, experience recurrent lower abdominal pain (predominantly in the left iliac fossa) and occasionally a change in bowel habit. These symptoms are similar to, and indeed can be indistinguishable from, the irritable bowel syndrome, and it is probable that the symptoms in these instances are due to the presence of concomitant irritable bowel. In severe diverticular disease, the colonic lumen is often distorted and narrowed in the sigmoid colon. Symptoms of partial bowel obstruction may then develop and produce recurrent lower abdominal, often left iliac fossa, pain. Diverticulitis is discussed in Chapter 4.

Lactose ingestion in *lactase-deficient* subjects can be associated with lower abdominal discomfort and diarrhoea, although such individuals usually need to ingest a significant amount of lactose before noting symptoms—even then, the symptoms may be more often a part of the irritable bowel syndrome.

Endometriosis, pelvic inflammatory disease and other gynaecological disorders can be associated with recurrent or chronic lower abdominal pain.

Endometriosis. Endometriosis may cause recurrent abdominal pain and bowel symptoms in women. Usually these patients are under the age of 45 years and two-thirds are nulliparous. Symptoms may sometimes occur with the period (because the endometrial implants are influenced by hormonal changes; at termination of the menstrual cycle, endometrial engorgement and sloughing occurs). However, in many cases symptoms do not coincide with periods. Common symptoms include abdominal pain, constipation or diarrhoea, proctalgia and lower back pain; gynaecological symptoms usually co-exist with the gastrointestinal symptoms (a clinical clue) and can include menstrual irregularity, dysmenorrhoea and dyspareunia. There may also be a history of infertility. Rectal examination may sometimes detect tender nodules or irregular induration. At sigmoidoscopy or colonoscopy, there may be findings of a submucosal mass, usually with overlying intact mucosa; biopsy may not be diagnostic because endometriosis is usually in the deeper layers. Barium studies may provide useful indirect evidence of the disease. Laparoscopy allows direct visualisation and biopsy of serosal lesions. In cases with complicated bowel disease, surgical resection may be required. Hormonal therapy (usually oral contraceptives) may be useful in mild disease. Danazol, a synthetic androgen, and gonadotrophin-releasing hormone agonists are more effective, but have a greater incidence of side effects. In incapacitating cases, a total abdominal hysterectomy and oophorectomy may be considered.

Pelvic inflammatory disease. This reflects ascending infection of the endometrium or fallopian tubes, and can be due to a number of pathogens including *Neisseria gonorrhoeae* and *Chlamydia trachomatis;* however, vaginal flora have also been implicated. With

TABLE 6.1: Differential diagnosis of chronic lower abdominal pain	
'Organic' disorders	**'Functional' disorders**
Common • Gynaecological disease • Lactase deficiency • Diverticulitis • Crohn's disease • Intestinal obstruction	*Common* • Irritable bowel syndrome • Functional abdominal bloating
Uncommon • Chronic intestinal pseudo-obstruction • Mesenteric ischaemia • Malignancy (e.g., ovarian carcinoma) • Abdominal wall pain • Spinal disease • Testicular disease • Metabolic diseases, e.g., diabetes mellitus, familial Mediterranean fever, C1 esterase deficiency (angioneurotic oedema), porphyria, lead poisoning, tabes dorsalis, renal failure	*Uncommon* • Functional abdominal pain

salpingitis, midline lower abdominal pain may be associated with a mucopurulent vaginal discharge and occasionally vaginal bleeding. Right iliac fossa pain and tenderness from peri-appendicitis can occur. Pelvic tenderness on bi-manual pelvic examination is typical (uterine fundal tenderness may be due to endometritis while adnexal tenderness may be due to salpingitis, which is frequently bilateral). Gynaecological referral is indicated and laparoscopy is the most definitive method for diagnosis.

Adhesive enteropathy. This is a controversial condition. Laparotomy is often followed by the development of some adhesions, and such adhesions are commonly encountered during a second laparotomy for some other reason. On most occasions these patients, when asked after that second operation, have had no symptoms referrable to these adhesions. There are, however, a small group of patients who have chronic abdominal pain that may be due to the adhesions. The pain described by these patients is not colicky, as occurs in intestinal obstruction; it may be lateralised to one side or other. It tends not to be associated with other features of bowel obstruction, such as vomiting and constipation. Physical examination nearly always reveals deep tenderness over the same area where the patient experiences the pain, and no signs of abdominal wall tenderness.

Investigation of these patients is usually not rewarding. The findings of standard haematological and biochemical screens are negative. Intra-abdominal imaging with ultrasound and CT is also negative. Colonic imaging with barium enema is negative. A small bowel series is negative or equivocal; some minor irregularity, but short of a definite obstruction, may be found and the clinician can be left wondering whether the symptoms and the radiological abnormality are related. Many patients will have taken or be taking oral or even parenteral analgesics for relief. Most have seen several clinicians for their problems.

Some will have been thought by their clinician to have a functional problem, not an organic disease. The clinical dilemma is: how much of the problem is organic and how much is functional? Unfortunately, there is no simple way of establishing the relative proportions. It is important that these patients be seen by a limited number of clinicians. It is also important that operation be left as the last resort because:

- dividing adhesions does not cure adhesions—they reform almost as soon as the abdomen is closed; and

- there is a risk of intra-operative perforation during adhesiolysis with possible progression to other infective complications in the post-operative period.

If division of adhesions is undertaken, the procedure is often time-consuming, because of the large number of adhesions that need to be divided.

Crohn's disease of the small intestine. This may produce pain from inflammation or symptoms of intermittent partial bowel obstruction (see Chapter 13).

Chronic intestinal pseudo-obstruction. This refers to a heterogeneous group of rare disorders affecting the neuromuscular apparatus of the bowel (Table 6.2). Recurrent symptoms of small or large bowel obstruction occur in the absence of luminal or extrinsic causes. Some cases can be associated with the ingestion of certain medications or secondary to rare metabolic or systemic disorders; others are idiopathic (Table 6.2). Therapies for the disorder are limited, and include symptomatic treatment, especially analgesia, nutritional support and treatment of complications. Drug therapy with prokinetic agents is not usually effective, especially in visceral myopathy. Antibiotics can be given for small bowel bacterial overgrowth. Surgical therapies include jejunostomy to facilitate enteral nutrition, venting gastrostomy or enterostomy to relieve abdominal distension, and resection of localised disease.

TABLE 6.2: Chronic intestinal pseudo-obstruction

Clinical features

- Abdominal pain—continuous or episodic
- Bloating and visible distension—continuous or episodic
- Vomiting—continuous or episodic
- Constipation (if predominant colonic involvement)
- Diarrhoea (if bacterial overgrowth from small bowel involvement)
- Dysphagia, chest pain (if oesophageal involvement)
- Weight loss (if reduced food intake or malabsorption)
- Palpable bladder (if megacystitis)
- Symptoms and signs of underlying cause (e.g., neurological, endocrine, connective tissue disease)

Diagnosis

- Imaging studies (plain films, barium contrast studies, endoscopy), e.g., air/fluid levels, dilated gut segments
- Functional studies (gastric and small bowel transit, oesophageal manometry, gastroduodenal manometry, cystometrogram)
- Diagnostic laparotomy or laparoscopy (plus full-thickness biopsy of intestine)
- Specialised histochemical staining techniques of full-thickness biopsy (enteric nerves and ganglia, interstitial cells of Cajal, smooth muscle layers)
- Evaluate for underlying cause

Causes

1. *Myenteric plexus disease*
   - Familial visceral neuropathies
   - Sporadic visceral neuropathies, e.g., paraneoplastic (small-cell lung cancer)
   - Hirschsprung's disease
2. *Smooth muscle disease*
   - Familial and sporadic visceral myopathies
   - Scleroderma
   - Polymyositis
   - Amyloid
3. *Endocrine disease*
   - Hypothyroidism
   - Hypoparathyroidism
   - Phaeochromocytoma
4. *Drugs*
   - e.g., phenothiazines, tricyclic antidepressants, clonidine, vinca alkaloids
5. *Neurological disease*
   - Parkinson's disease
   - Progressive muscular dystrophy
   - Myotonic dystrophy
   - Familial autonomic dysfunction

Abdominal angina (chronic mesenteric ischaemia). This is an important condition to recognise. Usually this is due to atherosclerosis but the condition can also occur with vasculitis or other lesions of the splanchnic vessels. Abdominal pain occurs 10–30 minutes after eating, gradually increasing in severity and then slowly resolving over one to three hours. The pain can occur in the periumbilical region or in the epigastrium. The patient becomes afraid to eat and reduces the meal size to avoid pain, leading to substantial weight loss. The pain may be due to an increase in gastric blood flow after food enters the stomach, leading to stealing of blood from the small intestine. On examination, there may be a systolic bruit in the abdomen but this is non-diagnostic. Doppler flow studies of the coeliac axis and superior mesenteric arteries are a useful screening test. Angiography is helpful to confirm the diagnosis if there is involvement of at least two of the three major arteries. However, as such abnormalities can occur in the absence of symptoms, this entity remains a largely clinical diagnosis.

Spinal disease. Referred abdominal pain from disorders affecting the spine or metabolic disease can also occasionally lead to diagnostic difficulties (Table 6.1). Spinal disease can cause abdominal pain, usually due to root irritation or compression. Coughing, straining or sneezing typically increases the pain.

Diabetes mellitus. This can cause abdominal pain due to diabetic radiculopathy or diabetic plexus neuropathy involving the thoracic nerve roots. Electromyography studies of the anterior abdominal wall muscles can assist in making this diagnosis.

Familial Mediterranean fever. This autosomal recessive disease is common in Europe and the Near East, and causes recurrent episodes of abdominal pain that may start in one quadrant and spread to involve the entire abdomen (due to peritonitis) associated with fever. There are often episodes of acute pleuritic pain with or without the abdominal pain; some patients have episodes of acute arthritis or painful erythematous areas of swelling, usually on the lower limbs. Leucocytosis and elevated C-reactive protein (CRP) are characteristic features during attacks. The MEFV (for MEditerranean FeVer) gene responsible for the disease has been identified, and many mutations reported. Renal amyloidosis can complicate this disease. Prophylactic long-term use of colchicine reduces the number of acute attacks, and prevents renal amyloidosis.

Angioneurotic oedema. This is an autosomal dominant disease associated with functional C1 esterase deficiency in which there are recurrent attacks of abdominal colic. There are no urticarial skin lesions but there may be episodes of laryngeal oedema. The diagnosis is suggested by a family history. In myeloproliferative disorders, an acquired form of C1 esterase deficiency has been reported.

Lead poisoning. In adults, abdominal pain associated with anaemia, renal disease, peripheral neuropathy, ataxia, memory loss and headache may occur in lead poisoning. Look for lead lines (a thin blue-black pigmented line along the gingival margin). The pain of lead colic, as well as porphyria, can be difficult to distinguish from intestinal obstruction.

Acute intermittent porphyria. This is a rare autosomal dominant condition. Abdominal pain is the most common symptom and is typically steady and poorly localised although it may be colicky in nature. Other symptoms include nausea and vomiting, constipation, tachycardia and hypertension, mental symptoms, pain in the limbs and elsewhere, sensory loss and muscle weakness, as well as urinary retention. Drugs, infections and surgery can precipitate attacks.

Tabes dorsalis. Acute attacks of pain may occur in the abdomen but pain in the legs is more common. Loss of position sense leads to gait ataxia in 50% of patients. Neurological signs in the legs (e.g., loss of reflexes and impaired position and vibratory sense) are usually present.

'Functional' bowel disorders

These disorders are the most common causes of chronic lower abdominal pain or discomfort. Based on characteristic symptom clusters, a number of functional bowel disorders can be recognised.

Irritable bowel syndrome (IBS)

Irritable bowel syndrome (IBS) is defined as at least three months of continuous or recurrent symptoms of abdominal pain or discomfort that has two of the following three features: 1) relieved with defecation; 2) onset associated with a change in frequency of stool; 3) onset associated with a change in consistency (form) of stool. The presence of the following symptoms increases confidence in the diagnosis: abnormal stool frequency; abnormal stool form (lumpy/hard or loose/watery stool); abnormal stool passage (straining, urgency or feeling of incomplete evacuation); passage of mucus; and bloating or a feeling of abdominal distension. These symptoms often occur in discrete episodes, varying in frequency and severity, and are present without abnormalities on radiological, endoscopic and laboratory investigations. IBS accounts for 5% or more of attendances to general practitioners and 20–50% of referrals to gastroenterologists. It is twice as common in females as males, and half of the patients are younger than 35 years of age.

Functional abdominal bloating

This disorder is defined as at least three days per month of symptoms of: 1) abdominal bloating or visible distension; and 2) insufficient criteria for diagnosis of functional dyspepsia, IBS or other functional gastrointestinal disorders. Symptoms are not usually constant or unremitting, and the abdominal bloating or distension may be visible and/or require clothing to be loosened, tends to be minimal on waking and to increase as the day goes on. There may be accompanying increased passage of flatus and, less often, borborygmi. Clearly, bloating or distension is also a criterion for IBS, in the latter case accompanied by abdominal pain and bowel dysfunction.

Functional abdominal pain syndrome

Functional abdominal pain syndrome (chronic idiopathic abdominal pain) occurs far less frequently than either of the above disorders. It is defined as at least six months of: 1) continuous or nearly continuous abdominal pain; and 2) no or only occasional relationship of pain with physiological events (e.g., eating, defecation or menstruation); and 3) some loss of daily functioning; and 4) the pain is not feigned (e.g., malingering); and 5) insufficient criteria for other functional gastrointestinal disorders that would explain the abdominal pain. The description of the pain does not fit a recognisable specific disorder and is reported to be present almost all of the time. The nature and site may change with repeated descriptions, but there are generally verbal and non-verbal indications of extreme severity. Abnormal illness behaviour is usually present.

CLINICAL EVALUATION OF CHRONIC LOWER ABDOMINAL PAIN OR DISCOMFORT

Similar principles apply to the clinical evaluation of chronic lower abdominal pain as to 'indigestion' (Chapter 5): the extent of the evaluation will depend on the age of the patient and the duration and severity of symptoms. Based on a detailed history and a general abdominal examination, the organ and disease process most likely to be involved should be defined. In the history, the presence of fever, weight loss, rectal bleeding or steatorrhoea are all strong pointers towards the presence of organic disease (Table 6.3). Further questions are often specifically required to elicit information, such as new exacerbating factors to the pain (e.g., dietary change, change in medication), worry about serious disease, especially cancer, new life stresses, presence of psychological or psychiatric disorders, or impairment in the patient's daily functioning. Because the functional bowel disorders cannot be established by any investigation, it is important to take a structured history, noting the features that support these diagnoses (see definitions earlier), as well as those that suggest another cause for the symptoms. In some of these disorders (e.g., IBS), upper gastrointestinal symptoms, such as heartburn, dyspepsia, nausea and excessive belching, are frequently present, and non-gastrointestinal symptoms such as fatigue, dysmenorrhoea, migraine, and symptoms of bladder irritability are also common. Moreover, in IBS for example, the history is often prolonged, with symptoms dating from a relatively early age and a course characterised by exacerbations and remissions.

TABLE 6.3: Clinical features against the diagnosis of a functional bowel disorder

---

- First onset of symptoms in an elderly patient
- Symptoms waking the patient from sleep
- New symptoms after a prolonged period of stable symptoms
- Progressive, steady worsening of symptoms
- Weight loss
- Dysphagia
- Evidence of bleeding or dehydration
- Evidence of steatorrhoea
- Recurrent vomiting
- Fever
- Elevated C-reactive protein
- Anaemia or leucocytosis
- Blood, pus or excess fat in stool
- Hypokalaemia or persistent diarrhoea during fasting
- Stool weight > 350 g/day

Physical examination

Abnormal findings, apart from abdominal tenderness, are not common. Tenderness is often present over the colon in IBS, especially the sigmoid, although this region can be palpable and tender in healthy subjects. Look for signs of abdominal wall pain that may be misdiagnosed as pain from IBS. The presence of an abdominal mass raises the possibility of complicated diverticular disease or Crohn's disease, while an abdominal aortic aneurysm should be palpable. External hernias should be excluded (Chapter 19). Enlarged lymph nodes (e.g., supraclavicular) may indicate the presence of malignancy. The testes should be palpated for tenderness and masses. Pelvic masses or tenderness present on rectal examination may indicate a gynaecological cause. Physical examination is usually normal in IBS; mild abdominal tenderness, a 'squelch' in the iliac fossae, or mild abdominal distension are features that may be present.

Investigations

Investigations are dictated by the findings on history and physical examination, and the age of the patient. These may be performed to exclude or confirm the likely diagnosis and may include colonic investigation with sigmoidoscopy, colonoscopy or barium enema. Abdominal and/or pelvic ultrasonography, small bowel radiology, abdominal CT scanning, or lactose tolerance testing may also be required. Screening blood tests are often performed, even if there are no specific causes discovered from the history and examination. Haematological tests include full blood count, blood film, CRP and, if indicated, iron studies, folate and vitamin B12 levels. Biochemical tests include liver function tests, serum albumin, electrolytes and urea—these are usually unhelpful. In cases of suspected IBS, however, coeliac serology, particularly tissue transglutaminase assay, is a recommended screening test.

If organic colonic disease is suspected, full colonic investigation by colonoscopy or sigmoidoscopy and barium enema is indicated. In patients 50 years of age or older, especially in those with a change in pre-existing symptoms, or in patients with a family history of colorectal carcinoma or colonic polyps, colonoscopy is the preferred investigation to rule out colorectal neoplasia. Highly specialised investigations, such as ultrasound with Doppler flow studies and mesenteric angiography, may be warranted (e.g., if symptoms such as postprandial pain and weight loss are suggestive of mesenteric angina).

Where an abnormality is detected by laboratory or radiological studies, it is always most important to consider whether this is likely to be the cause of the patient's symptoms. When functional bowel disease is suspected, a protracted or piecemeal approach to investigation should be avoided, as it is likely to increase patient uncertainty and anxiety. If the diagnosis remains in doubt, it may be useful to see and investigate the patient during an acute exacerbation of pain. Rare causes should be considered and checked at this stage and appropriate other investigations, e.g., plain abdominal X-ray during an attack of pain, performed if indicated. 'Diagnostic' laparoscopy or laparotomy is almost invariably non-contributory in cases of chronic abdominal pain already investigated as above. However, laparoscopy may, at times, be useful in this situation; occasionally it may enable the identification of recurrent intestinal obstruction from adhesions, which has escaped identification using other modalities.

IRRITABLE BOWEL SYNDROME (IBS)

Pathophysiology

The pathogenesis of IBS is unknown (Figure 6.1). No inflammation is present in the intestine and previous terminology such as 'mucus colitis' is inappropriate. A number of physiological factors, however, appear to be associated with the disorder.

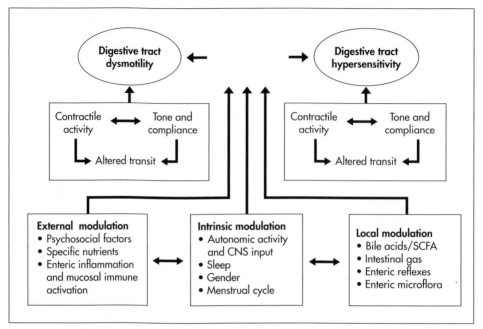

FIGURE 6.1: Potential pathophysiological mechanisms linked to functional bowel disorders, including irritable bowel syndrome. Digestive tract dysmotility and hypersensitivity are likely to underlie the gut symptoms in these disorders. A variety of modulatory factors, as shown, can affect the degree of digestive tract dysmotility and hypersensitivity.

Normal small bowel and colonic motility

In the small intestine, intermittent segmenting and propulsive contractions occur after ingestion of food, mixing it with digestive secretions and transporting the chyme aborally. Each propagated contraction is preceded by a propagated relaxation, a phenomenon termed the *peristaltic reflex*. The overall duration and intensity of postprandial motor activity depends upon the caloric content, and the proportion of fat, carbohydrate and protein in the meal. The jejunum acts primarily as a mixing and conduit segment, while the ileum, which has specialised absorptive properties, retains chyme until digestion and absorption are largely complete. The terminal ileum and ileo-colonic junction control the rate of emptying of ileal contents into the colon. In between meals, and particularly during sleep, motility in the stomach and small intestine undergoes regular cycles of activity every few hours, termed *migrating motor complexes*. These complexes migrate slowly along the small bowel, clearing away residual food and secretions.

In the colon, proximal colonic motor activity normally promotes the mixing of contents, absorption of water and electrolytes, and metabolism of colonic contents by bacteria. The recto-sigmoid region stores faeces and generates specific motor programs enabling convenient elimination. Contractions in the colon occur at irregular intervals; there are two main types: individual phasic contractions and high-amplitude propagated contractions or *giant migrating contractions*. The latter are the major propulsive motor events in the colon, producing the so-called *mass movements*. After eating, colonic motor activity and tone increases (gastro-colic reflex) in both the proximal and the distal colon. Intestinal gas originates from three sources: the majority (about 70%) from swallowed air, a proportion from gases (carbon dioxide, hydrogen and methane) produced by bacterial fermentation of incompletely absorbed food and fibre in the colon, and a very small amount by way of diffusion from the blood (Chapter 7). On an average diet, material takes up to three days to pass through the colon, accounting for about 90% of whole gut transit time in healthy subjects.

Gastrointestinal sensorimotor dysfunction

Up-regulation of the sensory pathways travelling from the gut to the central nervous system appears to account for a heightened perception of normal gut sensations arising from intestinal distension and contraction (*visceral hypersensitivity*). This phenomenon of hypersensitivity may result in abdominal discomfort or pain; it may also trigger disordered gut motility and/or alterations in gut secretion or absorption, resulting in an erratic bowel habit. Exaggerated patterns of contraction, especially postprandially, have been observed in the small and large intestine; the gastro-colic reflex can be delayed and prolonged.

Altered motor activity affects gut transit. Thus, delayed transit through the small and large intestine, and increased absorption of water, can lead to symptoms of constipation, while accelerated transit may result in diarrhoea. Uncoordinated or abnormally high pressure contractions may lead to distension of the intestinal lumen, or trap pockets of intestinal gas which distend the bowel and produce abdominal pain. Stools of small or 'normal' volume that are passed more frequently may result from the combined effect of rapid small bowel transit, colonic dysmotility and rectal hypersensitivity to distension. In the majority of patients a trigger factor producing gut hypersensitivity is not found.

In some patients (up to 25%), IBS symptoms appear to be precipitated by an attack of infective diarrhoea or gastroenteritis, perhaps due to occult damage to the enteric nervous system. Increased numbers of lymphocytes, mast cells and enteroendocrine cells have also been demonstrated in biopsies from the colon in this 'post-infective' irritable bowel syndrome. Altered permeability in the small intestine can occur. Symptoms in this disorder can persist for months, years or even a lifetime. There is no evidence that colonisation of the intestine with *Candida albicans* is a cause of IBS.

Behavioural factors

No specific personality type has been shown to be at special risk for development of IBS. Mental stress is associated with the onset and exacerbation of symptoms in some patients. It is not known, however, whether the common associations of depression and anxiety are cause or effect. Psychological factors are also important because they influence the individual's decision to seek medical attention as well as the ability to cope with the symptoms.

Dietary factors

Eating often provokes symptoms in patients with IBS. In general, meals high in fat move slowly through the gut, and in IBS this may exacerbate symptoms such as bloating and constipation. Foods such as baked beans, cabbage and brussel sprouts, and sugars such as fructose and sorbitol, may exacerbate symptoms in patients with complaints of excessive bloating and rectal flatus.

Patients frequently associate ingestion of specific food items with the development of symptoms. Although this may be a chance association, there is evidence that a non-immunological gut reaction may occur to a variety of foods such as dairy products, caffeine, onions, tomatoes and citrus fruits. Such food intolerance should be distinguished from the rare condition of true food allergy. Only a very small proportion of patients with IBS appear to have true allergic or immunological responses to specific foods (Chapter 16).

Treatment

Treatments are outlined in Table 6.4. Therapy begins at the initial consultation, where it is essential to establish rapport with patients and secure their confidence. This is achieved by a process of reassurance regarding the genuine nature of the symptoms. Many patients have been told that they are not suffering from a significant illness; the patient should be reassured that IBS is a well recognised and common, though benign and chronic, clinical entity.

The patient should be made aware at the outset that investigations will probably be negative, but that they serve to confirm the initial clinical diagnosis of IBS. An explanation about the possible mechanism of symptoms should be given. This depends on an assessment of the patient's level of sophistication, but always needs to be sympathetic and unhurried. Patient information leaflets and diagrams can be very helpful, but are not a substitute for individual explanation and discussion. At the follow-up visit the physician should check how much the patient has really understood.

A concise dietary history should focus on fibre intake, fat and specific carbohydrate ingestion, and any possible food intolerances (e.g., dairy products, soft drinks, some 'diet' confectionery, gas-producing foods, other specific foods). The pattern of symptoms in relation to the patient's day, including work, eating, exercise and sleeping habits can then be broadened into a discussion about stresses at work and at home.

The presence of psychological disorders, and, if possible, their onset in relation to the onset of gastrointestinal symptoms, should be ascertained. It is important to consider why the patient is seeking help now. A careful history to identify possible precipitating or contributing factors should lead to advice about simple lifestyle modifications. It is essential for the patient to understand that IBS is generally a chronic condition, in which exacerbations and remissions are often a feature. Notwithstanding this pattern of the disorder, the patient should be advised to report any changes in symptoms that develop over the years. A discussion of prognosis is important and is often overlooked; it is important to reassure patients that the condition does not predispose to other gut disorders, particularly malignancy, and to inform them that residual symptoms may persist despite therapy.

TABLE 6.4: Treatment of irritable bowel syndrome

- Complete history and examination are essential
- Avoid protracted investigation
- Reassure patient that:
  - diagnosis is correct
  - symptoms are produced by gut sensorimotor dysfunction
  - there is no predisposition to other bowel disorders such as cancer
- Use simple dietary modifications and non-drug therapy initially, according to predominant symptoms
- Assure patient that opportunity for review is available during difficult times, or if new symptoms develop
- Inform patient of likelihood of residual symptoms persisting or recurring from time to time

Diet and the role of fibre

Foods and beverages that clearly and consistently provoke symptoms should be avoided. If bloating and flatulence are prominent symptoms, the patient should be advised to eat slowly, to avoid smoking and chewing gum, and to try to avoid excessive air swallowing associated with belching.

Although it is controversial whether dietary fibre supplementation is of any greater overall benefit than placebo, a trial of stool bulking by a regular increased intake of fibre-rich foods (e.g., cereals, wholemeal bread, unprocessed wheat bran), and/or proprietary bulking agents, should be trialled in most patients. Fibre supplementation should be introduced gradually (e.g., a starting dose of one teaspoon of unprocessed bran daily), and continued for at least one month before its effect is judged. Patients should be made aware that too much fibre can produce excessive intestinal gas and cause bloating and flatus. Proprietary bulking agents (e.g., those containing psyllium or ispaghula) may be less likely to cause this problem than bran. A trial of stool bulking is less likely to be effective in patients with diarrhoea-predominant IBS. In selected cases, where there is a high suspicion of food intolerance, a symptom and food diary may enable the patient to recognise specific items more readily.

Medications

The decision to use a medication in IBS depends on the severity of symptoms and their impact on the quality of life of the patient. The choice of medication depends on the pattern of symptoms. Randomised, placebo-controlled trials of traditional pharmacotherapeutic agents in IBS have generally been disappointing. However, for predominant diarrhoea, antidiarrhoeal drugs such as loperamide have been shown to be effective. For predominant constipation—in addition to a trial of stool bulking, an increase in fluid intake, and regular exercise—osmotic laxatives such as magnesium-containing salts (e.g., Epsom salts), polyethylene glycol compounds or lactulose are safe and can be effective. Anticholinergic agents (such as hyoscine butylbromide or hydrobromide, hyoscyamine sulfate, or dicyclomine) or antispasmodic agents (such as mebeverine) may be helpful in some individuals with prominent abdominal pain, especially if it is meal-related. However, differentiation from the placebo response is difficult. Ideally, drugs such as those above should be used in the short term only, and the dose adjusted depending on the timing and severity of symptoms. Moreover, it should be appreciated that such medications target only one symptom—abdominal pain, diarrhoea or constipation—and may not improve (indeed in some cases can worsen) other aspects of the symptom complex.

A number of complementary medicine compounds have shown promise in the treatment of IBS. These include several types of probiotic agents and herbal preparations. Further studies are required to investigate other such compounds, and to determine the mechanism(s) of action of those agents exhibiting efficacy.

If there is no improvement

It is important to assess whether the patient can cope with ongoing symptoms, or still fears that some other underlying diagnosis is being overlooked. In this latter group, continued reassurance may be necessary. It is also important to re-emphasise to the patient the limitations of current therapies and that treatment strategies are not aimed at a cure, which in most is not achievable.

A small (non-antidepressant) dose of a tricyclic antidepressant (e.g., amitriptyline 10–25 mg in the evening) has been reported to be useful in some patients with resistant symptoms, probably by influencing central pain perception. When significant symptoms of depression are present, however, adequate therapy with full antidepressant doses should be employed. Minor tranquillisers (e.g., benzodiazepines) are not recommended for use in this chronic condition.

Recently, a number of high quality trials have established the efficacy of several novel drugs for the treatment of IBS. These include the serotonergic agents tegaserod and alosetron which, unlike other medications, can in some patients improve several symptoms of the IBS complex. Tegaserod, a serotonin (5-HT$_4$) agonist that is safe and well tolerated, can improve constipation, abdominal pain and bloating. Alosetron, a serotonin (5-HT$_3$) antagonist, can improve diarrhoea, abdominal pain and bloating. However, this latter drug can be rarely associated with ischaemic colitis and, hence, is reserved for severe and disabling IBS with predominant diarrhoea; it is not currently available in Australia. A variety of other compounds targeting different components of the enteric nervous system and its central connections are under development for the treatment of IBS.

If food intolerance is strongly suspected, trials of exclusion diets, and blind challenges to identify offending foods and additives have been reported to decrease symptoms in some patients, especially those with predominant diarrhoea. This is rarely necessary, and may be most appropriately carried out in an allergy clinic with a research interest in this field. There is no role for a gluten-free diet in IBS. If coeliac disease is suspected, serological testing and, if positive, small bowel biopsy are indicated (Chapter 13).

Relaxation therapy may be appropriate, and relaxation courses are becoming increasingly available. Individual psychotherapy or hypnotherapy, which have been reported to improve symptoms if other measures have not been helpful, can also be arranged by a psychologist, psychiatrist, or interested general practitioner.

When to review the diagnosis

If new symptoms develop or there is a change in the pattern of existing symptoms, it is important to review the diagnosis carefully or to consider the possibility that an additional problem has arisen. Other disorders that may need to be considered, depending on the individual case, include:

- development of colon cancer;
- an episode of diverticulitis or an intercurrent gastrointestinal infection;
- symptoms due to gallstones;
- peptic ulceration;
- development of pancreatic carcinoma;
- development or exacerbation of a psychological problem, such as depression.

Further reading

Drossman DA, Camilleri M, Mayer E, Whitehead WE. AGA technical review on irritable bowel syndrome. *Gastroenterology* 2002; 123: 2108–31.

Kellow JE. Small bowel disorders. In: Spiller R, Grundy D (eds). *Pathophysiology of the enteric nervous system*. Oxford: Blackwell, 2004: 134–46.

Kellow JE. Principles of motility and sensation testing. In: Mertz H (ed). Functional disorders of the gastrointestinal tract. *Gastroenterol Clin N Am* 2003; 32: 733–50.

Lembo A, Weber HC, Farraye FA. Alosetron in irritable bowel syndrome: strategies for its use in a common gastrointestinal disorder. *Drugs* 2003; 63: 1895–905.

Longstreth GF, Thompson WG, Chey WD *et al*. Functional bowel disorders. *Gastroenterology* 2006; 130: 1480–91.

Spiller RC. Postinfectious irritable bowel syndrome. *Gastroenterology*, 2003; 124: 1662–71.

Talley NJ, Spiller R. Irritable bowel syndrome: a little understood organic bowel disease? *Lancet* 2002; 360: 555–64.

Thompson WG, Longstreth GF, Drossman DA *et al*. Functional bowel disorders and functional abdominal pain. In: Drossman DA, Corazziari E, Talley NJ *et al* (eds). Rome II: Functional gastrointestinal disorders: diagnosis, pathophysiology, and treatment. McLean, VA: Degnon Associates, 2000; 351–432.

Wagstaff A, Frampton J, Croom K. Tegaserod: a review of its use in the management of irritable bowel syndrome with constipation in women. *Drugs* 2003; 63: 1101–20.

chapter 7

WIND AND GAS

Many patients present complaining of 'excess gas', which may mean excess passage of wind through the mouth or anus, abdominal bloating or audible bowel sounds (borborygmi). In population studies, 15–30% report bloating or abdominal rumblings. The term flatulence is sometimes used to describe such problems, but this term is variably defined and best avoided.

The causes of a sensation of excess gas include diet (e.g., excess ingestion of poorly digestible but fermentable foods, such as sorbitol in diet drinks or chewing gum, beans or bran), lactose intolerance (due to lactase deficiency), psychiatric disease (e.g., depression, anxiety, or somatisation disorder) or functional gastrointestinal disease. Visible distension can also occur in intestinal obstruction or pseudo-obstruction. Rarely, malabsorption (e.g., due to bacterial overgrowth) or giardiasis may cause a sensation of excess gas.

HISTORY

Ask the patient to describe the symptoms fully and when they commenced. Determine if the problem is excess belching (as occurs in air swallowing), excess flatus, a sensation of bloating or actual visible abdominal distension, or loud rumblings. Often in functional gastrointestinal disease many symptoms are reported, the symptoms are not constant or unremitting, and there are no alarm symptoms (e.g., absence of nocturnal complaints, weight loss, vomiting, fever or bleeding). A history of intermittent distension, vomiting, absolute constipation and abdominal pain suggests bowel obstruction.

Ask specifically about symptoms of irritable bowel syndrome, which can result in bloating or visible distension (Chapter 6). Air swallowing can be diagnosed by the history. Typically, the patient describes repetitive belching to relieve bloating, but only transient relief is obtained.

Ask about menstruation; bloating may occur premenstrually. Obtain a good diet history. Ascertain use of bran or bulking agents, dietary fibre intake, and milk or milk product ingestion. In adults, lactose intolerance is the normal state in non-Caucasian populations, so ascertain the patient's ethnic origin. Obtain a psychiatric history screening for symptoms of depression and anxiety.

PHYSICAL EXAMINATION

Observe the patient during the interview. You may directly observe gulping of air and repetitive belching in the air swallower.

Weigh the patient (obesity may explain distension). Examine the gastrointestinal system to exclude signs of organic disease (e.g., bowel obstruction, abdominal masses). Usually the examination findings are normal.

INVESTIGATIONS

X-ray and endoscopy

Plain abdominal X-ray examination is not normally required (unless bowel obstruction is suspected). Even in those with visible distension, the findings are usually normal.

An upper endoscopy should be considered if there are alarm features, such as weight loss or vomiting. A bezoar or evidence of gastric stasis may sometimes be found. Duodenal aspiration at endoscopy to exclude giardiasis should be considered in those at risk (e.g., those who live in or have travelled to endemic areas) where the endoscopic findings are normal.

Laboratory tests

Check haemoglobin levels (for evidence of anaemia that would suggest organic disease such as malabsorption of iron, folate or B12) and serum albumin levels (for evidence of hypoalbuminaemia). Other tests depend on the clinical setting but usually none are required.

Breath hydrogen testing for lactose intolerance

If this condition is suspected, a two-week trial of a lactose-free diet will help to confirm the clinical suspicion (Chapter 16). If a more definitive answer is deemed necessary, e.g., an equivocal response to diet or the patient wishes to have the diagnosis confirmed, then hydrogen breath testing can be performed.

The principle of the test is that non-absorbed carbohydrate is fermented by colonic bacteria with the production of hydrogen and its appearance in the breath within five minutes. In the lactose breath hydrogen test, to test for lactase deficiency, the subject is prepared by an overnight fast following a meal of meat and rice; smoking is prohibited. A baseline breath test is obtained and then a 50 g test load of lactose is administered. Breath samples are obtained at half-hourly intervals for four hours. An abnormal result is characterised by breath hydrogen exceeding 20 parts per million over the baseline (Figure 7.1). Lactose-intolerant patients may experience abdominal colic, bloating, borborygmi and excessive flatus (bacterial fermentation) as well as diarrhoea (osmotic effect) during or shortly after the test or on drinking milk. Remember, however, that the majority of adults with lactase deficiency have no symptoms (Chapter 16).

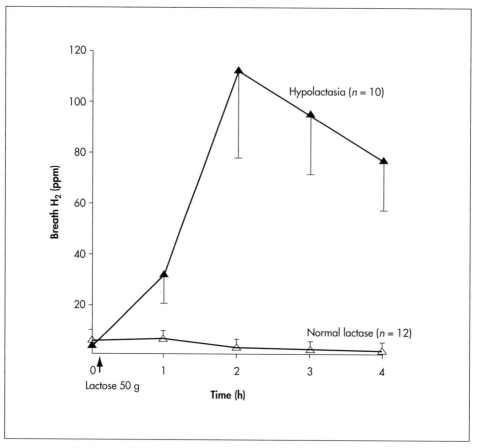

FIGURE 7.1: The lactose breath H_2 test.

PATHOPHYSIOLOGY

The limited available information about the content, composition and role of intestinal gases is due in part to the technical difficulties in obtaining data in humans. The information on intestinal gas is based on: 1) the 'washout technique' in which an inert gas (argon) is infused rapidly into the jejunum and gases are collected via a rectal tube for analysis; 2) analysis of colonic gas collected via a rectal tube; and 3) scattered observations have been obtained by sampling gases at various levels of the gastrointestinal tract. There are considerable differences between the composition of belched gas, gas collected at sites within the gut and flatus. Based on the washout technique, the normal gastrointestinal tract contains about 100 mL of gas. The rate of passage of gas per rectum ranges from 200–3000 mL/24 h. Based on observations in young healthy subjects, the normal frequency of passage of flatus is 14 times per day. The volume of flatus increases dramatically after ingestion of poorly absorbed carbohydrates, such as baked beans or brassica vegetables.

COMPOSITION

The composition of gases in the gut varies with the site of sampling. For example, nitrogen (N_2) concentration in the human stomach approaches atmospheric, suggesting that it originates from swallowed air. The five gases nitrogen, oxygen (O_2), carbon dioxide (CO_2), hydrogen (H_2) and methane (CH_4) compose about 99% of intestinal gas (Table 7.1, Figure 7.2). Nitrogen is the predominant gas and oxygen is present in low concentrations. Carbon dioxide in the upper small bowel reflects the interaction of gastric acid and bicarbonate secretion from the pancreas, biliary tree and small intestine. Most of the small bowel carbon dioxide appears to be absorbed. Carbon dioxide in the lower small bowel results from the interaction of bicarbonate and organic acids. Breath carbon dioxide can be studied by the use of isotopic labelling of the carbon atoms. Three gases, carbon dioxide, hydrogen and methane, are produced in the gut by bacterial action on unabsorbed carbohydrate. Hydrogen production is usually limited to the colon and is dependent on the ingestion of fermentable substrates, which escape absorption in the small intestine (Figure 7.3). In general, about 90% of most staple carbohydrate is absorbed in the small bowel but 10% escapes absorption and passes to the colon. Baked beans contain unabsorbable oligosaccharides such as stachyose and raffinose and these produce large quantities of gas after interaction with colonic bacteria. About 15% of hydrogen production in the colon is absorbed into the circulation and expired from the lungs. About 30% of normal individuals produce significant amounts of methane. The production is constant and unrelated to food intake.

All of the five major gases are odourless. The odour of flatus is due to trace quantities of other gases produced by colonic bacteria. Ammonia is due to urea breakdown, indoles and skatoles are produced by protein breakdown, and hydrogen sulphide (H_2S) and methane thiol result from amino acids with sulfur content. There are few published data on these odiferous gases.

TABLE 7.1: Gastrointestinal gas

Gas[1]	Origin
N_2 O_2	Swallowed air, diffusion from blood
CO_2	Secretion, diffusion, bacterial metabolism
H_2 CH_4	Bacterial metabolism

1. Plus traces of odiferous gases that are socially significant.

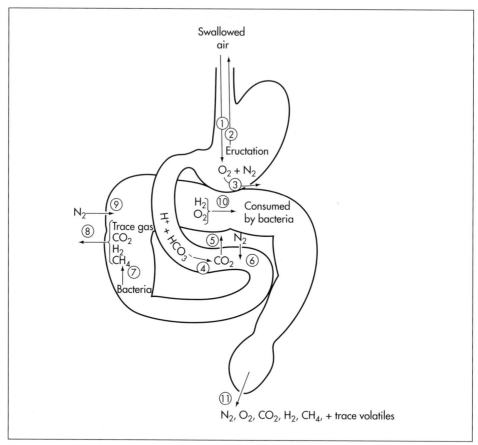

FIGURE 7.2: Mechanisms influencing rate of accumulation of gas in the gastrointestinal tract. Air is swallowed (1) and a sizeable fraction is then eructated (2). The O_2 of gastric air diffuses into the blood draining the stomach (3). The reaction of H^+ and HCO_3^- yields CO_2 (4), which rapidly diffuses into the blood (5) while N_2 (6) diffuses into the lumen down a gradient established by the CO_2 production. In the colon, bacteria produce CO_2, H_2 and CH_4 (7), which diffuse into the blood perfusing the colon (8). Bacteria also consume O_2 and H_2 (10). N_2 diffuses into the colon (9) down a gradient established by bacterial production of CO_2, H_2 and CH_4. The net result of all these processes determines the composition and rate of passage of gas per rectum (11).

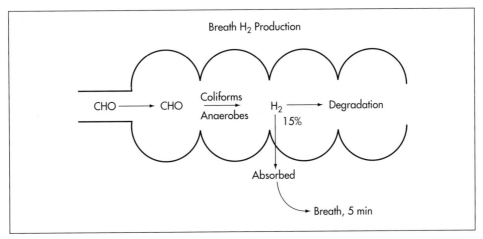

FIGURE 7.3: Schematic diagram showing presentation in the colon of carbohydrate (CHO) which has escaped digestion in the small intestine.

CONDITIONS ASSOCIATED WITH EXCESS WIND

Belching

Swallowed air is the major source of gas in the upper gastrointestinal tract. Some air is swallowed during routine meals and this is intensified by gulping when excited. At times, patients with troublesome, frequent and noisy belching are encountered. There is usually no detectable underlying pathology and the situation probably represents an acquired habit. The significance of an associated hiatal hernia or gastro-oesophageal reflux is unknown. This area has not been well studied, but the likely explanation is that air is sucked into the oesophagus during each act of belching. The most useful therapeutic option is to concentrate on avoiding the next belch.

Aerophagia

Aerophagia refers to the unconscious habit of swallowing air. This leads to repetitive air eructation, which may be audible and may be satisfying. Avoiding chewing gum, aerated drinks and smoking can be helpful. The situation may resolve with relaxation therapy. Anti-gas agents (e.g., simethicone, charcoal) are not of benefit.

Halitosis

The origin of odiferous breath gases after garlic ingestion has been studied. The halitosis initially originates from the mouth and subsequently from the gut (metabolism in the colon causing large concentration in alveolar air). Oral hygiene may reduce the halitosis from the mouth and manipulation of diet may limit the gas production from the gut flora.

Excess flatus

Based on observations in healthy young students the frequency of passage of flatus is 13.6 ($\pm$ 6) per day. The frequency and volume of flatus varies widely, and depends on the colonic flora composition. Maximum gas production occurs after poorly digested food, such as baked beans and brassica vegetables (cabbage and brussels sprouts), which should be avoided by those with excess flatus. Anti-gas drugs are of no benefit and diet is the mainstay of treatment. Least rectal gas follows ingestion of carbohydrate such as rice flour (which is fully absorbed in the small intestine).

Hydrogen and methane may reach combustible concentrations in the colon (> 4%). For this reason the use of electrocautery in the management of colonic polyps is restricted to the prepared colon (i.e., after washout of bowel content). Fermentable agents such as lactulose are best avoided in bowel preparation before electrocautery.

Buoyancy of stool

The buoyancy of stool is determined by the content of gas within the stool and not by the content of fat.

Bloating

The symptom of bloating, a subjective complaint of 'excessive gas', is frequent in patients with the irritable bowel syndrome (IBS) (Chapter 6). Abdominal X-ray films show normal or slightly increased quantities of gas in the intestines of patients with bloating. A washout technique has been applied to quantify intestinal gas volume and composition in patients with the irritable bowel syndrome and normal healthy control subjects; the collection of gas at the rectum demonstrated similar volumes and composition of gas in the two groups. Patients with irritable bowel syndrome, however, experienced increased symptoms in response to the infusion of gas and increased retrograde flow of gas as determined by aspiration by a gastric tube. This experiment supports the view that abnormal gut sensation occurs in some patients with irritable bowel syndrome, and this may explain their sensation of bloating. The proximal small bowel in other experiments seems to be the place where gas transit is impaired in IBS, probably related to deranged gut reflex responses. Visible distension may occur from a failure to contract the abdominal wall muscles to intra-abdominal volume change in IBS (an abnormal viscerosomatic reflex).

Further reading

Azpiroz F. Intestinal gas dynamics: mechanisms and clinical relevance. *Gut* 2005; 54: 893–5.

Azpiroz F, Malagelada JR. The pathogenesis of bloating and visible distension in irritable bowel syndrome. *Gastroenterol Clin North Am* 2005; 34: 257–69.

Chitkara DK, Bredenoord AJ, Rucker MJ, Talley NJ. Aerophagia in adults: A comparison with functional dyspepsia. *Aliment Pharmacol Ther* 2005; 22(9): 855–8.

Jones MP. Bloating and intestinal gas. *Curr Treat Options Gastroenterol* 2005; 8: 311–8.

CHAPTER 8

NAUSEA AND VOMITING

DEFINITION

Nausea and vomiting are common symptoms. *Nausea* is best considered a painless, unpleasant, subjective feeling of wanting to vomit. Vomiting, on the other hand, is the forceful expulsion of gastric or intestinal contents through the mouth, secondary to a pre-programmed series of motor and autonomic responses. *Vomiting* is not retching; retching describes contractions of the abdominal muscles that typically precedes vomiting, associated with laboured, rhythmic respiration, not the expulsion of the contents through the mouth. Vomiting must be distinguished from *regurgitation*, which is an effortless movement of gastric material into the mouth. Clinically, it is key to distinguish vomiting from *rumination*, as management is totally different. In the rumination syndrome, there is effortless regurgitation of recently ingested food back into the mouth that is not preceded by nausea or abdominal muscular contractions. The food tastes like it has not been eaten. Often the patient will re-chew or spit the food out, but this does not always occur. Rumination typically occurs within minutes of a meal and is almost always repetitive.

PHYSIOLOGY OF VOMITING

With the onset of nausea, there will be accompanying autonomic discharge of variable severity. This results in intense salivation, bradycardia, sweating, pallor and hypotension. The normal electrical activity of the stomach may become slow, fast or fluctuate wildly with nausea. It is unclear whether the same neural pathways that mediate vomiting also mediate nausea.

Just prior to vomiting, a large amplitude contraction in the small bowel is propagated retrogradely. Moderate amplitude phasic contractions may also occur in the small intestine, with these motor activities probably being mediated by the vagus nerve. These motor changes result in: small bowel contents entering the relaxed stomach where closure of the pylorus then occurs; and contraction of the abdominal muscles causing respiration to be suspended. Gastric contents are then forced against a contracted diaphragm, the lower oesophageal sphincter relaxes and the cardia elevates. Gastric contents are forced into the oesophagus that dilates. Protection of the airway occurs via the glottis closing and the soft palate rising, and then the vomitus is forcibly ejected from the mouth.

The vomiting centre is located in the dorsal portion of the medulla. The vomiting centre has afferent inputs via vagal fibres, which are rich in 5-hydroxytryptamine type 3 (5-HT_3) receptors. There is afferent input from sympathetic nerves. There is also input from the vestibular system, which is rich in histamine H_1 and muscarinic cholinergic fibres. The chemoreceptor trigger zone is in the area postrema in the floor of the fourth ventricle. This area, when stimulated, will activate the vomiting centre, and is responsive to drugs, hypoxia, toxins and acidosis; it is rich in dopamine D_2 and 5-HT_3 receptors. The presence of these receptor subtypes forms the rationale for drugs used to treat nausea and vomiting. Other trigger areas include the pharynx, coronary vessels, peritoneum and bile ducts, cortex, thalamus and hypothalamus, and the vestibular apparatus (motion sickness).

HISTORY

Nausea and vomiting are non-specific symptoms and may occur in many diseases. Table 8.1 lists the important causes of nausea and vomiting. When taking the targeted history, it is key to differentiate between vomiting, regurgitation and rumination.

It is very helpful to determine the duration, frequency and intensity of nausea and vomiting, and its relationship to eating. Self-limited symptoms will often occur with an acute infectious gastroenteritis, inflammatory disease such as cholecystitis or pancreatitis, or from drugs. Gastroenteritis is usually associated with headache, myalgias and diarrhoea and will settle within five days, so a longer duration of symptoms should raise the suspicion of another cause. An insidious onset of nausea without vomiting can occur with functional dyspepsia, gastroparesis, medication use, gastro-oesophageal reflux disease, pregnancy and metabolic disorders. Vomiting on waking in the morning may occur from excess alcohol use the night before. Early morning vomiting can also occur with pregnancy, renal failure and raised intracranial pressure.

The character of the vomit is useful to document. Undigested food in the vomit may occur from oesophageal disorders (e.g., achalasia or Zenker's diverticulum). Gastric outlet obstruction may result in partially digested food, free of bile. In small bowel obstruction, the vomitus is usually bile stained. Faecal vomiting indicates distal small bowel obstruction or a gastrocolonic fistula.

The presence of other gastrointestinal symptoms such as abdominal pain or diarrhoea suggests a primary gastrointestinal disease. In the presence of significant weight loss with nausea and vomiting, consideration needs to be given to a gastrointestinal tract malignancy, intestinal obstruction, or an eating disorder. An adolescent female with a history of repeated bouts of vomiting immediately after meals, particularly after binge eating, may have anorexia nervosa or bulimia nervosa; ask about accompanying weight loss, fear of gaining weight, impaired body image, amenorrhoea and binge eating. The vomiting is generally self-induced; laxatives, diuretics and vigorous exercise may also be used to prevent weight gain.

Diseases of the central nervous system can present with vomiting. This may manifest as sudden projectile vomiting without nausea. Emesis may also be triggered by an abrupt change in body position. It is unusual for a patient with a brain tumour to present with vomiting in the absence of other neurological symptoms such as headache, vertigo, deafness, tinnitus or visual impairment.

If the patient describes acute episodes of nausea and vomiting separated by intervening totally asymptomatic periods, this is suggestive of cyclical vomiting, which can occur in adults, but is much more common in children; a history of migraine may be present.

TABLE 8.1: Common causes of nausea and vomiting

1. Intestinal obstruction

- Anatomic:
  - Small bowel obstruction, e.g., adhesions
  - Gastric outlet obstruction, e.g., pyloric ulcer
- Functional:
  - Diabetic gastroparesis
  - Idiopathic gastroparesis
  - Chronic intestinal pseudo-obstruction

2. Infections

- Food poisoning
- Viral or bacterial diarrhoea
- Acute viral hepatitis

3. Central nervous system disorders

- Migraine
- Meningitis
- Increased intracranial pressure
- Ménière's disease
- Motion sickness

4. Metabolic disorders

- Renal failure
- Diabetic ketoacidosis
- Adrenal insufficiency (Addison's disease)
- Hyperthyroidism

5. Drugs

- Alcohol
- Digitalis
- Theophylline
- Narcotics
- Chemotherapeutic agents

6. Visceral pain

- Peritonitis
- Cholecystitis
- Pancreatitis

7. Psychiatric disorders

- Anorexia or bulimia nervosa
- Panic attacks

8. Other

- Pregnancy
- Conditioned reflexes
- Cyclical vomiting
- Functional vomiting

diseases that may cause nausea and vomiting, including diabetes ...ercalcaemia and hyperthyroidism, should be actively sought.

...'ux disease can present with recurrent vomiting in the ...ª acid regurgitation. Chronic nausea with little or no vomiting, ...ed by other symptoms or signs, presents a diagnostic challenge. ...s rarely cause chronic persistent nausea alone.

...ist trimester of pregnancy, nausea and vomiting are common. All women of ...earing age should have pregnancy excluded as a cause.

PHYSICAL EXAMINATION

An abdominal examination may reveal evidence of obstruction, malignancy or peritoneal signs, but is usually negative in the patient with chronic symptoms. Scars from previous surgery should be noted. Assessment of hydration status (skin turgor, mucous membranes, pulse, blood pressure lying and standing) is important in terms of management decisions. Look for the pigmentation of Addison's disease. Evidence of fever should be sought. Chronic vomiting can also cause dental erosions and caries. Self-induced vomiting can cause calluses or ulcers on the dorsum of the hand and dental erosions (from acid) and hypertrophied salivary glands. Pin-head sized red macules on the face and upper neck may occur with recurrent vomiting.

A careful neurological examination should be conducted. Evidence of nystagmus may occur in labyrinthitis. Focal neurological signs are usually present if there is a central nervous system cause for the nausea and vomiting, although the changes may be relatively subtle. Look in the fundi for evidence of raised intracranial pressure.

INVESTIGATION

Investigation is undertaken to:
1. define any derangements that may result from the loss of fluid and electrolytes during vomiting; and

2. determine the diagnosis of the underlying cause.

The investigations need to be guided by the initial history and physical examination. Serum electrolytes will exclude hypokalaemia, renal failure and metabolic alkalosis due to chronic loss of gastric contents. Serum albumin levels, if low, would suggest a chronic disease or malnutrition. Anaemia would suggest colonic or small bowel disease, while leucocytosis would suggest an inflammatory process. If there is upper abdominal pain, pancreatic and liver enzymes can be useful. Peripherally, eosinophilia can occur in eosinophilic gastroenteritis, which can present with recurrent vomiting. Pregnancy testing is mandatory before radiographic testing in any woman of reproductive age with new-onset nausea and vomiting.

A suggested management algorithm for chronic nausea and vomiting is shown in Figure 8.1. Supine and upright abdominal X-rays will document small bowel obstruction, although in 20% of cases partial small bowel obstruction can be missed with plain films. Upper endoscopy will exclude gastric outlet obstruction and significant gastroduodenal disease, such as peptic ulcer. If small-bowel follow-through fails to reveal evidence of obstruction, which can occur with a partial lesion, an enteroclysis (where barium and methylcellulose are infused into the proximal intestine

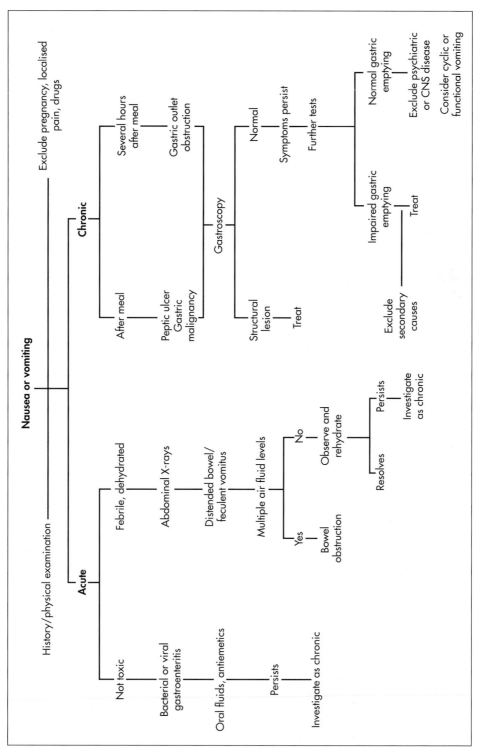

FIGURE 8.1: Diagnostic algorithm for nausea and vomiting.

via a nasojejunal tube in order to provide double-contrast pictures) or computed tomography enterography can be useful. If there is any suggestion of lower bowel obstruction, then barium enema or colonoscopy should be undertaken.

Endocrine disease may present with chronic vomiting and, therefore, testing should be done to exclude diabetes mellitus, hypothyroidism and, in particular, Addison's disease.

If the patient has normal structural evaluations and continues to be symptomatic, gastric emptying testing can be undertaken. An alternative is ^{13}C octanoic acid breath testing, which is non-radioactive and can be used in children or pregnant women. However, the value of documenting delayed gastric emptying is controversial. Symptom improvement on prokinetics correlates poorly with changes in gastric emptying, and abnormal emptying is not a reliable way to direct management of nausea and vomiting. Another controversial test is electrogastrography (EGG). Cutaneous electrodes can measure the gastric slow wave activity. In the setting of vomiting, there may be slow (bradygastria) or fast (tachygastria) myoelectric rhythms, but this has not been established to be useful for directing treatment of chronic nausea or vomiting. Antroduodenal manometry is valuable in specialised centres. Approximately 40% of patients with unexplained nausea and vomiting have normal results, and the test only alters management in about 10% of cases. It is useful to consider this test when symptoms continue to be very troublesome; if antroduodenal manometry is normal, this should direct evaluation outside the gastrointestinal tract, which is of value.

CONSEQUENCES OF NAUSEA AND VOMITING

The major complications with acute vomiting include trauma to the distal oesophagus as well as severe fluid and electrolyte disturbances.

Recurrent vomiting may result in laceration of the oesophageal mucosa at the gastro-oesophageal junction, and a small amount of blood may streak the vomitus, typically following repeated vomiting. Haemorrhaging may occur as a consequence of a laceration to the mucosa into the submucosa, termed a Mallory-Weiss tear. If the laceration extends through the submucosa and the serosa to result in an oesophageal perforation, this is called Boerhaave's syndrome. This perforation typically enters the left chest cavity producing intense pain. Acute severe vomiting, particularly in patients with neurological defects or impaired consciousness from alcohol intoxication, may result in aspiration of vomitus into the lungs.

Recurrent vomiting in young and elderly persons, particularly, may result in severe fluid and electrolyte disturbances. Most of these losses occur from the vomited secretions of the stomach and upper small intestine. As hydrogen, sodium, potassium and chloride irons are lost from gastric secretions, prolonged vomiting results in metabolic alkalosis, hypokalaemia and dehydration.

Occasionally, a patient who is vomiting will conceal it and present with unexplained hypochloraemic hypokalaemic metabolic alkalosis. Here, the differential diagnosis includes surreptitious diuretic use, primary hyperaldosteronism and Bartter's syndrome. The urine chloride is typically low with vomiting (or diuretics).

Chronic nausea and vomiting significantly impairs quality of life, and warrants appropriate therapy.

IMPORTANT DISEASES THAT MAY CAUSE NAUSEA AND VOMITING

Gastric and intestinal obstruction

The nature of vomiting and associated symptoms caused by intestinal obstruction depends on the level of the gut involved as well as the rapidity with which the obstruction occurs (Chapter 4). Acute small bowel obstruction is more likely to be associated with severe pain compared with obstruction of a more insidious onset. Bile is almost always present in the vomitus when the obstruction is below the duodenal ampulla. The vomiting of partially digested food one to several hours after eating would suggest obstruction at the pylorus. Malignant obstruction of any form is usually accompanied by anorexia and weight loss. Complete obstruction of the stomach or duodenum usually results in the loss of large volumes of fluid in the vomitus (Chapter 4).

Functional obstruction, as seen in diabetic gastroparesis or post vagotomy, differs from mechanical gastric obstruction in that intense nausea and anorexia are more common; signs of peripheral and autonomic neuropathy are usually present if diabetes mellitus is the cause. Postprandial fullness and early satiety are common symptoms with diabetic gastroparesis.

Physical examination of the abdomen varies depending upon the cause of the obstruction. In pyloric obstruction, upper abdominal distension and a succussion splash may be observed. Generalised abdominal discomfort may be noted. Distended loops of bowel are observed with peristaltic rushes early in intestinal obstruction but absent bowel sounds are noted later.

Infection

Acute viral gastroenteritis may result in vomiting. Bacterial gastroenteritis induces vomiting usually accompanied by fever and diarrhoea (see Chapter 12). Nausea and vomiting, which occasionally may be prolonged and result in dehydration, may be prominent characteristics of acute viral hepatitis (Chapter 22).

Central nervous system disorders

Space-occupying lesions with increased intracranial pressure are a cause of vomiting often without associated anorexia or nausea. The vomiting may be sudden and projectile in nature, and may occur early in the morning or with a sudden change in body position. Signs of raised intracranial pressure such as papilloedema on fundoscopy may not always be present. Radiological investigations including computed tomography or magnetic resonance imaging of the brain are important to perform if persistent or recurrent vomiting of unknown cause is being investigated.

Nausea and vomiting due to diseases of the vestibular apparatus are accompanied by vertigo and nystagmus. Tinnitus also accompanies Ménière's disease. Migraine headaches that are often unilateral and may be accompanied by a prodrome of visual disturbances are characteristically associated with nausea and vomiting.

Metabolic disorders

In certain metabolic disorders, vomiting is invariably present, such as in untreated uraemia and in diabetic ketoacidosis. Nausea and sometimes vomiting may accompany hypoadrenalism (Addison's disease) and less commonly hyperthyroidism.

Drugs

The potent emetic agent Ipecac is given as a therapeutic agent to induce vomiting. Morphine and opiate derivatives produce nausea and vomiting in some people when given in therapeutic doses, and in most patients when given in large doses.

Non-steroidal anti-inflammatory drugs may be associated with nausea and sometimes vomiting in susceptible individuals with or without accompanying peptic ulcer disease. Other gastric irritants such as iron preparations can also cause nausea. Erythromycin, despite its prokinetic actions, often induces nausea. Both digitalis and theophylline preparations may cause insidious nausea and occasionally vomiting; they may have been taken for months or years before symptoms occur because of a narrow margin between toxic and therapeutic levels.

Visceral pain

Vigorous stimulation of visceral afferent fibres either due to direct external pressure on certain organs such as the kidney and the testis or via unusual distension, as in obstruction of the intestine, ureter, cystic duct or common bile duct, result in nausea and vomiting. In addition, local inflammation in any of the above organs is frequently accompanied by nausea and vomiting (e.g., with mumps, orchitis, cholecystitis, or ascending cholangitis). Nausea and vomiting also occur with acute pancreatitis.

Infiltration of the gastrointestinal tract (e.g., eosinophils in eosinophilic gastroenteritis, amyloid in amyloidosis or malignant cells in carcinoma or lymphoma) may be associated with vomiting. Severe pain in other areas outside the abdomen may also be accompanied by nausea and vomiting (e.g., acute myocardial infarction).

Psychiatric disease

Nausea and vomiting are prominent symptoms in eating disorders including anorexia nervosa and bulimia nervosa (Chapter 15). Panic attacks can also cause nausea (Chapter 1). If nausea is not accompanied by anorexia or is associated with weight gain, an organic cause is rarely observed.

Pregnancy

In any woman of childbearing age who describes nausea of recent onset, a pregnancy test should be considered. Morning sickness may also be produced in susceptible women who use oral contraceptives. Morning nausea during the first 12 weeks of pregnancy is common and occurs in up to 90% of normal pregnancies. Accompanying vomiting, however, occurs in only 25 to 50%. The nausea usually resolves spontaneously as the day progresses with the appetite returning to normal in the afternoon and evening. In the majority of pregnant subjects, nausea and vomiting is self-limited and disappears spontaneously in the first trimester. If vomiting is severe and is associated with dehydration or electrolyte disturbances, it is termed hyperemesis gravidarum. The cause is unknown. This state can potentially threaten the fetus and mother because of electrolyte disturbances and nutritional deficiencies.

Conditioned reflexes

An offensive sight (e.g., blood) or unpleasant smell may result in immediate nausea and sometimes vomiting in susceptible people. Conditioning may occur in response to such sights or smells, such that nausea and vomiting is more easily precipitated by the same circumstances in the future. Such conditioning also applies to motion sickness and the vomiting induced by chemotherapy.

PRINCIPLES OF TREATMENT

Treatment involves successfully correcting any dehydration and electrolyte abnormalities. Malnutrition should also be corrected, if present. If clinically necessary, give intravenous fluids (normal saline with potassium) and place a nasogastric tube; measure the output, which should be replaced intravenously.

Dietary modification is particularly important if there is evidence of gastroparesis. Frequent small meals (six per day), a low-fat diet, avoidance of indigestible material to reduce the chance of bezoar formation and reduced fibre intake can all be useful. Splitting the ingestion of liquids and solids may reduce symptoms. Liquids are generally tolerated better than solids in this setting, and so use of a blender or liquid formulas can be helpful. Medical therapy (Table 8.2) may be necessary.

TABLE 8.2: Examples of drugs to control nausea and vomiting			
Drug	Site of action	Administration	Comment
Diphenhydramine	Antihistamine (H_1-blocker)	Oral/parenteral (25–50 mg x 3–4)	Sedative Motion sickness
Prochlorperazine	Phenothiazine	Oral/parenteral/ rectal (5–10 mg x 3)	Extrapyramidal side effects
Hyoscine	Anticholinergic	Transdermal	Motion sickness
Metoclopramide	Dopamine D_2 antagonist	Oral/parenteral (5–20 mg x 4)	Neurological side effects
Domperidone	Dopamine D_2 antagonist	Oral (10 mg x 4)	No neurological side effects
Ondansetron	Serotonin receptor 5-HT$_3$ antagonist	Oral/parenteral (8 mg x 3)	Cancer chemotherapy

Medical therapy

Antiemetics

Neuroleptic agents, such as prochlorperazine, chlorpromazine or haloperidol have both anticholinergic and antihistamine effects as well as blocking dopamine D_2 receptors in the chemoreceptor trigger zone. Sedation, blood dyscrasias, dystonia and jaundice are potential side effects. Prochlorperazine (5–10 mg three times a day) is most widely used and can be given orally, rectally or parenterally.

Motion sickness is treated with anticholinergic agents such as scopolamine. This can be given as a transdermal patch. Sometimes this will also help gastrointestinal causes of nausea and vomiting. H_1-receptor antagonists such as promethazine (25 mg four times a day) or diphenhydramine (25–50 mg three to four times a day) can be helpful in vestibular disturbances and motion sickness, and sometimes improve gastrointestinal-related nausea.

5-HT_3 antagonists (e.g., ondansetron, granisetron, dolasetron) are useful in postoperative vomiting, in prevention of chemotherapy-induced emesis and after radiation therapy, but appear to produce relatively little improvement in other forms of vomiting. Tetrahydrocannabinol and nabilone have proven useful in chemotherapy-induced emesis. These cannabinoids can produce drowsiness, orthostatic hypotension, dry mouth and tachycardia, as well as anxiety, depression and visual hallucinations.

The neurokinin-1 antagonist aprepitant is indicated for chemotherapy-induced nausea and vomiting. It is given orally (80–125 mg) and side effects include somnolence, fatigue and hiccups. Talnetant and osanetant are other neurokinin antagonists. Any benefit in gastrointestinal disease is uncertain.

Prokinetic agents

Metoclopramide (5–20 mg four times a day) is a substituted benzamide, and is a dopamine D_2-receptor antagonist. It has central anti-dopaminergic effects and stimulates cholinergic actions locally in the gut. It is associated with side effects including drowsiness, dystonia, parkinsonism and, rarely, cardiac arrhythmias or tardive dyskinesia, which can be irreversible despite ceasing the medication, particularly in the elderly. Metoclopramide is available both orally and parenterally. Domperidone is another substituted benzamide that poorly penetrates the central nervous system and so has fewer central side effects. It can cause cardiac arrhythmias and gynaecomastia (5%).

Tegaserod is a partial 5-HT_4 agonist that has been demonstrated to accelerate gastric emptying. However, any benefit in nausea and vomiting as well as gastroparesis remains inadequately documented.

Erythromycin is a macrolide antibiotic that, through motilin receptors, accelerates gastric emptying. However, it has a very narrow therapeutic window and high doses induce nausea. While the drug may accelerate emptying, it usually does not relieve symptoms when taken orally for nausea and vomiting. Other motilin agonists have proven disappointing in clinical studies of functional dyspepsia.

Benzodiazepines

Lorazepam and other benzodiazepines can reduce anticipatory nausea and vomiting prior to chemotherapy, although any benefit in other causes of nausea and vomiting is unclear. They may be a useful adjunctive treatment in combination with other therapy.

Tricyclic antidepressants

Limited data from primarily retrospective analyses suggest that low-dose tricyclics will reduce chronic nausea and vomiting in up to 80% of patients with functional bowel disease.

Botulinum toxin injection

Patients with gastroparesis may have temporary symptom reduction after injection of botulinum toxin into the pylorus, although data are limited.

Gastric electrical stimulation

Gastric electrical stimulation (GES) is emerging as a potentially useful therapy for refractory gastroparesis with nausea and vomiting. Applying stimulation parameters at four times the basal rate (12 cycles per minute), symptoms, but not gastric emptying, have been reported to improve. The neurostimulators are placed in the subcutaneous pouch and the electrodes are placed along the greater gastric curvature at laparotomy or laparoscopy. High-frequency GES is approved for patients with chronic intractable nausea and vomiting due to idiopathic or diabetic gastroparesis.

Alternative treatments

Accupressure or acupuncture, ginger, hypnosis, transcutaneous electrical nerve stimulation, behaviour modification treatments and psychological therapies are of some efficacy in selected clinical settings, but data remain limited particularly in terms of idiopathic nausea and vomiting.

SPECIFIC CLINICAL SCENARIOS

Gastroparesis

Start with an antiemetic and prokinetic agent in combination. Combination therapy tends to be more useful than in the clinical setting. If maximal medical therapy fails, options include gastric electrical stimulation, endoscopic placement of a percutaneous endoscopic gastrostomy (PEG), jejunostomy (PEG-J) or a subtotal gastrectomy in extreme cases. Gastric bypass procedures and less extensive gastric resection should be avoided as they give much poorer results.

Cyclical vomiting

This is a condition characterised by discrete acute episodes of nausea and vomiting with completely asymptomatic intervening periods. Migraine headaches, motion sickness and atopy may be positive on history taking. While primarily a condition of childhood, there are reports in adults. Typically in adults, the episodes of nausea and vomiting last for 3–6 days. Cyclical vomiting is often associated with abdominal pain (two-thirds of patients) and psychiatric diagnoses are uncommon (20%). In children, an association with mitochondrial DNA mutations has been described. Cannabis use is one cause and this should be excluded. Tricyclic antidepressants appear to be useful for this syndrome. Antimigraine therapy (e.g., beta-blockers, sumatriptan) may also be of some value, particularly if there is a family history of migraine.

Functional vomiting

This is a rare condition that has been defined by the Rome Committees (Table 8.3). If gastric emptying is delayed, it is important to exclude chronic intestinal pseudo-obstruction as well as mechanical intestinal obstruction. No medications have established efficacy in this group, but anecdotally, tricyclic antidepressants seem to be of value and can be tried at a low dose, but may require full dose to be efficacious.

TABLE 8.3: Functional vomiting diagnostic criteria

Diagnostic criteria

- Frequent episodes of vomiting, occurring on at least one separate day in a week over three months
- Absence of criteria for an eating disorder, rumination, or major psychiatric disease
- Absence of self-induced and medication-induced vomiting
- Absence of abnormalities in the gut or central nervous system, and metabolic diseases to explain the recurrent vomiting

(*Based on Rome III*, The Functional Gastrointestinal Disorders, 3rd edn. *2006: 331, with permission.* http://www.romecriteria.org)

Further reading

Abell TL, Bernstein RK, Cutts T *et al.* Treatment of gastroparesis: a multidisciplinary clinical reveiw. *Neurogastroenterol Motil* 2006; 18: 263–83.

Miller LS, Szych GA, Kantor SB *et al.* Treatment of idiopathic gastroparesis with injection of botulinum toxin into the pyloric sphincter muscle. *Am J Gastroenterol* 2002; 97: 1653–60.

Parkman HP, Hasler WL, Barnett JL, Eaker EY. Electrogastrography: a document prepared by the gastric section of the American Motility Society Clinical GI Motility Testing Task Force. *Neurogastro Motil* 2003; 15: 89–102.

Quigley EMM, Hasler WL, Parkman HP. AGA technical review on nausea and vomiting. *Gastroenterology* 2001; 120: 263–86.

Talley NJ. Diabetic gastropathy and prokinetics. *Am J Gastroenterol* 2003; 98: 264–71.

Acknowledgement

Much of the material in this chapter was originally written by J Lambert MMed, PhD and has been adapted for this new edition.

chapter 9

VOMITING BLOOD, BLACK STOOLS, BLOOD PER RECTUM, OCCULT BLEEDING

INTRODUCTION

Assessment and management of gastrointestinal bleeding is a challenging and exciting area of clinical practice. The problem is common and very diverse in its presentation, ranging from minor anal bleeding to massive, life-threatening haemorrhage from an ulcer or oesophageal varices. The doctor who is responsible for patients with gastrointestinal bleeding requires many skills; firstly a compassionate and empathetic approach to an often frightening experience for the patient; secondly, highly developed skills in emergency medicine and resuscitation principles; and thirdly, a good understanding of the causes of gastrointestinal bleeding and the appropriate investigations and treatments.

Five different clinical situations are commonly encountered:

1. Vomiting bright red blood or altered 'coffee grounds' blood. There may also be associated 'melaena' or passage of tarry black bowel motions;

2. Passage of melaena alone without any vomiting;

3. Passage of bright red blood per rectum. This may range from a trace on the toilet paper to a life-threatening massive bleed;

4. Iron-deficiency anaemia without any visible blood loss from the gastrointestinal tract; and

5. Blood loss detected only by a screening occult blood test.

The approach to management of these clinical situations forms the basis of this chapter.

VOMITING BLOOD

Haematemesis means vomiting blood, whether it is bright red, dark and clotted, or 'coffee grounds'. Vomiting blood is a frightening condition, which most patients recognise immediately as a serious problem and present urgently to their doctor or the local emergency department. The 'coffee grounds' appearance is due to gastric acid breaking down the haemoglobin in red blood cells to haematin. If the patient vomits 'coffee grounds', he or she may not recognise that this is due to internal bleeding and a delay in presentation to the doctor may occur.

The problem is common. Most large teaching hospitals in Australia will have at least 200 patients admitted each year with haematemesis. More than 50% of these patients are over 60 years of age, many have other medical problems and management is both urgent and complex. The overall mortality from haematemesis is of the order of 5%, though there are certain high-risk groups that can be identified and targeted for more intensive management.

The main causes of haematemesis are listed in Table 9.1. So how do these patients present? Firstly, they are often agitated by what has happened, so that history-taking can be difficult and the history of the event may be unreliable. They may feel nauseous, continue to vomit during the initial assessment or have symptoms related to blood loss including sweating, dizziness and confusion.

Management

The first goal in managing a patient with haematemesis is to resuscitate him or her and ensure that the haemodynamic state is stable. Limited time is available for detailed history taking and physical examination. The most important initial steps are:

- Ensure the patient's airway is clear;
- Check for shock/hypotension and organise blood/fluid replacement;
- Check if the patient is still actively bleeding; and
- Look for clues as to the source of bleeding.

These important steps will be considered in more detail below. Delays in assessment and institution of proper management may prove fatal.

1. Airway

The mental state should be noted carefully because a drowsy or comatose patient is at high risk of aspiration if he or she continues to vomit blood. The mental state may be impaired by a number of factors including:

- severe, acute blood loss leading to cerebral hypoperfusion;
- concomitant chronic liver disease or renal failure leading to encephalopathy; and
- alcohol or drug intoxication/overdose.

If the patient is unconscious or has an impaired gag reflex, the airway must be protected, especially if vomiting continues. The patient should be kept flat on his or her side. A cuffed endotracheal tube may need to be inserted.

2. Hypotension/shock

Assessment of hypovolaemia involves simple bedside clinical observations. The patient may be clammy and sweaty with cold peripheries and a fast thready pulse. There may be associated confusion. The blood pressure will be low, often < 90 mmHg systolic. If any of these signs are seen, resuscitation should commence immediately. At least two large bore intravenous cannulae should be inserted into large peripheral veins. A central venous line should be placed in high-risk cases (see below). Rapid infusion of isotonic saline followed by a plasma expander such as Haemaccel should commence and blood samples should be drawn urgently for full blood count, coagulation screen, blood group and cross matching of 4–6 units of packed cells, urea and electrolytes and liver function tests. A chest X-ray and ECG may be warranted.

As a rule of thumb, patients who have obvious signs of shock, with clammy peripheries and low blood pressure, may have lost up to 50% of their circulating blood volume. If these signs are not present, the patient may be sat up carefully and a check made for a postural drop in blood pressure. If this is present, it is likely that 10–20% of blood volume has been lost. Remember that with haemoconcentration immediately after a bleed, the haemoglobin may initially be near normal despite the loss of a considerable amount of blood.

Patients with a gastrointestinal bleed have lost 'whole blood' and there is, therefore, logic in transfusing them with whole blood (Table 9.2). In practice, however, donated blood is separated into packed cells and other products, such as platelets and plasma, which may be used in different clinical situations. Thus, in current clinical practice, patients with a significant bleed are given packed cells alternating with a plasma expander such as Haemaccel if they are hypovolaemic and packed cells alone if they are normovolaemic but anaemic. The aim of transfusion is to restore circulating blood volume so that the blood pressure is normal and to correct anaemia so that the oxygen carrying capacity of the blood is satisfactory. This generally means maintaining a haemoglobin level of approximately 100 g/L. One unit of packed cells will increase the haemoglobin level by 10 g/L (haematocrit by 3%).

In hypovolaemic patients, packed cells are transfused rapidly until the patient is haemodynamically stable. Rarely, group-specific uncrossmatched blood or O Rhesus-negative blood will be required. In haemodynamically stable patients, packed cells are transfused slowly, approximately one unit every 2 hours.

If the patient is coagulopathic or needs more than four units of packed cells, then fresh frozen plasma (two units initially) should also be given to provide clotting factors.

TABLE 9.1: Causes of haematemesis

Very common
- Gastric or duodenal ulcer or erosions

Common
- Mallory-Weiss tear (a laceration at the gastro-oesophageal junction)
- Ulcerative oesophagitis
- Oesophageal varices

Uncommon
- Vascular malformations
- Ulcerated gastrointestinal stromal tumour
- Carcinoma of oesophagus or stomach
- Aorto-enteric fistula

TABLE 9.2: Indications for blood transfusion in patients with gastrointestinal bleeding

Consider transfusing if:

- Blood pressure < 110 mmHg
  or
- Postural hypotension (> 10 mmHg)
  or
- Pulse > 110/min
  or
- Haemoglobin < 90 g/L[1]

1. May be a normal haemoglobin level with severe bleeds initially.

---

3. Active bleeding

As resuscitation is proceeding, it is important to consider if bleeding is still active. This is straightforward if the patient continues to vomit bright red blood or if the blood pressure keeps falling. Passing melaena does not necessarily signify active bleeding; it may simply be old blood that has worked itself through the bowel. However, if the patient starts to pass more 'fresh' melaena, which is maroon coloured or even bright red with visible clots, then active bleeding is likely. North American practice involves routine passage of a nasogastric tube in most apparently stable patients to check the gastric aspirate for signs of fresh bleeding. A false negative result may occur, especially with duodenal bleeding when the pylorus is in spasm, though a clear bile-stained aspirate has been shown to be a good prognostic sign. Nasogastric aspiration is much less commonly performed in Australian and British hospital practice though it should be considered, particularly if there are problems with obtaining urgent endoscopic assessment.

4. Source of the bleed

A targeted history should be obtained if possible from the patient or from the family. Particular attention should be given to:

- Amount of blood vomited and any obvious precipitant. Violent retching before the haematemesis suggests that bleeding may be from traumatised gastric mucosa such as a Mallory-Weiss tear.

- History of dyspepsia (often absent in older patients who have non-steroidal anti-inflammatory [NSAID]-induced ulceration) or previous peptic ulcer, liver disease, oesophageal varices or previous bleeds;

- Recent ingestion of aspirin, NSAIDs, warfarin, alcohol or selective serotonin reuptake inhibitors (SSRIs); and

- Other significant medical problems, such as recent myocardial infarction, cerebrovascular disease or chronic chest disease.

  The patient should be assessed, focusing on the following points:

- Close and repeated monitoring of haemodynamic state with pulse and blood pressure measurements—hourly initially. Central venous pressure monitoring may also be used, especially in high-risk, unstable patients and those with a history of cardiac failure for whom the problem of fluid overload from over-enthusiastic transfusion is nearly as much a concern as under-transfusion;

- Signs of chronic liver disease (e.g., spider naevi, palmar erythema) and, in particular, portal hypertension. Splenomegaly in a patient with signs of liver disease or a history of alcohol abuse suggests that portal hypertension may be present and that bleeding may be from varices;
- Consideration of some rare causes of bleeding. For example, check for signs of cutaneous or buccal telangiectasia, which may be a marker for hereditary haemorrhagic telangiectasia (Osler-Weber-Rendu syndrome). This condition is rare and associated with gastrointestinal bleeding from telangiectasia in the stomach or small or large intestine; and
- Obtain a baseline haemoglobin and measure it twice daily, initially, in more severe cases.

Endoscopy

Even if the history points to a likely diagnosis (e.g., past history of duodenal ulcer), remember that the cause of bleeding may be different on this occasion. Studies have shown that the clinical diagnosis as to the most likely cause of an upper gastrointestinal bleed is correct in only 60% of cases. Thus, investigation is necessary to establish a correct diagnosis.

Upper gastrointestinal endoscopy is the single most useful test. If performed within 24 hours of presentation, the cause of bleeding will be found in 90–95% of patients (Figure 9.1). Furthermore, it may allow therapeutic interventions to be performed by the endoscopist that may arrest the bleeding or minimise the chance of further bleeding. It requires considerable expertise, especially in the situation of an actively bleeding lesion and is not without some risk.

So who should be endoscoped and when should it be done? This decision is more easily made if we consider why we are doing the endoscopy. Firstly, the aim is to make an accurate diagnosis. Secondly, we may be able to give a prognosis for further bleeding, based on the endoscopic findings. Finally, we may be able to treat a bleeding lesion or one at high risk of re-bleeding. However, if the patient is not in a high-risk category, it may not be necessary to do an emergency procedure. In general terms, endoscopy should always be done within 24 hours but, for patients considered to be 'high risk', emergency endoscopy should be arranged once the patient has been adequately resuscitated.

Risk factors for greater morbidity and mortality from haematemesis are now well known and are listed in Table 9.3.

TABLE 9.3: High risk features in patients with haematemesis

- Older age (> 60 years old)
- Associated serious medical conditions (e.g., chronic lung disease, cerebrovascular disease, recent myocardial infarction)
- Coagulopathy
- Magnitude of bleed (patients presenting with hypotension/shock are a high-risk group)
- Re-bleeding after the initial bleed
- Endoscopic findings (variceal bleeding, peptic ulcer with arterial spurting, oozing, visible vessel or clot in the ulcer base)

These patients should be targeted for the most aggressive management with emergency endoscopy. Endoscopy for acute haematemesis requires a high level of skill and experience. The main risk to the patient is of aspiration of blood, especially if sedation is used and all staff must be aware of the need to protect the patient's airway with a cuffed endotracheal tube, if necessary. Recent reports have documented benefit from administration of intravenous erythromycin (approximately 250 mg) prior to endoscopy. The prokinetic effect of this drug clears blood from the stomach, thereby improving visualisation of bleeding lesions and probably also reducing aspiration risk.

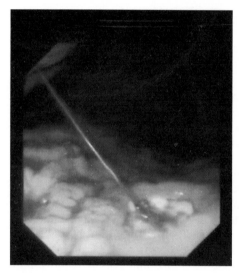

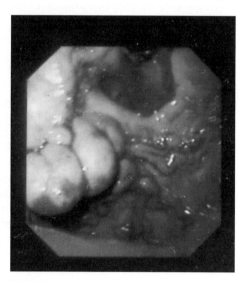

FIGURE 9.1A: Arterial spurting from a gastric ulcer.

FIGURE 9.1B: Gastric varices.

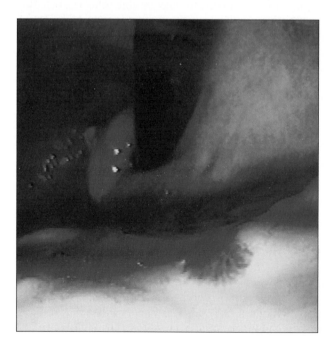

FIGURE 9.1C: Gastric arteriovenous malformation.

Common causes of haematemesis

Oesophageal varices

Oesophageal varices are dilated submucosal veins forming a portosystemic circulation anastomosis in patients with portal hypertension. They look like large varicose veins and bulge into the oesophageal lumen. Arising from these veins are very thin walled vascular channels, lined only by endothelium, extending into the squamous epithelium of the oesophagus. These have a high risk of rupture, which is considered to be mainly precipitated by sudden pressure rises.

About 30% of patients with cirrhosis of the liver have oesophageal varices, but only 30% of patients with varices ever bleed from them. Predictors of haemorrhage include the presence of very large varices and varices with 'cherry red spots'. These red spots represent the intraepithelial vascular channels arising from the varices. Ongoing alcohol ingestion and poor liver synthetic function are also predictors of variceal bleeding.

If bleeding oesophageal varices are found during endoscopy, rubber band ligation is the current treatment of choice. Bleeding can be controlled in 80–90% of cases with a relatively low risk of complications. If passage of the rubber band ligating device mounted on the tip of the endoscope is not feasible or if equipment and expertise for rubber band ligation are not available, then injection sclerotherapy may be performed (Figure 9.2). This involves direct injection of a sclerosant such as ethanolamine oleate or sodium tetradecyl-sulfate into the varices. Injection sclerotherapy has a very high success rate in controlling the bleeding, though with a greater risk of complications including sepsis, oesophageal stricture and mediastinitis.

Pharmacological treatment is also often used in the control of variceal bleeding. The safest and now most widely used drug in this situation is intravenous octreotide, which is an analogue of somatostatin. It can be given acutely in the emergency room if there is a high index of suspicion that varices are the cause of the bleed, even before endoscopic confirmation. It is given by an initial bolus injection of approximately 25–50 mcg, followed by an infusion of 25–50 mcg octreotide per hour in 5% dextrose. It works by decreasing portal venous blood flow and has been shown to control variceal bleeding in over 70% of cases. If variceal bleeding has been fully controlled by endoscopic banding or injection sclerotherapy, there may not be any need for concomitant octreotide infusion. However, if there is any doubt about adequacy of bleeding control, it is appropriate to give the drug.

Sometimes, the above approaches fail and the patient continues to bleed. This is a very high-risk situation and a long-term management plan must be prepared. Important questions are:

- What other methods of bleeding control are available?

- Is the patient suitable for an urgent liver transplant?

- Is the patient's general condition so poor and severity of underlying liver disease so advanced that ongoing resuscitation is inappropriate?

If ongoing aggressive management is decided upon, the next step should be to insert a Minnesota or Sengstaken-Blakemore tube into the oesophagus and stomach (Figure 9.3). This can be passed through the nose, preferably with the patient anaesthetised, though in practice the tube is often inserted in an emergency situation without a general anaesthetic.

Once the position of the tube has been confirmed by X-ray examination to be in the stomach, the gastric balloon is inflated to 300 mL with air or with water and the tube withdrawn so that the gastric balloon is snug against the cardia. This can be maintained in position by gentle traction using a weight of approximately 0.5 kg. Most variceal bleeding will stop since the oesophageal varices are 'fed' from veins passing up across the cardia and these are compressed by the gastric balloon. If bleeding continues, the oesophageal balloon should be inflated to a pressure of 30–40 mmHg using a sphygmomanometer to monitor the pressure achieved.

Patients who have a Minnesota or Sengstaken-Blakemore tube in situ need special monitoring in an intensive care environment and have a nurse dedicated to the care of the tube. It is imperative that the nurse watch carefully for displacement of the tube and regularly check the pressure in the oesophageal balloon. This technique may stabilise the patient until alternative treatments can be given. A further attempt at endoscopic sclerotherapy or rubber band ligation is the next step. If this fails to control the bleeding, then other strategies must be considered.

TIPS (transjugular intra-hepatic portosystemic stent) is a radiological procedure that involves creation of a fistula within the liver substance between the hepatic and portal veins, followed by insertion of an expandable metal stent. This forms a portosystemic shunt and lowers the pressure in the portal venous system. The technique is being increasingly used after failed banding or sclerotherapy and buys time for definitive long-term management such as liver transplantation. If a patient has a good life expectancy but is not suitable for a liver transplant, there may still be a place for a more definitive surgical shunt, for example the 'Warren shunt' which involves a surgical anastomosis between the splenic and renal veins.

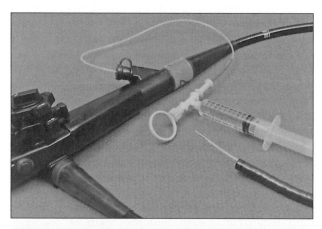

FIGURE 9.2: Injection sclerotherapy equipment for variceal bleeding.

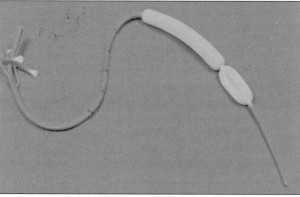

FIGURE 9.3: Sengstaken-Blakemore tube.

Oesophageal transection is the other surgical procedure not uncommonly used in the past as a 'rescue' operation in the recurrent bleeder. The mortality of this approach is 50% in an emergency setting and TIPS is now regarded as the safer option if the expertise is available.

Mortality from bleeding oesophageal varices is of the order of 30% despite the advances in endoscopic and radiological management. The severity of the underlying liver disease is the main determinant of outcome. For those patients who do respond well to the initial banding or sclerotherapy, careful follow-up is required with ongoing endoscopic treatment at 1–3 weekly intervals until the varices are obliterated. These treatments can be given on a day-case basis.

Gastric or duodenal ulceration

Ulcers bleed when an artery or other vessels in the base of the ulcer are eroded. If the bleeding is arterial in origin, it may be very brisk and rapidly lead to shock. In a young patient, there is good arterial contractility, which can cause spasm of the damaged vessel and bleeding may cease spontaneously. In an elderly patient with atherosclerotic arteries, this ability to induce arterial spasm is impaired and bleeding is more likely to continue.

Endoscopic interventions may be used if a gastric or duodenal ulcer is found at endoscopy. These are particularly appropriate if there is active bleeding with oozing or arterial spurting, or if there is a visible blood vessel in the base of the ulcer crater. These are stigmata, which predict a high risk of ongoing or recurrent bleeding. An adherent clot over the base of an ulcer signifies a moderate risk of re-bleeding and the application of endoscopic interventions in this situation is more controversial. Two recent small studies support aggressive management combining adrenaline injection therapy, clot removal and thermal ablation. The most widely used agent for injection is 1:10,000 adrenaline, which probably works by causing spasm of any feeding arteriole or artery and encourages platelet plugging and thrombosis.

For actively spurting vessels or visible vessels in a peptic ulcer, thermal ablation therapy using a heater probe or bipolar electrocoagulation probe alone or in combination with adrenaline injection is now the most widely utilised technique. Other endoscopic treatments include argon plasma coagulation, clipping techniques and Neodymium Yag laser treatment.

After endoscopic diagnosis of peptic ulceration with stigmata indicative of a high risk of re-bleeding, many clinicians will also treat with an intravenous infusion of a protein pump inhibitor (e.g., omeprazole). Several studies have shown a clear reduction in the risk of re-bleeding when omeprazole is used as primary therapy for bleeding ulcers without concomitant endoscopic therapy. Best results appear to occur with high-dose infusion (e.g., omeprazole 8 mg per hour) over a period of 3–5 days. There is also theoretical evidence to support high-dose intravenous infusions, which elevate gastric juice pH to above 6, a level at which fibrinolysis of adherent clots is inhibited. Both regular and high-dose intravenous infusions of omeprazole have been shown to be effective at preventing re-bleeding in patients whose peptic ulcers have been treated initially by endoscopic therapy.

After bleeding has stabilised, definitive ulcer healing treatment is introduced and this comprises avoidance of ulcerogenic medications, such as aspirin, administration of oral proton pump inhibitor therapy at standard dosage and eradication of *Helicobacter pylori* if identified on initial assessment (gastric histology, urease testing, breath testing or serology). An endoscopy to document healing is often performed 4–6 weeks after treatment has been given, especially in a high-risk patient whose ulcer has bled without warning symptoms.

The discovery that most peptic ulcers are caused by an infection in the stomach, *H. pylori*, has led to the routine adoption of antibacterial therapy (Chapter 5). Treatment of *H. pylori* in patients with peptic ulcer markedly reduces the risk of subsequent ulcer relapse and associated bleeding, without the need for long-term maintenance drug treatment. The current regimens will work in about 80–90% of patients, eradicating the infection, healing the ulcer and markedly reducing the risk of ulcer recurrence. In the immediate aftermath of a haematemesis, clinicians may choose to use the simpler drug regimen of an H_2-receptor antagonist or proton pump inhibitor alone to heal the ulcer and then, when the patient has stabilised and out of hospital, follow on with *H. pylori* eradication, or treat the infection as soon as the patient can eat at the same time as giving acid suppression drug therapy.

The success of the treatment can be documented in the patient with a bleeding ulcer by taking gastric biopsies to look for the organism during a subsequent endoscopy four or more weeks after stopping therapy. Alternatively, a ^{14}C or ^{13}C urea breath test or a stool antigen test, which are less invasive, can be done.

If a peptic ulcer is found in a patient receiving NSAID therapy, these drugs should be discontinued at least in the short term and, ideally, long term. Ulcer healing can then proceed along the lines outlined above. Some patients cannot manage without regular NSAIDs and, in that case, long-term prophylactic treatment with a proton pump inhibitor should be considered. Misoprostol can also be used to protect against recurrent gastric ulceration in a patient on NSAIDs. The COX-2 inhibitors can be used in these patients in place of traditional NSAIDs but the risk of further bleeding is only reduced, not abolished, by this substitution.

Other causes of haematemesis

Acute gastric erosions and a Mallory-Weiss tear are usually self-limiting lesions that will heal fully over a matter of days. In the case of erosions, withdrawal of gastric irritants such as aspirin or NSAIDs should be done. A short course of a proton pump inhibitor is often prescribed though it may not be needed.

Ulcerative oesophagitis that bleeds sufficiently to cause an overt haematemesis is usually severe and requires aggressive acid suppression. Rarely, a chronic ulcer in a Barrett's oesophagus may bleed (Chapter 1). By far the most effective treatment for oesophageal ulceration is with the proton pump inhibitors such as omeprazole, lansoprazole or pantoprazole. Long-term therapy is likely to be needed. Laparoscopic fundoplication may also be considered as an alternative to long-term medical treatment.

Role of surgery in bleeding peptic ulcers

Modern endoscopic treatments have reduced the need for surgical intervention in bleeding peptic ulcers. Nonetheless, some patients will be bleeding so massively at presentation that endoscopic therapy cannot be applied due to poor visualisation of the lesion. A major arterial bleed (e.g., from the gastroduodenal artery in a posterior wall duodenal ulcer) is unlikely to respond to endoscopic therapy. Therefore, it is imperative that all high-risk patients be assessed *early* by a gastrointestinal surgeon, preferably in an established Haematemesis and Melaena unit.

For patients with uncontrollable massive bleeding, emergency surgery can be life-saving and the decision to operate is usually straightforward. For patients whose bleeding continues at a slower rate or who have episodic re-bleeds despite initial endoscopic treatment, the timing of surgical intervention is more difficult and requires careful consideration of the risks of ongoing conservative management and blood transfusion balanced against the risks of an anaesthetic and operation. An experienced surgeon can give far better input to this decision-making if they have been reviewing the patient from admission rather than being called in at the last moment.

The choice of operation will vary according to the clinical circumstances. In most instances, an oversewing of the bleeding artery is all that is performed since it is assumed that medical therapy afterwards will deal with the ulcer effectively. In some instances, especially if there is a history of recurrent bleeding or ulceration despite medical therapy, a more definitive operation will be performed. A selective vagotomy and pyloroplasty is appropriate for a duodenal ulcer and a partial gastrectomy for a gastric ulcer (Chapter 5).

Discharge from hospital

As a general rule, patients with bleeding should be admitted to hospital. There is a growing body of literature supporting same-day discharge in carefully selected patients following clinical and endoscopic evaluation. This would be an appropriate strategy for young, otherwise healthy individuals with clinically small bleeds in whom endoscopy shows minor erosive gastritis, mild oesophagitis or peptic ulceration without any high-risk stigmata. These patients can resume eating normally after the endoscopy. A long-term management strategy should be considered and communicated to the local general practitioner.

Patients with bleeding varices are the highest risk group and these patients should remain in hospital for at least a week, during which time the risk of massive re-bleeding is highest. Treatment also has to be directed to the underlying liver disease and its complications (Chapter 22). Patients with high-risk peptic ulcers are at increased risk of re-bleeding for at least 72 hours after the initial bleed. Discharge from hospital is reasonable after 4–5 days if the patient's course in hospital has been uncomplicated.

PASSING MELAENA ALONE

This is a common clinical situation, sometimes badly managed, because the patient or the doctor underestimates the seriousness of the complaint. The patient may blame the colour of the motions on something eaten and not appreciate that the black colour is due to altered blood. The characteristic strong odour of melaena should help the clinician distinguish it from other causes of black coloured motions (e.g., use of iron, bismuth or liquorice).

Most cases of melaena are due to bleeding from the upper gastrointestinal tract, mainly from peptic ulceration. Oesophageal varices rarely present in this way because they bleed so briskly that bright red haematemesis occurs long before melaena is seen. However, some patients with portal hypertension ooze blood more slowly from dilated blood vessels in the stomach (portal gastropathy, Figure 9.1B) or intestine (portal enteropathy) and melaena may be the first sign.

Therefore, all patients with active melaena should be assumed to have an upper gastrointestinal cause and be managed in exactly the same way as the patient who presents with haematemesis. Admission to hospital is warranted, even if the patient is haemodynamically stable, since the melaena from a mild initial bleed may herald a more severe life-threatening bleed to follow. If the melaena has been transient and is over a week old, it may be safe to investigate on an outpatient basis, though endoscopic evaluation should be done urgently, within a few days, so that an accurate diagnosis can be made and definitive treatment started.

Some patients with melaena will not be bleeding from the upper gastrointestinal tract and the endoscopy will fail to show a lesion. Blood loss from the right colon or the small intestine may also present as melaena. Colonic lesions such as polyps, cancer, angiodysplasia and diverticula are much more common than small bowel lesions and the next step should, therefore, be a colonoscopy. If polyps are found, these can be removed by polypectomy during the examination. Bleeding angiodysplastic lesions can be treated by argon plasma coagulation or by injection sclerotherapy.

If no abnormality is found on upper endoscopy and colonoscopy, a decision to investigate the small bowel has to be made. The yield from small bowel evaluation is low, however, and many clinicians will elect to observe the situation and only investigate the small bowel if melaena recurs. If there are any associated small bowel symptoms, then small bowel evaluation with enteroscopy or capsule endoscopy should be considered. These tests can identify vascular lesions and angiodysplasia, small bowel tumours and inflammatory bowel disease. In some cases, more extensive evaluation with enteroclysis, Meckel's scanning and angiography will be required. This will be discussed further in the next section.

If patients with melaena have associated iron deficiency anaemia secondary to chronic blood loss, iron replacement therapy may be necessary. It is important to warn the patient that oral iron will colour the motions black and mimic the appearances of melaena. Iron containing stools, though black in colour, do not have the characteristic odour of melaena and most patients will be able to distinguish at least a more severe melaena stool from the effects of iron tablets.

BRIGHT RED BLOOD PER RECTUM

This is also an extremely common clinical complaint affecting patients of all ages. In the vast majority of cases, the bleeding is trivial in quantity though in some patients a large volume of blood is passed and, rarely, the bleeding is massive and associated with hypotension or shock.

Causes of rectal bleeding in young patients under the age of 40 years are listed in Table 9.4. In older patients, the differential diagnosis is wider, and more serious conditions such as colorectal cancer are much more prevalent (Table 9.4).

A careful history should be taken, focusing on the following points:

- Amount of bleeding and colour of blood;
- Blood on toilet paper only (suggesting anal pathology) or blood mixed in with the stool;
- Associated perianal pain suggesting local anal pathology;
- Pattern of bowel habit—constipation and straining at stool point towards haemorrhoids or anal fissure; diarrhoea and mucus per rectum suggest ulcerative proctitis; and
- Family history of colorectal diseases such as carcinoma.

TABLE 9.4: Causes of rectal bleeding

In patients < 40 years old

Very common:
- Haemorrhoids
- Anal fissure
- Inflammatory bowel disease (mainly proctitis)

Less common:
- Polyps (hamartomatous or adenomatous)
- Infective colitis
- Meckel's diverticulum
- Intussusception

Rare:
- Colorectal cancer

In patients > 40 years old
- Haemorrhoids
- Anal fissure
- Colorectal cancer
- Colorectal polyps (mostly adenomas)
- Angiodysplasia
- Diverticular disease
- Inflammatory bowel disease
- Ischaemic colitis
- Infective colitis

Examination should include a check for an abdominal mass arising from the colon and a careful inspection of the anal area, stretching apart the tissues to look for any signs of an anal fissure. A rectal examination should be done, feeling with the finger for any palpable lumps and any local tenderness. A proctoscopy and/or rigid or flexible sigmoidoscopy should next follow. This is an extremely useful test in this situation, especially if done acutely. If a bleeding source is clearly identified, such as bleeding haemorrhoids or fissure, then further investigation may be avoided. If no lesion is found or if a *possible* source is seen but with no evidence of recent bleeding (e.g., non-bleeding haemorrhoids), then further investigation will be necessary in most instances. Remember that haemorrhoids are common and it is dangerous to assume that they are the source of the bleeding, especially in a more elderly patient, if no evidence of recent bleeding is seen at the time of the examination.

For patients over the age of 40 years, a colonoscopy should be arranged if the initial local inspection and sigmoidoscopy have not clearly identified the source of bleeding. A barium enema is not an appropriate investigation in this situation. It is less accurate than colonoscopy, especially in the detection of vascular lesions such as angiodysplasia. Barium also obscures the views if subsequent colonoscopy or angiography is required, and therapeutic interventions, such as polypectomy, cannot be performed.

For younger patients, discretion and clinical judgment are needed if the initial work-up is negative. The yield from colonoscopy in this group is small and serious pathology, such as colorectal cancer, is very rare. If the bleeding is persistent or recurrent, a colonoscopy is clearly warranted.

Causes of rectal bleeding

Specific points related to the individual causes of rectal bleeding are given below.

1. Haemorrhoids

These are particularly associated with constipation and straining at stool. They are vascular cushions which form in the venous plexuses at the anorectal junction. Bleeding is typically intermittent. Blood is seen on the toilet paper, as a splash in the toilet bowl or on the outside of the stools. For minor bleeding, reassurance is all that is necessary after the clinical evaluation has been performed. Attention to diet and treatment of associated constipation is appropriate. If bleeding is more persistent or recurrent, then local treatment of the haemorrhoids can be given. Options include injection of the haemorrhoids with sclerosant, rubber band ligation and stapling. For more severe prolapsing haemorrhoids, haemorrhoidectomy is appropriate (Chapter 11).

2. Anal fissure

Treatment again is directed towards the underlying constipation. Fibre supplements and stool softeners are used and the patient is encouraged to avoid straining at stool. Glyceryl trinitrate ointment will relax anal spasm and allow some fissures to heal. This conservative approach will work in many cases but for more chronic recurrent fissures, surgical intervention is necessary (Chapter 11).

3. Rectal polyps

If these are seen at sigmoidoscopy, the patient should be fully prepared for a colonoscopy so that a search for more proximal polyps can be made. Most polyps can be removed at colonoscopy using a snare or hot biopsy forceps. Since approximately 90% of colorectal cancers arise from pre-existing adenomatous polyps, the rationale for polyp excision is not only control of the rectal bleeding but also cancer prevention. If the polyps are found at histology to be adenomatous, colonoscopic surveillance is warranted, especially in patients with multiple polyps or large polyps, as there is an increased risk of new polyp formation and colorectal cancer. Repeat examinations should be done at three- to five-yearly intervals in most cases (Chapter 20).

4. Angiodysplasia or vascular ectasia of the bowel

These vascular lesions are increasingly common with advancing age. About 25% of patients over the age of 60 years have angiodysplasia but only a small proportion bleed. They are most commonly found in the caecum and ascending colon though are occasionally found in the small intestine or left colon. They may present with occult bleeding leading to iron deficiency anaemia or with more brisk bleeding leading to moderate or even massive rectal bleeding. The cause of these lesions is unclear. They are dilated thin-walled vascular lesions in the submucosa of the colon and may develop in response to chronic pressure changes, especially in the right colon. Bleeding is typically intermittent and ceases spontaneously, only to recur at a later date in most patients. Sometimes the bleeding is torrential and emergency intervention is required. If detected at colonoscopy, argon plasma coagulation, injection therapy or laser may be used to stop the bleeding. At angiography, injection of vasopressin or embolisation techniques may be used successfully. In some patients, surgical intervention, often a right hemicolectomy, may prove necessary. Delineation of the extent of angiodysplasia by investigation, such as capsule endoscopy for small bowel involvement, is appropriate before surgical intervention is planned.

5. Diverticulosis

These are pseudodiverticula or mucosal herniations through the colonic wall, at sites of relative weakness caused by penetrating blood vessels. They become increasingly common with age; 5% of 50-year-old persons and more than 50% of 90-year-old persons have colonic diverticula. It is widely believed that the Western refined diet, low in fibre, is a major predisposing cause for diverticula formation. They develop most commonly in the sigmoid colon though, for reasons that are not understood, bleeding is more commonly seen with right colonic diverticula. In the vast majority of patients, bleeding settles spontaneously and management is conservative. Fewer than 25% of patients will have further episodes of bleeding, though those patients that do have further episodes tend to continue with bleeding and require surgical resection. Diagnosis is usually presumptive, made at colonoscopy when other colonic causes have been excluded. Active bleeding is rarely seen at colonoscopy though it can be treated using thermal ablation or injection therapy.

6. Inflammatory bowel disease

Ulcerative proctitis may present as rectal bleeding without any associated change in bowel habit, though most patients also have diarrhoea. The condition may be due to ulcerative colitis or Crohn's disease and is easily diagnosed by sigmoidoscopy (Chapter 13). If there are other symptoms suggesting the presence of more proximal disease, the patient may need a colonoscopy. Local treatment of proctitis with steroid enemas, 5-aminosalicylic acid enemas or oral sulfasalazine treatment works well in most patients. Resistant cases need more aggressive immunosuppression with high-dose oral steroids.

7. Ischaemic colitis

This usually occurs in the setting of widespread peripheral vascular disease or cardiac disease. The rectal bleeding is often associated with mild lower abdominal cramps. Characteristic changes are seen on colonoscopy or barium enema usually at the level of the splenic flexure and descending colon because this is a watershed area in the blood supply to the colon (Figure 9.4). Treatment is conservative and the condition settles spontaneously in most cases. Some patients develop a stricture at the site of the ischaemia, which rarely requires subsequent excision (Chapter 4).

Massive rectal bleeding

This is a relatively uncommon clinical problem and needs some additional comment as the clinical management is more complex and acute. The patient may be hypotensive or in shock and require urgent resuscitation, as has been described above for patients with haematemesis. The most frequent causes of this clinical presentation are massive bleeding from colonic diverticula or angiodysplasia. However, the site of bleeding may be virtually anywhere in the gastrointestinal tract since massive bleeding even from the stomach or duodenum may pass rapidly to the rectum without becoming discoloured to form melaena. *History taking should focus not only on colorectal symptoms but on any symptoms that might suggest an upper gastrointestinal origin for the bleeding.*

A rectal examination and rigid sigmoidoscopy should start the diagnostic work-up because occasionally a local perianal cause will be found. If the findings are negative, it is appropriate to proceed to an upper gastrointestinal endoscopy so that a gastroduodenal cause is fully excluded. This can be accomplished quickly and prepares the way for more complex and invasive investigation of the small and large intestine.

Recent studies have demonstrated that it is safe to give these patients bowel preparation and to proceed to emergency or urgent colonoscopy within 12–24 hours. Since most colonic lesions will stop bleeding spontaneously, there is still debate about the appropriateness of emergency, as opposed to urgent, colonoscopy. If a bleeding lesion is identified during emergency colonoscopy, it can be treated using similar techniques to those described for upper endoscopy. Adrenaline injections, argon plasma coagulation, thermal probes and endoscopic clips all have a role.

The next step in the work-up depends on the clinical condition. If the patient is haemodynamically stable and colonoscopy fails to identify the source of bleeding, a technetium-labelled red cell scan is often performed. In this test, a sample of the patient's blood is taken and labelled with a radioisotope before being injected back into the patient's blood stream. Abdominal scans can then be taken at intervals, looking for

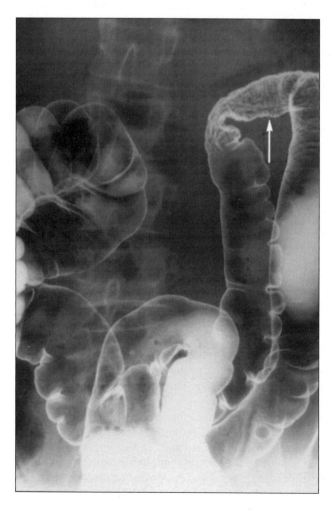

FIGURE 9.4: Ischaemic colitis of the splenic flexure on barium enema.

extravasation of radiolabelled blood into the bowel. The technique can detect bleeding at rates as low as 0.1 mL per minute. If bleeding is intermittent, the patient can be sent for repeated scans over the next 24–48 hours in the hope of catching a fresh bleed. The object is to localise the source of bleeding to small or large bowel and give some indication to the surgeon of the precise site in the event of surgery being necessary. The accuracy of the test has been questioned by some clinicians and false localisation of the site of bleeding is a problem in some cases.

A Meckel's scan (^{99}Tc pertechnetate) should be considered in young patients with massive rectal bleeding. The ^{99}Tc is taken up by the ectopic acid-secreting gastric mucosa of a Meckel's diverticulum, which rarely ulcerates and bleeds.

A positive red cell scan may lead on to a mesenteric angiogram, which may be both diagnostic and therapeutic. The radiologist may identify not only the site of bleeding but also the cause. Vascular lesions such as angiodysplasia may be seen. There may be an abnormal tumour circulation identified.

Active bleeding may be controlled by vasopressin infusion into the appropriate feeding artery or by embolisation with alcohol or with small beads, and thus obviate the need for surgery.

Growing experience with capsule endoscopy has highlighted a beneficial role for this procedure in patients with large-volume rectal bleeds who are relatively stable. The capsule test provides the best mucosal imaging of the small intestine and is particularly useful for the detection of vascular lesions such as angiodysplasia. A capsule endoscopy study takes many hours to perform and then report. Accordingly, the patient must be in a stable condition to allow the procedure to be performed. Small bowel endoscopy can now be performed by using a colonoscope (push enteroscopy) or special small bowel scopes (e.g., double-balloon enteroscope).

If the above techniques identify the lesion but fail to control the bleeding, an operation will be necessary. In some instances, a laparotomy is combined with an on-table endoscopy or colonoscopy as the endoscopist may be able to assist the surgeon in the precise localisation of a small bleeding point, particularly in the case of angiodysplasia.

IRON DEFICIENCY ANAEMIA

In all patients over the age of 40 years, this should be assumed to be due to gastrointestinal bleeding. Investigation gives a high yield of gastrointestinal lesions in this age group, even if the anaemia is not associated with any gastrointestinal symptoms. Young menstruating women, however, have a very high incidence of iron deficiency and pathology in the gastrointestinal tract is rarely found. Thus, empirical treatment of the anaemia without full investigation in the absence of gastrointestinal symptoms is usually the correct approach.

The presentation may be vague with ill-defined symptoms, such as lethargy, dizziness or depression. Some patients will present with shortness of breath or angina. A careful search for signs of anaemia is warranted though often none is found. The skin creases, buccal mucosa and conjunctivae should be examined for pallor. There may rarely be spooning of the fingernails present (koilonychia) if the condition is chronic. Blood tests confirm the presence of anaemia and show that it is iron deficient.

The key elements are:

- microcytic hypochromic anaemia; and
- low serum iron and serum ferritin with decreased transferrin saturation.

Sometimes a high platelet count occurs in patients with chronic active blood loss. A wide range of gastrointestinal lesions may be responsible for the anaemia, from ulcerative oesophagitis to colonic angiodysplasia. A major concern in elderly patients is the possibility of a caecal carcinoma. Usually, distal colonic lesions or oesophageal lesions present with overt blood loss from respective ends of the gastrointestinal tract leading to haematemesis or rectal bleeding and are uncommon causes of isolated iron deficiency anaemia. Non-bleeding lesions should also be considered. Malabsorption of iron in patients with coeliac disease, previous gastrectomy or atrophic gastritis may occur.

Unless there are specific symptoms pointing to a particular region of the gastrointestinal tract, investigation should focus initially on the large intestine and, in most instances, also include an upper gastrointestinal evaluation. If the findings are negative, most clinicians would treat the anaemia with oral iron and observe the response. If the haemoglobin fails to rise or if anaemia recurs, more detailed investigation should be considered. Enteroclysis (small bowel enema) was the preferred next step in the past but, today, capsule endoscopy and/or enteroscopy should be performed. These endoscopic techniques will identify vascular lesions that cannot be detected by enteroclysis and are also more sensitive at detecting benign and malignant tumours of the small intestine. Other tests that may help in some cases include a Meckel's scan in younger patients and angiography of the mesenteric vessels.

POSITIVE OCCULT BLOOD TEST

Faecal occult blood testing is only recommended in the context of population screening for colon cancer. It is *not* an appropriate test for the assessment of patients with colonic symptoms such as rectal bleeding or anaemia. These patients should have more definitive investigations performed.

The most widely used occult blood test is the Hemoccult test. This is a guaiac test, which detects the pseudoperoxidase activity of haem. It is generally recommended that three spontaneously passed stools are tested twice to give a total of six possible reactions. A positive reaction is seen as a blue colour on any one of the specimens and is interpreted as a positive test result for the battery. This implies blood loss from the colon of the order of 1–2 mL/day or blood loss from the stomach of 10–20 mL/day. This test will likely detect 40–80% of asymptomatic colorectal cancers and 30–40% of large colorectal adenomas.

False positive results can be caused by the presence of peroxidase activity in certain foods or from the haemoglobin content of red meat. Antioxidants such as vitamin C may produce a false negative result. Aspirin and NSAIDs may cause excessive bleeding from the gastrointestinal tract causing a true but unrelated positive result. Thus, the following conditions should apply when performing occult blood testing with the Hemoccult test:

- Dietary restrictions for three days before and during the testing;
- No red meat;
- No high peroxidase-containing vegetables such as cantaloupe (rock melon) and other melons, raw radishes, turnips, horseradish, broccoli or cauliflower; and
- No vitamin C and NSAIDs.

Newer occult blood tests are also now available. These include more sensitive versions of the guaiac test such as Hemoccult SENSA and immunological tests that utilise antibodies to human haemoglobin.

Occult blood tests have been used in a number of major population trials in an attempt to diminish the mortality from colorectal cancer in the screened population. The tests have been offered to asymptomatic people over the age of 50 years in most of these studies. When positive results were obtained, the subjects were offered colonoscopy and, if appropriate, polypectomy. These studies have shown a 20–33% reduction in mortality from colorectal cancer in the screened population when compared with the control group. In these programs, about 60% of the subjects accepted the invitation to do the test and about 2% had a positive result. When these were investigated, 3–5% of the positive results were found to be associated with a colorectal cancer and 30–45% with an adenoma. The other positive results may have reflected bleeding from a wide range of gastrointestinal tract lesions or false positive reactions from peroxidase-containing foodstuffs.

If the tests are done correctly with appropriate dietary restrictions, then high specificity is achieved with 98–99% of healthy subjects being occult-blood negative. Thus, if an asymptomatic patient, aged 40 years or more, is found to have a positive occult blood test, they should be referred for a colonoscopy. If polyps are found, these should be removed at the time of the colonoscopy. Any cancer found should be biopsied and the patient referred on for surgical resection. If the colonoscopy findings are negative, investigation of the upper gastrointestinal tract by upper endoscopy should be considered. In practice, the yield from this is very small except in patients with upper gastrointestinal symptoms, such as dyspepsia, or in patients with frank iron deficiency anaemia.

When should occult blood testing be performed? At present, in Australia, NHMRC guidelines support annual occult blood testing for all asymptomatic people over the age of 50 years. Pilot schemes looking at the mechanics of implementing a population-based occult blood testing programme are underway. In the USA, annual occult blood testing has been endorsed as one of a number of bowel-cancer-prevention strategies that can be offered to asymptomatic people of 50 years and over.

More invasive screening with colonoscopy may be appropriate if there is a strong family history of bowel cancer. One first-degree relative in the family with bowel cancer at age < 55 years or two first-degree relatives with bowel cancer at any age increases the chance of your patient getting bowel cancer by 3–4 fold, compared with the general population. A colonoscopy in those with a strong family history is recommended every five years from the age of 40 years, or from the age of onset of cancer in the family member less 10 years (Chapter 20).

Further reading

Bleau BL, Gostout CJ, Sherman KE et al. Recurrent bleeding from peptic ulcer associated with adherent clot: a randomised study comparing endoscopic treatment with medical therapy. *Gastrointest Endosc* 2002; 56: 1–6.

Church NI, Palmer KR. Ulcers and nonvariceal bleeding. *Endoscopy* 2003; 35: 22–6.

Frossard JL, Spahr L, Queneau PE et al. Erythromycin intravenous bolus infusion in acute upper gastrointestinal bleeding: a randomised controlled double blind trial. *Gastroenterology* 2002; 123: 17–23.

Grace ND. Diagnosis and treatment of gastrointestinal bleeding secondary to portal hypertension. American College of Gastroenterology Practice Parameters Committee. *Am J Gastroenterol* 1997; 92: 1081–91.

Hadithi M, Heine GD, Jacobs MA et al. A prospective study comparing video capsule endoscopy with double-balloon enteroscopy in patients with obscure gastrointestinal bleeding. *Am J Gastroenterol* 2006: 101: 52–7.

Lamberts SWJ, van der Lely A-J, de Herder WW, Hofland LJ. Drug therapy – octreotide. *N Engl J Med* 1996; 334: 246–54.

Lau JY, Sung JJ, Lee KK *et al.* Effect of intravenous omeprazole on recurrent bleeding after endoscopic treatment of bleeding peptic ulcers. *N Engl J Med* 2000; 343: 310–6.

McCormick PA, Burroughs AK, McIntyre N. How to insert a Sengstaken Blakemore tube. *Br J Hosp Med* 1990; 43: 274–7.

Pennazio M, Santucci R, Rondonotti E *et al.* Outcome of patients with obscure gastrointestinal bleeding after capsule endoscopy: report of 100 consecutive cases. *Gastroenterology* 2004; 126: 643–53.

Rockall TA, Logan RF, Devlin HB, Northfield TC. Selection of patients for early discharge or outpatient care after acute upper gastrointestinal haemorrhage. National Audit of Acute Upper Gastrointestinal Haemorrhage. *Lancet* 1996; 347: 1138–40.

Rockey DC, Koch J, Cello JP *et al.* Relative frequency of upper gastrointestinal and colonic lesions in patients with positive fecal occult-blood tests. *N Engl J Med* 1998; 339: 153–9.

Young GP, St John DJ, Winawer SJ *et al.* Choice of fecal occult blood tests for colorectal cancer screening; recommendations based on performance characteristics in population studies: a WHO (World Health Organization) and OMED (World Organisation for Digestive Endoscopy) report. *Am J Gastroenterol* 2002; 97: 2499–507.

chapter 10

CONSTIPATION

INTRODUCTION

Constipation is a very common symptom. When a patient presents with constipation, they must be asked what they mean by this term. They may mean that they have a decreased bowel frequency, hard stools or some difficulty or pain with bowel evacuation. In surveys of the general population not seeking health care, 10–17% of people strain at stool on more than a quarter of occasions, but only between 1 and 4% report bowel frequency of fewer than two stools per week.

Constipation is often dismissed as a minor symptom by doctors, although for some patients it can be the source of considerable anxiety and disability, and is frequently associated with general malaise and a sense of poor health. A list of the causes of chronic constipation is presented in Table 10.1. While the majority of patients who complain of constipation have a benign disorder of colorectal function associated with faulty diet, drugs or bowel habit, called simple constipation, it should always be remembered that constipation may be the presenting symptom of a serious colonic disorder, such as carcinoma, or a generalised metabolic disorder, such as hypothyroidism or hypercalcaemia. Chronic constipation can occur in the absence of structural or metabolic disorders because of abnormally slow intestinal transit (slow transit constipation), obstructed defecation (pelvic floor dysfunction), or both. The irritable bowel syndrome, (IBS), characterised by abdominal pain and a variable bowel habit, is also an important cause of constipation (Chapter 6). A careful history and examination to ascertain the likely mechanism producing constipation allows investigations to be correctly chosen, which in turn should determine management.

CLINICAL APPROACH TO PATIENTS WITH CONSTIPATION

History

First, take the history. Determine if the problem is a chronic one, and ask why the patient has sought help on this occasion. They may have fears about the possibility of malignancy or the chronic use of laxative drugs. Details of bowel frequency, stool consistency and colour, presence of blood or mucus and accompanying features such

---

TABLE 10.1: Classification of constipation in adults

No gross structural abnormality

- Inadequate fibre intake
- Irritable bowel syndrome (associated with abdominal pain) or functional constipation
- Idiopathic slow-transit constipation
- 'Obstructed defecation'—pelvic floor dysfunction (or dyssynergia)

Structural disorders

- Anal fissure, infection or stenosis
- Colon cancer or stricture
- Aganglionosis and/or abnormal myenteric plexus:
  - Hirschsprung's disease
  - Chagas' disease
  - Neuropathic pseudo-obstruction
- Abnormal colonic muscle:
  - Myopathy
  - Dystrophia myotonica
  - Systemic sclerosis
- Idiopathic megarectum and/or megacolon
- Proximal megacolon

Neurological causes

- Diabetic autonomic neuropathy
- Damage to the sacral parasympathetic outflow
- Spinal cord damage or disease, e.g., multiple sclerosis
- Parkinson's disease
- Blunting of consciousness, mental retardation, psychosis
- Pain induced by straining, e.g., sciatic nerve compression

Endocrine or metabolic causes

- Hypothyroidism
- Hypercalcaemia
- Porphyria
- Pregnancy

Psychological disorders

- Depression
- Anorexia nervosa
- Denied bowel habit

Drug side effects

---

as abdominal pain, bloating or weight loss are therefore relevant questions. Stools that feel hard to the patient usually are not when objectively tested!

Ascertain the onset of the complaint. Constipation dating from the neonatal period may suggest Hirschsprung's disease (congenital aganglionosis causing absent peristalsis in a part of the rectum or colon), while symptoms dating from the time of toilet training or early childhood may suggest childhood megarectum or stool withholding (often with soiling and overflow). Severe constipation (with a defecation frequency of less than once a week off laxatives) in young women dating from adolescence or following pelvic surgery may indicate slow transit constipation; these patients typically lack the urge to defecate. In older patients, progressive constipation may indicate a colorectal neoplasm or diverticular stricture.

Some patients with a disorder of pelvic floor function complain of a sense of difficulty with evacuation and feeling of anal blockage or obstruction; they may manually disimpact themselves by pressing in or around the rectum or vagina. A history of obstetric trauma in such patients may be relevant. However, symptoms cannot distinguish pelvic floor dysfunction with sufficient accuracy from IBS or functional constipation.

Constipation may be induced by certain drugs, such as narcotics, antihypertensives or antidepressants. Thus, it is very important to ask about the use of drugs and whether their introduction corresponded to recent alterations in bowel habit. A lack of dietary fibre is a common cause of constipation and a full dietary history should be taken. Slow transit constipation, and occasionally simple constipation, may run in families and a history of other family members being similarly affected may provide useful information.

If the problem is chronic, it is important to find out whether previous investigations have been performed and what previous treatment regimes have been employed, including alternative medicine treatments.

Physical examination

An important part of the assessment of patients with chronic constipation is the physical examination. The general demeanour of the patient may give information regarding anxiety or depression. Look for signs of neurological or endocrine diseases, such as hypothyroidism or Parkinson's disease. Abdominal palpation may reveal faecal masses in young patients with rectal impaction or a tender spastic colon in a young anxious patient with irritable bowel syndrome. A craggy abdominal mass may indicate a colonic neoplasm.

A rectal examination is important. The perineum should be inspected for painful anal fissures, fistulae, abscesses or local neoplasm. The patient should be asked to bear down to demonstrate perineal descent due to pelvic floor weakness, haemorrhoidal prolapse or the formation in women of a rectocoele or uterine prolapse. Occasionally, rectal mucosal or full-thickness prolapse may be seen (Chapter 20). An anal fissure will be very painful on trying to put your finger in the anal canal. Obvious fistula suggests Crohn's disease. A rectal examination can detect if there is any evidence of anal canal stenosis. An obvious rectal mass may represent a cancer. Obvious faecal impaction may be present in very severe constipation particularly in the elderly. To complete the rectal examination, ask the patient to try to push your finger out by straining. If the puborectalis and anal sphincter contract and increase pressure in the anal canal rather than relaxing to widen the canal this suggests (but is not diagnostic of) pelvic outlet obstruction. Next, turn your finger to the anterior position. Try and feel if there is any evidence of a rectocoele, which pushes through the anterior rectal wall when straining. Sigmoidoscopy should be performed if adequate rectal emptying can be achieved.

INVESTIGATIONS

Generally, constipation can be divided into those with no apparent structural abnormality of the anus, rectum or colon and into those with recognised structural disease such as cancer, a stricture or megacolon. A third group of patients have

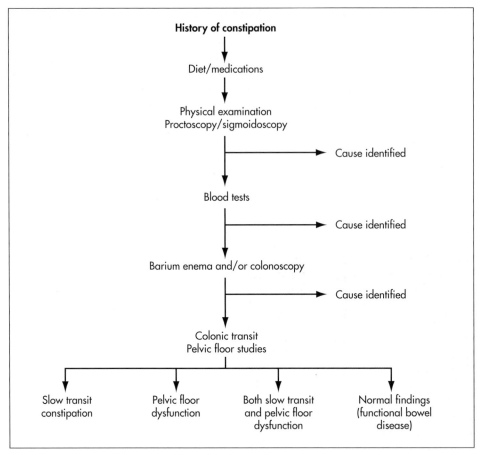

FIGURE 10.1: Diagnostic approach to chronic constipation.

generalised metabolic, neurological or endocrine diseases, which may produce constipation as a secondary event (Table 10.1).

The extent of investigations for the individual patient with constipation depends very much on the clinical assessment (Figure 10.1). In young patients in whom suspicion of serious underlying disease such as colon cancer is low, a trial of therapy without investigation is reasonable. In most other patients it is logical to first assess that the colon is structurally normal. In those patients who do not respond to initial simple therapy, further investigations may be necessary.

Haematology and biochemistry

It is reasonable to check for anaemia (especially iron deficiency) and a raised erythrocyte sedimentation rate or C-reactive protein result. Biochemical tests to check thyroid function and serum calcium levels may also be performed.

Radiology

A plain abdominal X-ray examination often gives useful information about colonic loading and the presence of distended loops or fluid levels if obstruction is a possibility.

The plain X-ray examination is also often helpful in children in whom megarectum is suspected. The rectum or colon is of increased diameter in adult patients with megacolon (due to Hirschsprung's disease or chronic idiopathic intestinal pseudo-obstruction). An unprepared barium enema is useful to assess the size, shape and configuration of the distal colon, especially in cases where rectal impaction or Hirschsprung's disease is suspected. A double-contrast barium enema after bowel preparation can assess a structural disorder, such as stricture, volvulus or megacolon.

Colonoscopy

Colonoscopy can exclude significant structural colonic disease. It is an alternative to sigmoidoscopy and barium enema. Melanosis coli may be evident in patients who use laxatives regularly (Figure 10.2). Colonic stricture and neoplasm can usually be effectively diagnosed by this technique.

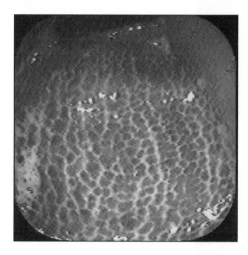

FIGURE 10.2: Melanosis coli.

Bowel transit studies

An increased stool consistency is correlated with slower colonic transit. Total gut transit time (to which the colonic transit time is the greatest contributor) may be simply measured by giving radio-opaque shapes by mouth and recording their course through the colon by abdominal X-ray or stool collection. It is known that normal subjects pass 80% of administered shapes by five days.

One clinically useful quantitative test is to give 24 radio-opaque markers by mouth on three consecutive days and obtain a plain abdominal X-ray examination on day 4; the number of markers is counted to calculate total and regional colonic transit times (Figure 10.3). A transit time of 70 hours or longer is abnormally slow. Laxatives should be stopped two days prior to the test and a high-fibre diet should be continued throughout.

More sophisticated techniques involve radioisotope labelling of food material, such as bran, to allow isotope scanning to measure colonic clearance. This can provide information regarding specific emptying times for different segments of the colon.

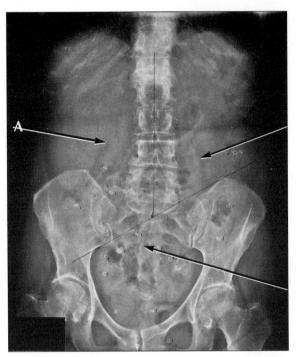

FIGURE 10.3A: Normal colonic transit.

FIGURE 10.3: Colonic transit time assessed by radio-opaque markers: 20 markers were taken on each of 3 days, and the X-ray film was taken on day 4. To calculate colonic transit time (in hours), add up the number of markers visible on day 4 and multiply by 1.2. Regional colonic time (right colon (A), left colon (B) and rectosigmoid colon (C)) can be determined in the same way by dividing the X-ray film into regions as shown.

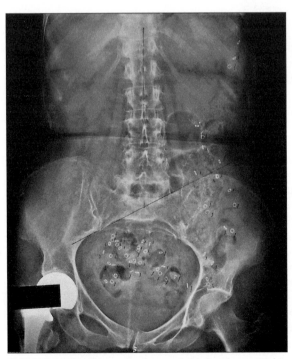

FIGURE 10.3B: Slow colonic transit (defined as > 70 h).

Ano-rectal manometry, sensation and balloon expulsion

Pressure within the anal canal may be recorded by perfused tubes, micro balloons, or strain-gauge transducers (see Chapter 14). Resting anal tone and the response to voluntary contraction and straining at defecation give useful information about the state of the pelvic floor muscles. The recto-sphincteric reflex may be elicited by rectal distension with simultaneous recording of anal pressure. A positive reflex consists of a relaxation of the internal anal sphincter (lowered resting anal tone) following rectal distension (Figure 10.4). The reflex is mediated by the myenteric plexus and is characteristically *absent* in those with Hirschsprung's disease (because of congenital aganglionosis).

Rectal sensation can be tested by inflating a rectal balloon with increments of air, noting the onset of initial sensation and the maximum tolerated volume. Using more sophisticated equipment, a pressure volume curve may be obtained. These tests are useful in distinguishing the hypertonic rectum of the irritable bowel syndrome from the large, insensitive rectum of megacolon.

Assessment for pelvic outlet obstruction may be made with a very simple screening test, the expulsion of a 50 mL filled balloon. If the patient is unable to expel the balloon within one minute, this strongly suggests there is pelvic outlet obstruction. In some laboratories, additional weights are added to the balloon and patients are still unable to expel it even with 500 g or more of weight on the balloon, which is further evidence of outlet obstruction.

Dynamic proctography

Video radiographic recording of defecation with contrast material in the rectum (by a defecating proctogram or magnetic resonance imaging) will demonstrate perineal descent, rectal intussusception and paradoxical sphincter contraction in some patients with obstructed defecation (Chapter 14).

Motility studies

Small bowel motility can be measured by placing a manometric assembly through the mouth in the upper small intestine. Chronic intestinal pseudo-obstruction, a rare but important cause of slow transit constipation, can be diagnosed by this test (Chapter 6). Recording of colonic motility is, at present, a research tool and is not routinely used to base diagnosis and management.

Rectal biopsy

In rare cases where the history, X-ray findings and results of physiological studies suggest the possibility of Hirschsprung's disease, a rectal biopsy is usually necessary for confirmation. Traditionally, this has been of the full-thickness type, requiring general anaesthesia. More recently, suction biopsies with special stains have been shown to be useful, especially in children.

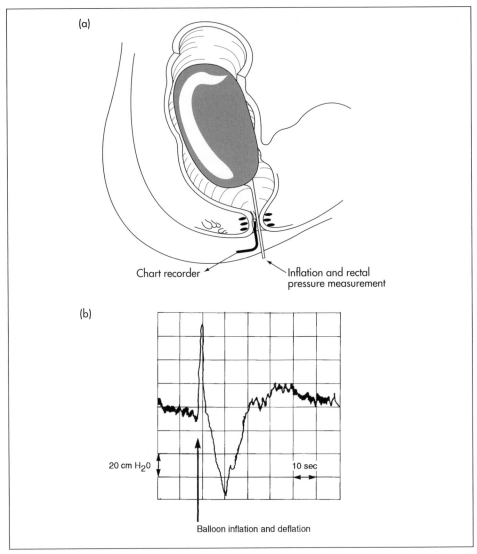

FIGURE 10.4: To elicit the rectoanal reflex, a balloon is inserted into the rectum and a pressure measuring device (in this case a microballoon connected to a pressure transducer and chart recorder) is placed in the anal canal (a). Distension of the balloon causes an initial rise in pressure, due to the external anal sphincter contraction, followed by a more prolonged fall in anal pressure due to internal anal sphincter relaxation (b). This latter fall in pressure confirms the presence of intact intramural nerves, excluding Hirschsprung's disease. A false negative result is sometimes seen in patients with an idiopathic megarectum.
(Based on Kamm MA, Lennard-Jones JE (eds), Constipation, *Wrightson Biomedical Publishing, 1994, with permission.)*

APPROACH TO MANAGEMENT

Once structural and metabolic disease has been excluded by appropriate investigations, it is important to reassure patients that their symptoms of constipation are not due to serious organic disease. This often has a positive effect in relieving anxiety.

General measures

In general terms, many patients with constipation may be managed by a high-fibre diet containing 20–30 g of fibre. This can be achieved by adding cereal, unprocessed bran, and fruit and vegetables (especially root vegetables and legumes) in conjunction with an increased fluid intake. Bulk-forming agents are useful supplements. There are three types: those derived from ispaghula, sterculia (a plant gum) or methylcellulose. Instructions should be given on regular toilet habit and exercise. A review of intercurrent drug therapy should be undertaken and, if possible, drugs promoting constipation should be stopped.

Therapeutic agents

Therapeutic agents available for the treatment of constipation are listed in Table 10.2.

1. Hydrophilic bulk-forming agents

These substances are grain fibre products or pharmaceutical preparations of processed plant fibre, gums or resins. They consist of varying amounts of complex carbohydrate moieties; cellulose, the hemicelluloses, pectins; and the non-carbohydrate polymer, lignin.

TABLE 10.2: Therapeutic agents in constipation and major side effects	
Agents	Side effects
Hydrophilic bulk-forming agents	
Psyllium mucilloid, sterculia, ispaghula, methylcellulose, unprocessed bran	Inadequate fluid intake may result in intestinal obstruction
Osmotic laxatives	
Polyethylene glycol, magnesium sulfate/hydroxide, mannitol, lactulose, sodium salts	May cause electrolyte imbalance
Stimulant laxatives	
Bisacodyl, senna, cascara, danthron	Damage to the myenteric plexus with prolonged use now appears very rare after the withdrawal of phenolphthalein
Stool-softening agents	
Paraffin oil, dioctyl-sodium sulfosuccinate	May cause mineral oil aspiration and pneumonia
Per rectum evacuants	
Glycerine suppositories, phosphate enemas	May cause rectal or anal sphincter damage if incorrectly used

These agents bind water, increase stool weight and act as a substrate for colonic bacteria. Increased intake in constipated patients usually results in larger stools and reduced colonic transit time. Small bowel absorption of other substances (e.g., zinc, iron, glucose and bile salts) may be affected, but this is rarely of clinical significance. It should be remembered that severely constipated patients sometimes do not respond to these agents. In some cases, symptoms may be made worse because of the increased flatus produced. Patients with slow transit constipation generally do not respond to fibre (and may get worse).

2. Osmotic laxatives

These are non-absorbable compounds that produce loose or liquid stool by a direct water-binding effect. Laxatives of this type include sodium and magnesium salts and sugars, lactulose and sorbitol. Polyethylene glycol (PEG) is a larger polymer and a very effective osmotic laxative that is safe. It causes less bloating and gas than other osmotic laxatives.

These agents are among the safest to use on a long-term basis. Some patients find magnesium salts unpleasant and sometimes intolerable. The non-absorbed sugars often increase pain and flatus. These agents should be used on a once- or twice-daily basis to produce the necessary effect and may be continued long term if necessary.

3. Stimulant laxatives

These agents stimulate peristalsis and net fluid secretion by a direct irritant effect on the nerve, muscle or mucosa of the gut. Long-term use of these laxatives may produce tolerance, often leading to an escalating dose regimen. However, these agents are safe and modestly effective for limited periods.

4. Stool-softening agents

Paraffin oil has been used for many years as a stool lubricant. It is sometimes combined with other laxative agents in compound preparations. There is debate about its long-term safety and effectiveness. The detergent dioctyl sodium has an effect on bile salt activity and is sometimes used as a 'stool-wetting agent' in combination with stimulant laxatives or alone.

5. Per rectum evacuants

Suppositories and enemas have a mild irritant effect and stimulate peristalsis. Glycerine suppositories are cheap and effective. Enemas should generally be administered by staff skilled in their use because local complications can occur.

6. Neuromuscular agents

Tegaserod, a serotonin type 4 receptor agonist, stimulates peristalsis and stimulates fluid secretion. Randomised controlled trials have shown the drug is efficacious in functional constipation in men and women under the age of 65. The usual dose is 6 mg twice daily. The drug is usually well tolerated but can cause diarrhoea (to be expected) and headaches. Bethanechol can increase cholinergic stimulation of smooth muscle in the colon but little data exist on its use in constipation. Neostigmine is sometimes used but has significant side effects (it is effective for acute colonic pseudo-obstruction). Opiate antagonists can be helpful in opioid-induced constipation.

In difficult cases unresponsive to usual therapy, some doctors have tried prescribing colchicine (a mucosal poison) or misoprostol (a prostaglandin analogue) in chronic constipation.

Surgical treatment

Colectomy

Surgical therapy should be regarded as a measure of last resort in patients with very severe constipation and documented slow colonic transit without other disease. The surgical procedure of choice in slow transit constipation is subtotal colectomy with ileorectal anastomosis. Extensive resection is required as lesser resection is usually associated with recurrence of constipation.

While the majority of patients have increased bowel frequency after ileorectal anastomosis, some have persistent symptoms of pain and bloating, and a few develop megaileum after surgery and continued constipation. In those with documented obstructed defecation such as mucosal prolapse, perineal descent, or paradoxical contraction of the anal sphincter on straining (called anismus), difficulty with rectal evacuation may persist postoperatively and occasionally patients complain of diarrhoea and incontinence. Hence, pelvic floor dysfunction and small intestinal dysmotility must be excluded before colectomy is considered. Even so, currently it is still difficult to predict the outcome of surgery based upon preoperative physiological studies.

Other surgical approaches

Sphincter division. Internal sphincter myotomy has been reported to help selected constipated patients, although the procedure has failed to become popular. It may be most useful in those with ultrashort-segment Hirschsprung's disease. In those with anismus (paradoxical voluntary sphincter contraction during defecation), voluntary sphincter division either posteriorly or laterally has failed to improve bowel frequency or ease evacuation in the small number of patients studied.

Pelvic floor repair. In those patients with a disorder of defecation characterised by mucosal prolapse or perineal descent, repairing a rectocoele or posterior pelvic floor repair may help, but often does not. In women, it is prudent to only consider repair if better rectal evacuation can be demonstrated after placing pressure on the posterior wall of the vagina. Prolapsing anterior rectal mucosa may be injected with sclerosants, but this procedure rarely improves difficult evacuation.

Stoma. In some patients, the creation of a permanent stoma, either as a loop or end-ileostomy or colostomy, may be useful when all other therapeutic modalities have failed and difficult symptoms persist.

Biofeedback

This technique has been used in patients with chronic constipation and pelvic floor dysfunction on the basis of failure of rectal evacuation. Those who appear to have a paradoxically contracting anal sphincter during evacuation may be retrained to relax the sphincter during defecation straining to allow easy rectal evacuation, with a 70% success rate. This approach is superior to standard care if laxatives and per rectum evacuants have failed.

Other treatment modalities

Botulinum toxin injected into the anal sphincter may help some with paradoxical anal sphincter contraction but is not long lasting. New drug approaches include chloride channel activators and use of neuronal growth factors. Electrical stimulation is also being tried.

Much research is being directed towards the complex interaction between the central and enteric nervous symptoms. In some patients with chronic constipation, there may be a psychological abnormality and alternative approaches to therapy, such as relaxation and behavioural therapy or hypnotherapy, may have a role to play, although no strong scientific evidence supports their use.

CLINICAL APPROACH TO SPECIFIC TYPES OF CONSTIPATION

Simple constipation

This may be defined as that caused by faulty diet, bowel habit, travel or drugs. Once organic disease has been satisfactorily excluded, treatment of this group should be along the lines outlined in the general measures above. Dietary manipulation should be used initially and laxative agents only used if the problem does not respond to simple means.

Constipation in elderly persons

Approximately 50% of elderly patients in primary care will complain of a disturbance of bowel function, more commonly constipation. Drug treatment given for other conditions often leads to constipation. Other factors include a low fibre intake because of poor nutrition and relative immobility producing difficulties with toilet access.

Many elderly nursing home patients develop rectal impaction and this sometimes produces spurious diarrhoea. This diagnosis can be made by rectal examination. Treatment consists of cleaning out the rectum completely by digital fragmentation, lavage, or PEG (for three days), then prescription of an osmotic laxative, increasing the dose as needed to induce a stool every second day. Occasionally, elderly patients present with obtundation or delirium, which improves as the constipation is treated.

Idiopathic slow-transit constipation

This is a rare disorder mainly seen in young women, and the history usually dates from childhood or adolescence. Typically these patients go for weeks between bowel actions! Occasionally, the problem follows abdominal or pelvic surgery.

It is now recognised that the majority of these patients have loss of the interstitial cells of Cajal (ICC), which drive intestinal smooth muscle activity as pacemakers (producing myogenic electrical slow waves). Sometimes this disorder is part of a widespread inherited or acquired defect in intestinal muscle or nerve that causes symptoms of bowel obstruction (chronic idiopathic intestinal pseudo-obstruction). There may be diffuse abnormality of smooth muscle function with abnormalities in oesophageal motility, gastric emptying, small bowel transit and bladder function. Dietary manipulation and other simple measures are ineffective, and usually these patients only manage bowel evacuation with laxatives or enemas.

Other patients may have an abnormality of rectal evacuation producing a hold-up in transit. This could be due to a sensory defect in the rectum as many of these patients appear unable to satisfactorily expel liquid or solid content from the rectum due to paradoxical contraction of the pelvic floor striated muscles during defecation. Pelvic ultrasonography has not demonstrated any significant anatomical abnormality, but many of these women have descending perineum syndrome due to chronic straining at defecation. If pelvic floor dysfunction can be corrected by biofeedback, in true slow-transit constipation, the abnormal colonic function persists.

Medical treatment of this group of patients remains difficult. Osmotic laxatives should be tried in the first instance but often are unpredictable and are associated with bloating, nausea and frequent loose stools. Occasionally, per-rectal evacuants are useful. The efficacy of tegaserod is unknown, but this agent is often tried.

Surgical treatment should be reserved for those with disabling symptoms that have been present for many years when all medical treatment options have been exhausted. In general terms, surgery should be performed only after appropriate physiological and psychological assessment in units with a particular surgical interest in this area. Ileorectal anastomosis has been reported to be successful in a small number of patients.

Megacolon

Megacolon is a rare disorder characterised by an increased rectal or colonic diameter on X-ray examination. Hirschsprung's disease is an important cause. Multiple genetic mutations have been identified in Hirschsprung's disease, mainly in the RET proto-oncogene. It may present for the first time in adult life and can usually be diagnosed by radiological and physiological tests. An unprepared barium enema will usually show a cone-shaped rectosigmoid transition zone (from narrowed to dilated; the narrowed segment is where there is a lack of colonic ganglion cells). The rectosphincteric reflex on anorectal manometry is absent. Rectal biopsy is needed to confirm the diagnosis. The treatment for Hirschsprung's disease in adults is surgery.

Chagas' disease is endemic in tropical South America, particularly Brazil. The disease is caused by the organism *Trypanosoma cruzi* and causes neuronal damage to cells in the autonomic nervous system, most particularly affecting the hollow organs and heart. Megacolon occurs during the chronic phase of the disease and is associated with a dilated, aperistaltic segment of intestine—often the sigmoid colon. Megacolon and mega-oesophagus often occur together. Patients whose symptoms are uncontrolled by medical measures require surgical resection of the dilated colonic segments.

Those with non-Hirschsprung's or idiopathic megacolon may be subdivided into patients whose symptoms develop in childhood and patients whose symptoms develop in later life. In the former group, faecal impaction and soiling are usually the presenting symptoms. The initial step is to disimpact the rectum as described above and then maintain the patient on regular oral laxatives. Encouragement regarding regular defecation is important. Sometimes regular per-rectum evacuants are needed to maintain an empty rectum.

Those whose symptoms develop in later life are usually troubled by pain and bloating and respond poorly to laxatives. Many have taken antidepressants, antipsychotics or antiparkinsonian drugs for prolonged periods. Some evidence suggests that these people may have an inherited or acquired defect in nerve or muscle of the colonic wall. Some patients have idiopathic intestinal pseudo-obstruction. If symptoms are severe and unresponsive to medical treatment and the patient is otherwise fit, colectomy usually gives good results.

Endocrine and metabolic causes

Constipation is common in hypothyroidism; megacolon has been reported, which improves if the patient becomes euthyroid on treatment. Hypercalcaemia and acute porphyria can present with constipation and again respond to appropriate therapy.

Autonomic neuropathy

The most common cause is diabetes mellitus. These patients appear to lack the normal gastrocolic response following food ingestion. Prokinetic drugs may be useful in therapy.

Spinal cord lesions

Damage to the sacral cord leads to a distensible atonic distal colon. Constipation is thus a major problem in paraplegia. Usually, a bowel regimen with a bulk-forming agent, stimulant laxatives and per-rectal evacuants twice or thrice weekly helps to maintain regular bowel patterns.

Other neurological diseases

Constipation may accompany multiple sclerosis, Parkinson's disease and psychosis or dementia. Constipation may be seen in depression or anorexia nervosa. Treatment should be along the usual lines in a stepwise fashion as outlined.

Further reading

Bharucha AE. Treatment of severe and intractable constipation. *Curr Treat Options Gastroenterol* 2004; 7: 291–8.

Brandt LJ, Prather CM, Quigley EM *et al.* Systematic review on the management of chronic constipation in North America. *Am J Gastroenterol* 2005; 100 Suppl 1: S5–21.

Di Palma JA, Smith JR, Cleveland M. Overnight efficacy of polyethylene glycol laxative. *Am J Gastroenterol* 2002; 97: 1776–9.

Emison ES, McCallion AS, Kashuk CS *et al.* A common sex-dependent mutation in a RET enhancer underlies Hirschsprung disease risk. *Nature* 2005; 434: 857–63.

Johanson JF. Review article: tegaserod for chronic constipation. *Aliment Pharmacol Ther* 2004; 20 Suppl 7: 20–4.

Jones MP, Talley NJ, Nuyts G, Dubois D. Lack of objective evidence of efficacy of laxatives in chronic constipation. *Dig Dis Sci* 2002; 47: 2222–30.

Kamm MA, Muller-Lissner S, Talley NJ *et al.* Tegaserod for the treatment of chronic constipation: a randomized, double-blind, placebo-controlled multinational study. *Am J Gastroenterol* 2005; 100: 362–72.

Lembo A, Camilleri M. Chronic constipation. *N Engl J Med* 2003; 349: 1360–8.

Muller-Lissner SA, Kamm MA, Scarpignato C, Wald A. Myths and misconceptions about chronic constipation. *Am J Gastroenterol* 2005; 100: 232–42.

Prather CM. Subtypes of constipation: sorting out the confusion. *Rev Gastroenterol Disord* 2004; 4 Suppl 2: S11–6.

Ramkumar D, Rao SS. Efficacy and safety of traditional medical therapies for chronic constipation: systematic review. *Am J Gastroenterol* 2005; 100: 936–71.

Rao SS, Ozturk R, Laine L. Clinical utility of diagnostic tests for constipation in adults: a systematic review. *Am J Gastroenterol* 2005; 100: 1605–15.

Talley NJ. Definitions, epidemiology, and impact of chronic constipation. *Rev Gastroenterol Disord* 2004; 4 Suppl 2: S3–10.

Talley NJ. Management of chronic constipation. *Rev Gastroenterol Disord* 2004; 4: 18–24.

Talley NJ, Jones M, Nuyts G, Dubois D. Risk factors for chronic constipation based on a general practice sample. *Am J Gastroenterol* 2003; 98: 1107–11.

chapter 11

PERIANAL PAIN

CLINICAL APPROACH

In a patient presenting with perianal pain, the important points in the history are:
- the severity of the pain;
- the duration of the pain;
- whether the pain has been constant or fluctuating;
- the relationship of pain to defecation; and
- associated bowel symptoms (e.g., rectal bleeding, prolapse at the anus).

The causes of perianal pain are listed in Table 11.1.

HISTORY

A patient presenting with severe unrelenting pain over recent hours to days is likely to have either perianal sepsis or thrombosed haemorrhoids. These patients are usually totally distracted from other activities by the pain. Some patients will complain of episodic severe perianal pain with intervening periods without pain.

Typically the pain from an acute fissure-in-ano is severe and is precipitated by defecation; it may take minutes to hours to gradually settle. Thrombosed haemorrhoids cause severe, acute pain, while non-thrombosed haemorrhoids are usually not associated with pain although there can be discomfort during defecation if the haemorrhoids prolapse. The pain associated with pruritus ani can be moderately severe. The pain is specifically associated with the presence of faecal soiling over a raw area and is relieved by effective cleaning of the soiled surface.

The pain of anal fistula tends to be mild, dull and aching. Associated symptoms such as perianal discharge or leakage of pus are clues. The pain of proctalgia fugax is of short duration, often waking the patient from sleep, with a rapid onset over seconds and resolution over 15–20 minutes. There are long periods without any pain. There are a number of chronic perianal pain syndromes associated with a vague dull throbbing ache.

The presence of associated bowel symptoms or systemic symptoms may clearly point to the diagnosis. Ask about any *rectal bleeding*. There may be minor perianal bleeding with fissure-in-ano, usually apparent on the toilet paper after defecation or occasionally on the bowel motion. With internal haemorrhoids, bleeding can be a more prominent feature than pain; the bleeding tends to be related to defecation and is most commonly noted on the toilet paper after wiping (haematochesia) or in the toilet bowl. Pruritus ani can be associated with minor bleeding associated with wiping the perianal region after defecation. Perianal abscess should not be associated with bleeding unless the abscess has erupted spontaneously or has been drained. There may be a minor degree of perianal bleeding with anal fistula. There should not be significant rectal bleeding with any of the chronic pain syndromes or with proctalgia fugax.

Symptoms of constipation are commonly associated with a number of painful perianal conditions (Chapter 10). This is because in some cases patients are reluctant to defecate because it induces or exacerbates pain. This can occur with a fissure-in-ano or thrombosed haemorrhoids. Excessive straining can also cause a fissure in some cases. The conditions causing perianal pain should not themselves be associated with diarrhoea. Therefore, the presence of diarrhoea suggests another disease process (e.g., Crohn's disease).

TABLE 11.1: Causes of perianal pain

- Fissure-in-ano
- Anal sepsis
  - Anal abscess
  - Anal fistula
- Haemorrhoids
  - Internal haemorrhoids
  - External haemorrhoids
- Pruritis ani
- Proctalgia fugax
- Chronic perianal pain syndromes
  - Coccygodynia
  - Descending perineum syndrome
  - Levator ani syndrome
  - Idiopathic perineal pain

EXAMINATION

Inspection

While the history will commonly give vital clues as to the cause of the perianal pain, local examination will usually confirm the diagnosis. The examination clearly needs to be focused in the perianal region. A general abdominal examination, however, is also necessary.

The easiest and most comfortable position for inspection is with the patient in the left lateral position with the hips and knees flexed. The buttocks are parted with gentle pressure from the palm of the hand so that the perianal skin can be closely scrutinised. Red excoriated, weeping skin suggests that the pain is due to pruritus ani. The presence of a sinus means an anal fistula should be sought. The presence of a spot of pus or blood in the perianal region, particularly if this returns after a gentle wipe, can point one to the external opening of a fistula. A perianal abscess can be associated with a perianal swelling depending upon the proximity of the abscess to the external skin. The skin over an abscess may be red, depending on the proximity of the abscess to the skin, and such swellings are usually diffuse and greater than 2 cm.

There may be irregular flaccid tags of skin, which are asymptomatic, but may be associated with a fissure or haemorrhoids. The presence of a small, tense, often bluish swelling, just beyond the anal verge is suggestive of a thrombosed external haemorrhoid. A fissure-in-ano is commonly not obvious on external examination, except in very chronic cases because, in the acute case, the patient will not allow the buttocks to be parted sufficiently to allow adequate inspection due to the pain that is induced. A thrombosed internal haemorrhoid that has prolapsed may be evident at the anal verge as an oedematous 1–2 cm swelling.

Internal haemorrhoids are usually not apparent on external examination. The chronic pain syndromes are not associated with perianal stigmata on inspection.

Palpation

The features to be sought on palpation are:

- the presence of a lump;
- tenderness with or without an obvious palpable lump;
- the presence of a submucosal cord; and
- associated abnormality of sphincter tone.

A *perianal abscess* presenting as a perianal lump with associated overlying erythema will always be focally extremely tender. Focal tenderness to palpation is also present with thrombosed internal as well as external haemorrhoids.

The patient with an *anal fissure* will usually not tolerate perianal examination because of the pain. Do not part the buttocks vigorously since this will be very painful. Insert the finger very gently, applying pressure anteriorly, as most fissures are posterior (see below). The perianal regions should be gently palpated looking for a subcutaneous or submucosal cord leading from the opening of an *anal fistula*. This cord should be followed internally and its position in relation to the anal sphincter noted. A prolapsed thrombosed internal haemorrhoid can be distinguished from a thrombosed external haemorrhoid by a cord extending inside the anus to the upper part of the internal haemorrhoid.

Deeper rectal examination may demonstrate focal tenderness associated with abscess formation inside the anus in the intersphincteric space (between internal and external sphincter) or laterally in the ischiorectal fossa. If the cause of the perineal pain is not clear at this stage, gently rocking the coccyx with posterior pressure may elicit sharp pain suggesting the diagnosis of *coccygodynia*. None of the conditions that cause chronic perianal pain are associated with an abnormality of sphincter function on digital rectal examination.

If an adequate rectal examination is not possible because of perianal pain, then it may be necessary to perform this examination under anaesthesia. This examination should be performed by an experienced person capable of dealing with any perianal pathology found on examination.

Proctoscopy

Proctoscopy will be possible in an office setting for most patients (Chapter 20). It may not be possible in patients with a fissure-in-ano, anal abscess or thrombosed haemorrhoids. Proctoscopy will allow a diagnosis of internal haemorrhoids, which will become more prominent or evident as the proctoscope is withdrawn.

Sigmoidoscopy

This examination is commonly performed and provides useful information in cases where more proximal bowel disease is suspected, based on the history.

FISSURE-IN-ANO
Aetiology

Primary fissures. The majority of anal fissures are primary fissures without any predisposing cause. Although more than 50% of patients are constipated, this precedes the fissure in only 25% of cases; in other patients, the constipation results from the fissure because of a fear of defecating; 5% of fissures follow childbirth. In children, fissures are caused by constipation in the majority of cases and will heal when the constipation is treated. The condition is most common between 20 and 40 years of age, and occurs slightly more often in males.

Secondary fissures. These are caused by Crohn's disease, ulcerative colitis, immunosuppression (e.g., AIDS) and, rarely, tuberculosis or syphilis.

Site

Eighty per cent of fissures are in the posterior midline; 10%, anterior midline; 7%, both posterior and anterior midline; 3%, lateral.

Pathology

The acute fissure is a superficial split with soft edges. A chronic fissure evolves through several phases:

- Superficial—longitudinal muscle fibres of musculus submucosae ani may be seen in the base;
- Deeper fissure—the edges may be indurated; transverse fibres of internal sphincter are seen;
- Advanced fissure—edges are indurated and may be undermined; a skin tag (sentinel pile) develops at the lower edge; a hypertrophied anal papilla may form at the upper end of the fissure at the dentate line;
- Finally, an abscess may form in the submucosal plane or between the internal and external sphincters (intersphincteric) or in the skin tag.

Secondary fissures may be broad or long. If a fissure extends into the upper anal canal above the dentate line then it is usually a secondary fissure. These are sometimes called anal ulcers.

Pathophysiology

Chronic anal fissures are almost always associated with intense spasm of the internal anal sphincter muscle. There was much debate about which came first, but it is now known that the spasm precedes the fissure, although it is not the actual cause of the fissure. The fissure is initially produced by trauma from the passage of hard faeces. Why do chronic fissures often then fail to heal? Under normal circumstances a small split like a fissure would rapidly heal, but in patients where there is underlying spasm, the pressure generated in the mucosa by the internal sphincter spasm exceeds arteriolar blood pressure resulting in ischaemia in the anal mucosa. Reversal of the sphincter spasm results in rapid healing in most cases.

Clinical features

History

Pain is the most common symptom. It occurs during defecation and may persist for some hours after. Some patients describe a feeling of 'passing razor blades' or 'splitting'. Bleeding occurs commonly and is bright red, usually just on the toilet paper but occasionally the blood may drip into the toilet bowl. Itching or a lump at the anus (skin tag) may be reported.

A secondary fissure resulting from inflammatory bowel disease may be associated with symptoms of proctitis or colitis. Some fissures or ulcers caused by inflammatory bowel disease produce little pain and tenderness. Syphilitic fissures are very rare, but are typically painless. When a fissure is caused by acquired immune deficiency syndrome (AIDS) or tuberculosis, there may be systemic features of those conditions.

Examination

In most cases the diagnosis should be made without a full digital examination since this produces severe pain. Gentle bilateral traction on the anal verge reveals tight spasm in most cases and the fissure is usually visible. If the fissure cannot be seen, then gentle pressure just inside the posterior midline will produce tenderness. Only if this is not found should a deeper digital examination be done. The examining finger is inserted pushing firmly anteriorly away from the posterior midline (since most fissures occur posteriorly), and then gentle pressure in a posterior direction is applied. This may produce the classical tenderness, or the induration associated with a deep fissure may be palpated.

A small proportion of primary fissures are not associated with internal sphincter spasm, particularly post-partum fissures. However, if spasm is not present then underlying pathology (secondary fissure) should be suspected. A sigmoidoscopy should then be done to look for evidence of proctitis. Serum should be collected for HIV and syphilis serology, when indicated.

Treatment

Conservative

In 75% of cases of acute fissure and up to 30% of chronic fissures healing will be spontaneous if constipation is treated. Initial conservative (non-surgical) treatment is always indicated unless pain is so severe that immediate surgery is required. A bulking agent, such as psyllium husk or sterculia, should be used regularly. Adequate fluid intake (1.5 L in the healthy adult) should be taken in order to allow the additional fibre bulk to work effectively. If this does not soften the stool, then an osmotic laxative such as Epsom salts should be added. Warm baths have a soothing effect and have also been shown to reduce internal sphincter spasm. Recent studies have found that the substance mediating internal sphincter function is nitric oxide. If a nitric oxide donor, such as 0.2% glyceryl trinitrate, is applied to the anal mucosa, this produces rapid internal sphincter relaxation, with improved blood flow in the mucosa and resultant healing of a high proportion of chronic fissures. Treatment should continue for at least four weeks. If the fissure fails to heal with glyceryl trinitrate then inactivated botulinum toxin is injected into the sphincter. This paralyses the muscle for about three months and allows a further proportion of fissures to heal. There is no evidence that other topical agents, including steroids or local anaesthetics, have any effect on fissure healing or pain, and these should be avoided since allergy may occasionally occur. Use of an anal dilator is very painful and should be avoided.

Surgery

Surgery is only indicated if the fissure fails to heal and remains painful despite all the above measures, because a small percentage of patients will develop faecal incontinence after sphincterotomy. The basis of surgical treatment is to disrupt the spasm in the lower part of the internal anal sphincter. Anal dilatation successfully achieves this aim but can lead to incontinence in up to one-quarter of cases, and has therefore been abandoned in favour of the more controlled method of sphincter division (sphincterotomy). Sphincterotomy was initially performed posteriorly together with excision of the fissure, but this may cause a keyhole deformity with resultant seepage of stool. Sphincterotomy is therefore now carried out laterally. It may be done as a closed or open technique, and the recurrence rate is less than 2%.

ANAL SEPSIS

The majority of cases of anal abscess develop from a primary infection in an anal gland (Table 11.2). This infection results in formation of an abscess in the intersphincteric space, which in turn may spread to form a perianal abscess, ischiorectal abscess, or supralevator abscess. If an abscess communicates with the anal canal, and also discharges or is surgically drained through the perianal skin then a fistula has formed. Anal abscess and fistula are therefore part of the same pathological process.

Anatomy

The anal canal is surrounded by two concentric muscle rings. The inner circular layer (internal anal sphincter) consists of smooth muscle, and is formed from the downward continuation of the circular muscle of the rectum. The outer layer (external anal sphincter) consists of striated muscle, which is continuous at its upper border with the levator ani muscle. The space immediately above the levator ani is called the supralevator space. The space between the internal and external sphincters is called the intersphincteric space. On the outer side of the internal sphincter is a layer of longitudinal smooth muscle, which is the downward continuation of the longitudinal muscle of the rectum. This muscle sends strands laterally through the external sphincter to reach the ischiorectal fossa, and infection may spread along this plane.

TABLE 11.2: Aetiology of anal abscess and fistula

1. Primary anal gland infection
2. Secondary abscess:
   - Inflammatory bowel disease
     - Crohn's disease
     - Ulcerative colitis
   - Infection
     - Tuberculosis
     - Actinomycosis
     - Threadworm
   - Trauma
   - Leucopoenia
   - Immunosuppression
     - HIV
     - Drugs
   - Rectal cancer
   - Diabetes mellitus

The lining of the anal canal consists of an upper mucosal half and a lower cutaneous half. The upper mucosal lining may be either stratified cuboidal epithelium or columnar epithelium, and this ends caudally as the dentate (pectinate) line which consists of a series of mucosal folds. Below the dentate line is the cutaneous region, consisting of modified skin containing squamous epithelium with no hairs or sebaceous glands. The mucosa at the junction of the two regions contains four to eight glands, the ducts of which open into the anus at the level of the dentate line. The glands extend into the submucosa where they have several branches, some of which penetrate the internal anal sphincter to end blindly in the intersphincteric space. The glands appear to have no important secretory function, and their significance is that they are the focus of infection, which leads to anal abscess formation.

Pathology

1. Primary anal gland (cryptoglandular) abscess and fistula

Abscess

Infection in an anal gland starts after faecal bacteria gain entry via the anal duct, resulting in an *intersphincteric abscess*. This may then spread:

- downward to the perianal skin to form a perianal abscess;
- upward to the supralevator region to form a supralevator abscess;
- laterally along the longitudinal muscle strands which penetrate the external sphincter, or down and around the lower edge of the internal sphincter, in both cases to reach the ischiorectal fossa to form an ischiorectal abscess (Figure 11.1).

An intersphincteric, ischiorectal or supralevator abscess may spread circumferentially to form a 'horseshoe' abscess.

Microbial culture of pus from an anal abscess yields Gram-negative organisms and anaerobic organisms (mainly *Bacteroides*) originating from the bowel.

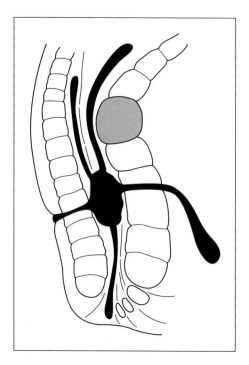

FIGURE 11.1A: Spread of anal infection. Infection starts in an anal gland which leads to an intersphincteric abscess. This may spread downwards, upwards, or outwards across the external sphincter.

(Based on Parks et al, Brit J Surg 1976, 63: 1–12, John Wiley & Sons Ltd, with permission.)

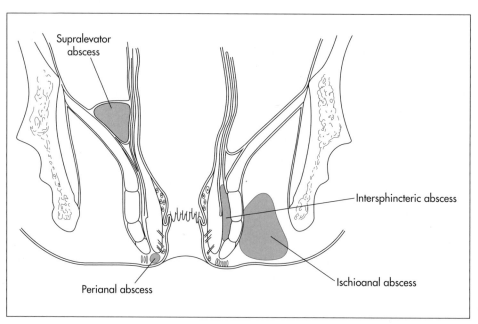

FIGURE 11.1B: Spread of anal infection. As a result of this spread, an abscess forms in a perianal, supralevator or ischiorectal position.

(Based on Gordon and Nivatvongs, Principles and Practice of Surgery for the Colon, Rectum and Anus, 2nd edn, Routledge/Taylor & Francis Group, LLC, with permission.)

A cryptoglandular abscess should be distinguished from:

- an abscess originating in the perianal skin from infection in a hair follicle. Culture of pus shows skin flora, particularly *Staphylococcus aureus,* and the abscess is never associated with an anal fistula;
- hidradenitis suppurativa: apocrine sweat glands are found in the axilla, groin, areola and perianal region. Infection may result in abscess and chronic sinus formation; and
- pilonidal sinus: a pilonidal sinus usually occurs in the natal cleft, beginning as an ingrown hair which results in a chronic infection in the subcutaneous tissues. Occasionally, a pilonidal sinus may occur in the perianal region and appear very similar to a true cryptoglandular abscess or fistula.

Fistula

A cryptoglandular abscess may progress to form a fistula (Figure 11.2).

Intersphincteric fistula (40% of fistulae). This forms from a *perianal abscess* which discharges spontaneously through the perianal skin or is surgically drained through the perianal skin to form a communication between the skin and the anal canal.

Trans-sphincteric fistula (50%). This forms in a similar way to an *ischiorectal abscess.* The fistula encloses a variable amount of external sphincter muscle, and the amount of muscle enclosed will determine the correct surgical treatment.

Suprasphincteric fistula (6%). This forms when a *supralevator abscess* discharges downwards through the levator ani muscle into the ischiorectal fossa and then through the skin.

Extrasphincteric fistula (2%). In most cases there is a history of attempted surgical drainage of a fistula. Iatrogenic damage results from probing an ischiorectal abscess or trans-sphincteric fistula, creating a passage into the rectum instead of along the correct course into the anal canal. Very rarely an extrasphincteric fistula results from spontaneous discharge of a rectal or sigmoid abscess resulting from diverticular disease, Crohn's disease or from perforation of the bowel by a fish or chicken bone.

Subcutaneous fistula (2%). This is a superficial fistula that begins as an abscess in an oedematous skin tag usually associated with an anal fissure. The abscess discharges through the mucosa of the lower anal canal and through the perianal skin to form a small subcutaneous fistula.

2. Secondary abscess and fistula

Inflammatory bowel disease

Crohn's disease is the most common cause of secondary abscess formation, which in turn may lead to fistula formation. Complicated, circuitous or multiple fistulae may form. Ulcerative colitis is a less common cause.

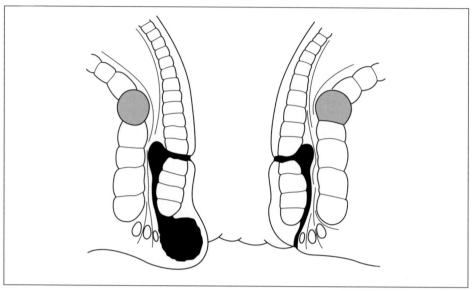

FIGURE 11.2A: Intersphincteric fistula—infection does not cross the external sphincter. Perianal abscess (left) results in the fistula (right). Note that the fistula opens internally in the anal canal at the position of the infected anal gland at the dentate line.

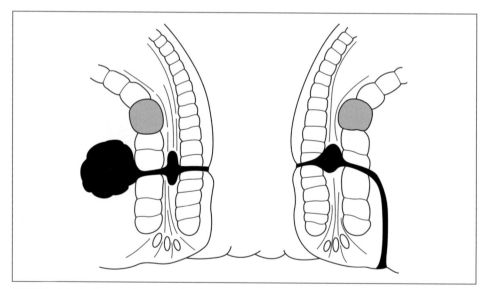

FIGURE 11.2B: Trans-sphincteric fistula—infection crosses the external sphincter to form an ischiorectal abscess (left), which then discharges to form the fistula (right).
(Figures 11.2 A–D based on Parks et al, 1976; 63: 1–12, John Wiley & Sons Ltd, with permission.)

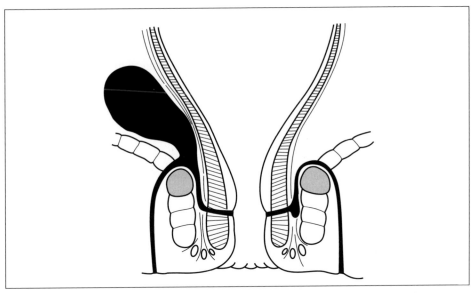

FIGURE 11.2C: Suprasphincteric fistula—infection spreads upwards in the intersphincteric plane to form a supralevator abscess (left) which discharges downwards through the levator ani to reach the ischiorectal fossa and then through the skin to form a fistula.

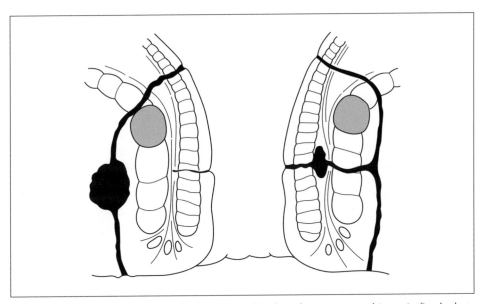

FIGURE 11.2D: Extrasphincteric fistula (right)—develops from a trans-sphincteric fistula that is incorrectly probed so that the probe is pushed upwards through the levator ani into the rectum. Rarely the fistula forms spontaneously from pathology in the rectum (left).

Leucopaenia

Leukaemia or other cause of pancytopaenia may result in anal sepsis. Pain and spreading perianal infection occur. Since there is a paucity of white blood cells, an abscess does *not* form. Treatment is therefore with antibiotics rather than surgical drainage.

Immunosuppression

Drugs causing immunosuppression, or AIDS predispose to infection in the anal glands, with abscess and fistula formation.

Infection

Tuberculosis, actinomycosis and occasionally threadworm infestation may cause abscess formation.

Trauma

Trauma to the rectum by a penetrating injury, or by insertion of a sharp object per anum, may pierce the rectum and cause a supralevator abscess and extrasphincteric fistula.

Rectal carcinoma

Advanced rectal cancer may undergo tissue necrosis and abscess formation, usually in the ischiorectal fossa. Another rare variety of malignant fistula occurs when a rectal cancer seeds malignant cells into an established primary fistula.

Diabetes mellitus

The incidence of diabetes mellitus is higher in patients with anal sepsis than in the rest of the population. Occasionally, anal sepsis is the presenting feature of occult diabetes.

Clinical features

Abscess. The cardinal feature of an anal abscess is severe pain. A perianal abscess usually causes a tender red swelling near the anal verge (Figure 11.3). An ischiorectal abscess is placed more deeply and there is usually less tenderness and swelling, but there may be high fevers if the abscess is large. An intersphincteric abscess produces marked tenderness on digital examination of the anal canal.

    Fistula. Usually the external opening of a fistula is easily identified (Figure 11.4). The position should be noted in order to predict where the internal opening will be found (Figure 11.5). Supralevator extension is easily palpated on digital examination (Figure 11.6).

Principles of surgical treatment

Incorrect surgical treatment of anal sepsis can have devastating consequences, with faecal incontinence resulting from division of excessive amounts of sphincter muscle. An abscess requires immediate drainage. This is best done under general anaesthetic, both for patient comfort as well as to optimally assess the extent of the abscess. An internal opening is found in 30–50% of cases. If an internal opening is not present and culture of pus yields a growth of *Staphylococcus* and other skin flora, then no further treatment is needed. If bowel flora are cultured, then an internal opening may be present and examination under anaesthesia should be carried out 10 to 14 days later. If an internal opening is present at the time of abscess drainage, then the fistula should be laid open (fistulotomy).

An intersphincteric or trans-sphincteric fistula can be laid open if there is sufficient muscle remaining above the fistula track. If the track is too high, or if it is suprasphincteric or extrasphincteric, then it should be treated either with a Seton technique (where a rubber drain is placed around the fistula and gradually tightened, Figure 11.7) or by placing a flap of mucosa and internal muscle to close the internal opening of the fistula.

Recurrent fistula requires careful assessment under anaesthesia, with fistulotomy when appropriate. Intra-anal ultrasound may identify a track that had not been detected during initial surgical treatment. Underlying inflammatory bowel disease should be excluded.

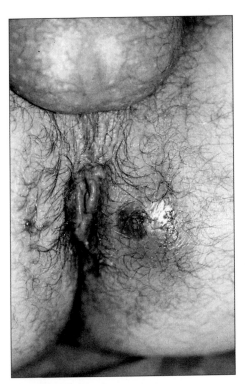

FIGURE 11.3: Perianal abscess.

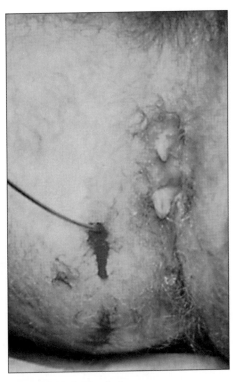

FIGURE 11.4: Fistula-in-ano.

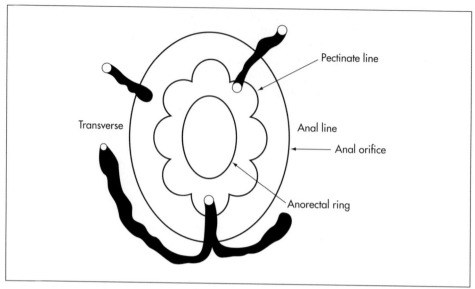

FIGURE 11.5: Goodsall's rule—a posterior fistula passes around to open internally at the posterior midline. An anterior fistula passes radially to open directly at a corresponding internal position.
(Based on Goligher, with permission from Baillière Tindall.)

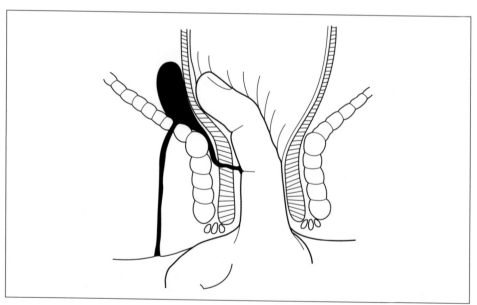

FIGURE 11.6: Supralevator induration is palpated on rectal examination. This indicates proximal extension of an abscess or fistula, and should raise suspicion of a suprasphincteric fistula.
(Based on Parks et al, 1976; 63: 1–12, John Wiley & Sons Ltd, with permission.)

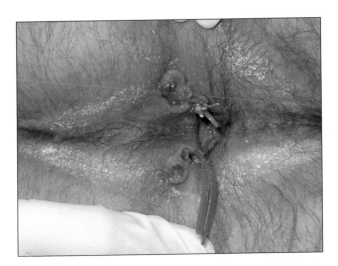

FIGURE 11.7: Multiple external openings from a complex anal fistula. A seton has been placed around the main fistula.

HAEMORRHOIDS (PILES)

Uncomplicated haemorrhoids are usually a painless condition and, although haemorrhoids may cause discomfort, severe anal pain should not be attributed to haemorrhoids unless thrombosis of the haemorrhoids is found.

Anatomy

The submucosa of the anal canal is expanded at three sites to form the submucosal cushions, located in the 3, 7 and 11 o'clock positions. The submucosa is supported by muscle fibres of the musculus submucosae ani. Within the submucosa is a plexus of vessels that joins arteries to veins without capillaries. This plexus of vessels is called the *internal haemorrhoidal plexus* above the dentate line, and the *external haemorrhoidal plexus* below the line.

Pathophysiology

The anal cushions are central to the development of haemorrhoids. During normal defecation there is a slight downward movement of the cushions together with their submucosal vasculature. If there is excessive prolapse or pressure on the cushions, such as occurs with prolonged straining at stool or with hard stools, then the cushions become oedematous and the submucosal vascular plexus becomes engorged. Damage to the musculus submucosae ani caused by chronic straining at stool results in loss of support of the anal cushions, which worsens the prolapse of the cushions. In addition, in the majority of patients with haemorrhoids there is a hypertonic internal sphincter muscle, producing very high intra-anal canal pressure. This leads to trapping of the prolapsing anal cushions outside the sphincter. All these factors result in progressive prolapse, oedema and engorgement of the submucosal plexus of vessels, with rupture of the vessels connecting arteries directly to veins. Bleeding then is bright red.

It can therefore be seen that many traditional theories about the pathophysiology of haemorrhoids are incorrect. Haemorrhoids are not varicose veins of the anal canal, bleeding from which would be venous and hence dark red in colour. Haemorrhoids occur at 3, 7 and 11 o'clock because of the position of the anal cushions, not because the blood supply is distributed mainly at those three sites. Haemorrhoids are not accounted for by a simple rise in venous pressure, and the incidence is no higher in patients with portal hypertension. The incidence of haemorrhoids is higher in men than women, and only slightly higher in parous than nulliparous women, so that pregnancy is not the main causal factor. Similarly, lifting heavy objects or engaging in other strenuous activities does not produce haemorrhoids since there is reflex contraction of the external sphincter muscle during these actions, which supports the anal cushions. Prolonged sitting, or sitting on cold or hard surfaces also has no relation to the development of haemorrhoids.

Clinical features

Bleeding

Bleeding is the most common symptom. The blood is bright red and noted on the toilet paper. When the haemorrhoids prolapse externally beyond the hypertonic internal sphincter then there may be a large amount of blood dripping into the toilet bowl during defecation. Occasionally, there may be streaks of blood on the surface of the stool, but this symptom should always raise suspicion of more serious rectal pathology. When the haemorrhoids are continuously prolapsed then spontaneous bleeding unrelated to defecation may occur with blood seeping through to the clothes. Anaemia uncommonly results from haemorrhoidal bleeding, but may occur with profuse bleeding over a prolonged period.

Prolapse

Haemorrhoids are classified according to the degree of prolapse of the anal cushions:

First degree: Prolapse within the anal canal so that the subject is not aware of any external prolapse. Bleeding is the only symptom.

Second degree: Prolapse outside the anal canal on defecation, with spontaneous reduction immediately after defecation.

Third degree: Prolapse that requires manual reduction. If the patient chooses not to reduce the haemorrhoids, they remain external for some hours and then reduce spontaneously.

Fourth degree: Haemorrhoids that cannot be reduced (Figure 11.8A).

Discomfort

External prolapse of large haemorrhoids may cause discomfort. There may be further discomfort when attempting to reduce the haemorrhoids. Severe pain is only experienced if thrombosis occurs.

Thrombosis

Prolapse beyond the anal sphincter may result in thrombosis. There is swelling and severe pain. The prolapsed haemorrhoids are easily visible and very tender. If thrombosed haemorrhoids are not treated surgically there is usually gradual resolution, but symptoms persist for up to 2–4 weeks. Necrosis and infection may result. Occasionally, thrombosed haemorrhoids may return into the anal canal and are not visible externally, but if thrombosis is established, then severe pain persists and a tender lump is palpated on digital examination.

Incontinence

Minor seepage of faeces or mucus may occur. The perianal skin may become excoriated with resulting pruritus and pain.

Treatment

Initial advice about adequate dietary fibre and fluid intake should be given. This may be supplemented with daily fibre in the form of either unprocessed wheat bran (one tablespoon) or psyllium (two teaspoons), which can be slowly increased. Improved compliance is achieved if written instructions are given. Randomised trials, however, show only a slight advantage of fibre over placebo. Defecation habit should be improved by avoiding excessive straining at stool. The initial call to stool should be obeyed as soon as possible. Taking reading material into the toilet should be strongly discouraged. Adopting the squatting position to defecate does not reduce strain on the anal muscles and there is no evidence that this practice offers protection from developing haemorrhoids.

The majority of patients with symptomatic haemorrhoids will require other treatment. Treatment involves:

- reducing the prolapse of the mucosal cushions containing the haemorrhoids; or
- removal of the haemorrhoids.

Reducing the prolapse is achieved in several ways. The most common method is injection of a solution of 5% phenol in almond oil into the submucosa at the base of the haemorrhoid, 1 cm above the dentate line. This produces fibrosis in the submucosa which stops the haemorrhoid prolapsing and becoming engorged. Injection is suitable for first-degree and small second-degree haemorrhoids. Other methods that prevent prolapse in a similar way, but are used much less commonly, are infrared photocoagulation and cryotherapy.

Larger second-degree haemorrhoids and some third-degree haemorrhoids are treated by rubber band ligation. This involves placing a small rubber band around the base of each haemorrhoid about 1 cm above the dentate line. If the band is placed lower than this within the sensitive zone of the anal mucosa then it produces severe pain. Rubber banding works by two mechanisms: it produces a full-thickness mucosal ulcer, which fixes the base of the anal cushion and prevents prolapse, and it removes the proximal part of the prolapsing anal cushion.

If patients are carefully selected, then 80% will be successfully treated by injection or banding. Less than 5% of patients require haemorrhoidectomy. The indications for haemorrhoidectomy are continued bleeding or prolapse after injection and banding; large third-degree haemorrhoids, particularly where there is a substantial component in the lower sensitive part of the anal canal; or fourth-degree haemorrhoids.

Thrombosed external haemorrhoids

This condition is considered separately. It occurs as a result of thrombosis of the lower part of the external haemorrhoidal plexus of submucosal vessels. The term 'perianal haematoma' is incorrect, since the clot is contained within an endothelial-lined blood vessel and is therefore not a haematoma (Figure 11.8B).

It presents as a characteristic purple, tense, tender haemorrhoid at the anal verge, not extending any distance into the anal canal. It must be clearly distinguished from a prolapsed thrombosed internal haemorrhoid.

If the haemorrhoid is small and the pain level is tolerable, then treatment is conservative with analgesics and warm baths. Resolution will occur in 1–2 weeks. If pain is severe, then the haemorrhoid should be widely incised under local anaesthesia. Rapid relief and full resolution occur if the clot is fully evacuated. Patients should be discouraged from straining at stool, and constipation should be treated with dietary fibre or a bulk-forming laxative (psyllium or sterculia).

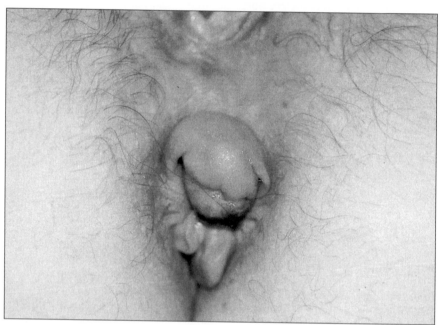

FIGURE 11.8A: Strangulated haemorrhoid.

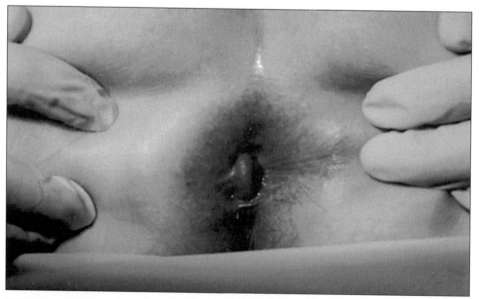

FIGURE 11.8B: Thrombosed external haemorrhoid.

PRURITUS ANI

Pruritus ani is a common condition varying from mild itching to severe intractable itching and pain. The true prevalence is unknown since many sufferers do not seek medical advice, but one study found that 45% of people surveyed had symptoms of pruritus within a 5-year period.

Aetiology

In a minority of cases a definite cause is found. The majority of cases are idiopathic. In those cases where the perianal skin is cracked and excoriated, the cause for the itch and pain is obvious; but in many cases the perianal skin appears normal and the precise cause for the itching is unknown.

Predisposing causes

Faecal seepage. Minor degrees of soiling may cause irritation of the perianal skin. Underlying anal pathology such as haemorrhoids, mucosal prolapse or anal fissure should be identified and treated. Some patients are not aware that minor seepage is occurring.

Anal disease. Primary anal conditions must always be excluded. These include anal warts, skin tags, haemorrhoids, fissure, fistula, anal cancer, Bowen's disease, and generalised skin conditions such as eczema and psoriasis, which may also affect the perianal skin.

Infection. Organisms known to be associated with pruritus ani include:

- fungi—*Candida albicans*, tinea;
- bacteria—*Corynebacterium minutissimum*; and
- parasites—threadworm (*Enterobius vermicularis*), a common cause in children but a rare cause in adults.

Allergy. Hypersensitivity of the perianal skin may result from:

- topical creams or suppositories containing steroids or local anaesthetic agents; and
- underwear, particularly nylon; washing powders for clothing.

Management

Pruritus ani is a difficult condition to treat and several steps must be followed if success is to be achieved.

1. A careful history about symptoms of local pathology and faecal seepage should be obtained. Examination for local pathology is made and any condition which predisposes to seepage is treated. Threadworms are seen at the anal verge or in the anal canal and are treated with a single dose of pyrantel.

2. If the skin is excoriated then scrapings are obtained for microscopic examination and culture. A scalpel blade is used and several scrapings are placed onto a glass slide which is sealed in a container. If *Candida* is present, then topical nystatin cream is used. Tolnaftate is used for tinea.

3. If there has been a recent change to nylon underwear or a change of washing powder, then these should be eliminated as a cause.

4. If no predisposing cause is found, then idiopathic pruritus ani is present. Vigorous efforts at perianal hygiene are needed since seepage and collection of moisture are sometimes present. Washing the area once or twice daily may not be adequate. Washing may need to occur at least three to four times daily. Thereafter, the area is dabbed dry (Table 11.3).

TABLE 11.3: Instructions to patients with anal irritation (pruritus ani)

1. The area must be kept clean and dry. This means cleaning as instructed below at least three times in the day and once at night, and after every bowel action. It is not sufficient to clean once or twice a day only.
   a. Use soft toilet paper only.
   b. Wipe the area with cotton wool and warm water. 'Baby wipes' can be used if preferred.
   c. Gently dab the area completely dry with soft toilet paper.
   d. Apply a zinc oxide powder to the area. Smooth the powder onto the skin. Do not use other powders, or any cream or ointment unless prescribed by your doctor.

2. Use a pH-balanced soap for bathing or showering.

3. Do not scratch the skin. If irritation is severe, pinch the skin outside the clothes.

4. If there is minor seepage of mucus or bowel motion, report this at your next visit.

5. Continue treatment strictly for three months after the itching stops, or the irritation may return.

CHRONIC PERIANAL PAIN SYNDROMES

There are a number of conditions of uncertain aetiology that produce chronic perianal and pelvic pain. They may produce significant morbidity, and treatment is often unsuccessful.

Coccygodynia

This presents with an ache in the lower sacrum and coccyx. The pain may radiate to the buttocks and is worse on sitting. Eighty percent of cases are in women, usually over 50 years of age. Sometimes there is a history of trauma to the coccyx. X-ray findings are normal. Rocking the coccyx on rectal examination may elicit pain.

Treatment

Local points of tenderness are infiltrated with local anaesthetic; the injection of alcohol or phenol has been reported to be successful in up to 50% of cases. This treatment is best carried out in a specialised pain clinic. Coccygectomy is usually unsuccessful.

Proctalgia fugax

This is an unmistakable clinical condition, most commonly affecting young men, although it occurs at all ages, consisting of severe pain in the anal canal or slightly higher in the pelvis, lasting 5–30 minutes. It may occur during the day or night, sometimes waking the sufferer. It is occasionally relieved by flexing the thighs up against the chest. The pain is not relieved by inducing a bowel action with suppositories. The frequency of episodes varies from a few times weekly to once every few months. It is thought to be due to spasm in the levator ani muscles.

Treatment

There is no effective treatment. The hip flexion manoeuvre should be attempted. Galvanic electrostimulation of the puborectalis muscle has been reported to be successful, but this technique is not widely available. Patients should be reassured that there is no serious pathology in the rectum.

Descending perineum syndrome

Abnormal descent of the pelvic floor as a clinical sign was first recognised in 1970, and a clinical syndrome consisting of pelvic discomfort or pain, abnormal perineal (pelvic floor) descent, marked difficulty with defecation (obstructed defecation), and straining at stool was subsequently described. The pain is felt as a dull ache in the anal area and perineum, sometimes worse after defecation.

There are a variety of clinical conditions in which perineal descent and straining at stool are found including haemorrhoids, neurogenic faecal incontinence, urinary stress incontinence, solitary rectal ulcer syndrome, uterovaginal prolapse, and rectocoele. This group of conditions arises as a result of a functional obstruction to rectal evacuation, which causes excessive straining during defecation.

The importance of this concept is that treatment of any of these conditions (e.g., haemorrhoidectomy) often will not cure the anal pain, which is caused by pelvic muscle weakness rather than by the associated condition. It is therefore important to decide in each case whether the pain is due to the muscle weakness or to the associated condition, such as the haemorrhoids. Treatment should be directed at changing defecation habits and avoiding straining at stool.

Levator ani syndrome

This condition presents with intermittent pain, generally lasting up to an hour, but sometimes persisting through the day. It is usually felt in the anorectal region but sometimes slightly higher in the pelvis. It is associated with a history of straining at stool, a feeling of incomplete rectal evacuation. The condition is distinct from the descending perineum syndrome since there are no signs of perineal descent or pelvic floor muscle weakness in the levator ani syndrome.

Treatment

Treatment is difficult but should be directed to encouraging the patient to avoid straining at stool. Initial treatment is with *biofeedback therapy*, in which patients are taught to evacuate the rectum by contracting the abdominal muscles effectively while relaxing the anal sphincter muscles. Muscle function is demonstrated to the patient during biofeedback using pressure sensors.

Idiopathic perianal and perineal pain

Sometimes called perineal neuralgia, this is a condition of unknown aetiology affecting women in 80% of cases. The pain is characteristic and usually easily diagnosed on history; it is described as constant and unremitting, often with a feeling in the perineum like 'sitting on a ball'. In 75% of cases, the pain has been found to radiate into various places from its position of maximal intensity in the anal area, including the sacrum, pelvis and back of the thighs. In 50% of cases the pain is exacerbated when sitting. It is not worse during defecation. Patients have often undergone a variety of unsuccessful operations in the anal area including excision of skin tags, anal dilatation or treatment of haemorrhoids.

The cause of the pain is unknown. Clinical examination of the anal area and pelvic floor muscles, the pelvic gynaecological organs, and neurological examination provide normal findings. Investigations including X-ray examination of the spine and sacrum, and endoscopic examination of the rectum and sigmoid are all unhelpful. A neuralgia affecting the sacral or pudendal nerves has been postulated. Pelvic nerve ischaemia has also been considered. Although the absence of any weakness of the pelvic floor muscles is against the neuralgia hypothesis, it is possible that the injury is not sufficiently severe to lead to muscle weakness.

Management of chronic pain conditions

It is very important to exclude other causes of chronic pain, including chronic intersphincteric or supralevator abscess, endometriosis of the pelvis or rectovaginal septum, and pelvic or spinal lesions compressing the sacral plexus. A CT scan of the pelvis and CT myelography of the lumbosacral area should be carried out. To ensure that none of the above is overlooked, the diagnosis should be confirmed by a specialist. Treatment is very unsatisfactory. Standard analgesics or tricyclic antidepressants are usually not effective. Anticonvulsant drugs have been tried, without success. Transcutaneous or spinal cord stimulation has had poor results. Psychological counselling is sometimes required to assist the patient to cope with the pain.

Further reading

Allan A, Samad AJ, Mellon A, Marshall T. Prospective randomised study of urgent haemorroidectomy compared with non-operative treatment in the management of prolapsed thrombosed internal haemorrhoids. *Colorectal Dis* 2006; 8: 41–5.

Hancock BD. Anal fissures and fistulas. *Brit Med J* 1992; 304: 904–7.

Hancock BD. Haemorrhoids. *Brit Med J* 1992; 304: 1042–4.

Heard S. Pruritis ani. *Aust Fam Physician* 2004; 33: 511–3.

Keighley MRB. Anorectal abscess. In: Keighley MRB, Williams NS (eds), *Surgery of the Anus, Rectum and Colon*. London: WB Saunders, 1993: 397–417.

Lawler LP, Fleshman JW. Hemorrhoids. In: Pemberton JH, Swash M, Henry MM (eds), *The Pelvic Floor: its Function and Disorders*. London: WB Saunders, 2002: 371–84.

Loder PB, Kamm MA, Nicholls RJ, Phillips RK. Haemorrhoids: pathology, pathophysiology and aetiology. *Brit J Surg* 1994; 81: 946–54.

Lubowski DZ. Anal fissures. *Aust Fam Physician* 2000; 29: 839–44.

Mazier WP. Hemorrhoids, fissures, and pruritis ani. *Surg Clin Nth Am* 1994; 74: 1277–92.

Parks AG, Gordon PH, Hardcastle JD. A classification of fistula-in-ano. *Brit J Surg* 1976; 63: 1–12.

chapter 12

ACUTE DIARRHOEA

INTRODUCTION

Diarrhoea remains a common problem around the world in both developing and industrialised countries. It is usually mild and self-limiting but may develop into an overwhelming life-threatening illness. It is arbitrarily defined as acute if it is of less than two weeks duration.

Definition

Diarrhoea is defined as a change in bowel habit with an increase in stool frequency or fluidity or both. It is the change from normal for that individual that is significant, with a normal range being from one bowel motion every three days to three times daily.

Normal physiology

In the non-fasting state, approximately 9 L of fluid pass into the small intestine, of which only 1–2 L pass into the colon and 100 mL is present in the stool. The colon has an absorptive capacity of 3–5 L a day, and an ileal flow of greater than this will result in diarrhoea.

Water is absorbed passively in both the small and large intestine because of an osmotic gradient created by active sodium transport. The co-transport of glucose with sodium in the small intestine has been well documented. Both sodium and glucose must be bound to the carrier before transport can occur. Active transport is promoted by a Na^+ gradient created by a Na/K ATP-ase in the basolateral membrane. Co-transport of other sugars and amino acids in the small intestine is also recognised. Advantage can be taken of these co-transport systems by using oral rehydration solutions containing both sodium and glucose to enhance water absorption in patients with diarrhoea.

Pathophysiology

The pathophysiological mechanisms resulting in acute or chronic diarrhoea can be divided into major groups: osmotic, secretory, exudative and abnormal motility (see Table 12.1).

Osmotic diarrhoea results when a non-absorbable solute accumulates within the small intestine. The osmolality of the small intestine is adjusted to that of plasma by water influx across the small bowel and watery diarrhoea results. Examples of osmotic diarrhoea include carbohydrate malabsorption (such as lactase deficiency) and ingestion of magnesium salts. Osmotic diarrhoea ceases when the poorly absorbed solute is removed from the diet.

Secretory diarrhoea results from reduced ion absorption or increased intestinal ion secretion. Bacterial toxins are a common cause, and of these, cholera toxin has been the most intensively studied. Non-osmotic laxatives, bile salts and short chain fatty acids are other agents that can damage electrolyte transport and result in watery diarrhoea. Hormonal secretion from tumours can also cause secretory diarrhoea (e.g., gastrin, vasoactive intestinal polypeptide).

TABLE 12.1: Pathophysiological mechanisms in diarrhoea

1. Osmotic (non-absorbable solute)
- Carbohydrate malabsorption
- Magnesium salts
- Lactulose
- Sorbitol
- Malabsorption syndromes
- Postsurgical, e.g., gastrojejunostomy

2. Secretory (impaired electrolyte transport)
- Bacterial endotoxins
- Laxatives (non-osmotic)
- Bile salts (e.g., terminal ileal resection or disease)
- Fatty acids
- Hormone-producing tumours (e.g., gastrinoma, vasoactive intestinal polypeptide)

3. Exudative (intestinal mucosal damage)
- Bacterial/viral/parasitic infections
- Inflammatory bowel disease
- Colonic cancer
- Gluten-sensitive enteropathy
- Drug-induced colitis
- Irradiation
- Ischaemia
- Diverticulitis

4. Motility (increased transit)
- Laxative abuse
- Diabetic diarrhoea
- Thyrotoxicosis
- Irritable bowel syndrome

The third major pathophysiological cause of diarrhoea is inflammatory damage to intestinal mucosal cells: *exudative diarrhoea*. When the large bowel is involved, blood is commonly present in the stool. Apart from invasive organisms, mucosal damage may result from inflammatory bowel disease, gluten-sensitive enteropathy and irradiation damage.

The fourth major cause is increased transit in the small bowel or colon: *abnormal intestinal motility*. Increased transit may occur with thyrotoxicosis (due to excess thyroid hormone), diabetes mellitus or in the irritable bowel syndrome (Chapter 6).

It is common for a single agent to cause diarrhoea by more than one patho-physiological mechanism. For example, malabsorbed carbohydrates are fermented in the colon to short chain fatty acids, which impair colonic absorption of the water and electrolytes. Similarly, invasive enteric bacteria may also secrete toxins resulting in secretory diarrhoea.

Some generalisations can be made about clinical syndromes arising from different pathophysiological causes of diarrhoea. Osmotic diarrhoea will usually stop when the poorly absorbed solute is omitted from the diet. Secretory diarrhoea will usually continue during fasting and the stools are of large volume (> 1 L). Invasive organisms will cause inflammation, which often results in blood in the stool. However, considerable overlap exists, such as when secretory diarrhoea results from laxatives. This may cease during fasting if the laxative is also omitted. Similarly, diarrhoea due to invasive organisms may begin as watery diarrhoea when the inflammation is mild.

CLINICAL APPROACH TO ACUTE DIARRHOEA

The causes of diarrhoea vary depending on the type of practice, but in all settings gastrointestinal infections are a common cause of acute diarrhoea (Table 12.2). It is clinically useful to divide acute causes of diarrhoea into clinical syndromes, watery (non-inflammatory) diarrhoea, bloody (inflammatory) diarrhoea, food poisoning, diarrhoea in the traveller, diarrhoea associated with recent antibiotic or other drug use and diarrhoea in the HIV-positive or male homosexual patient. Overlap may occur between the categories. Of course, an illness may begin as watery diarrhoea, only to progress to bloody diarrhoea later.

The clinical approach to those with acute diarrhoea should focus initially on:

- separating minor from severe illness;
- selecting patients who need further investigation; and
- instituting specific therapy, where appropriate.

History

A careful history is important in evaluating patients with acute diarrhoea and in separating minor from severe illness. Features that suggest the diarrhoea may not be self-limiting include severe diarrhoea, blood in the stool, severe abdominal pain or a high fever (Table 12.2).

TABLE 12.2: Features favouring medically important diarrhoea

- Severe prolonged diarrhoea
- High fever/systemic toxicity
- Severe abdominal pain
- Blood in the stool
- Signs of volume depletion
- Immunocompromised host

Ask about the duration of symptoms as well as severity. An abrupt onset of diarrhoea, which then gradually improves suggests an infective process. Systemic features with infectious diarrhoea include fever, myalgia, malaise, nausea and vomiting. The onset of diarrhoea with food poisoning is often severe but short lived. With prolonged watery diarrhoea, volume depletion is more likely to develop, especially when there is associated vomiting. Large volume watery diarrhoea may be of small bowel origin. The presence of blood in the stool is usually due to an intestinal inflammatory process (see Table 12.3).

TABLE 12.3: Causes of acute watery and bloody diarrhoea

---

1. Acute watery diarrhoea

- Gastrointestinal infections
  - Protozoal, e.g., *Giardia*
  - Bacterial, e.g., enterotoxigenic *Escherichia coli*, cholera
  - Viral, e.g., rotavirus, Norwalk virus
- Drugs
- Toxins
- Dietary constituents (e.g., lactose intolerance)
- Onset of chronic diarrhoeal illness

2. Acute bloody diarrhoea

- Infectious colitis
  - Confluent proctocolitis (e.g., *Shigella*, *Campylobacter*, *Salmonella*, *Entamoeba histolytica*)
  - Segmental colitis (e.g., *Campylobacter*, *Salmonella*, enteroinvasive *E. coli*, *Aeromonas*, *E. histolytica*)
- Drug-induced colitis (e.g., non-steroidal anti-inflammatory drugs [NSAIDs])
- Inflammatory bowel disease
- Ischaemic colitis (usually elderly patient with underlying heart disease or arrhythmias)
- Antibiotic-associated colitis

The setting in which diarrhoea occurs also provides clues as to the diagnosis. Recent travel or consumption of food eaten from fast-food outlets suggests infective diarrhoea or food poisoning, especially if other members of the party are affected. A drug history is important with particular attention to antibiotics (*Clostridium difficile* infection), over-the-counter and herbal preparations. A dietary history including dairy products (lactose intolerance) and sorbitol ingestion may be helpful.

Chronic illnesses may first present with acute diarrhoea. Recent bloody diarrhoea, for example, may be the initial onset of inflammatory bowel disease.

Physical examination

The physical examination will help assess the effects of the diarrhoeal illness and may provide clues as to its cause.

Effects may include volume depletion (dry mouth, orthostatic hypertension) and signs of toxicity (high fever, tachycardia, shock).

The abdominal examination may reveal tenderness (inflammatory bowel disease, diverticulitis) a mass or visceromegaly (e.g., colon cancer deposits in the liver). The stool should be examined and the presence of blood noted. A rectal examination is mandatory and may document faecal impaction (overflow diarrhoea in the elderly) or a tumour.

Investigations

The history and physical examination will help differentiate those with minor diarrhoea from those with a more severe illness.

Those with minor resolving diarrhoea need no investigations and no specific therapy beyond maintenance of hydration. Those with features outlined in Table 12.2, where a definitive diagnosis is likely to alter management and outcome, should usually be further investigated. The diagnostic tests should be targeted, where possible, towards a specific diagnosis according to clues from the history and physical examination.

Blood screen

A full blood count may document anaemia secondary to underlying disease or neutrophilia in bacterial infections. Atypical lymphocytes may be noted in viral illnesses.

The creatinine and urea may be elevated in severe diarrhoea with volume depletion.

Stool examination

The presence of red or white cells helps to differentiate inflammatory from non-inflammatory causes of diarrhoea, although the specificity and sensitivity are variable.

Stool cultures are often useful in patients with severe or prolonged acute diarrhoea to help target those who may respond to specific antibiotic therapy.

Specific testing for various pathogens should be requested where appropriate. If the epidemiological settings suggest the possibility of *C. difficile* infection, a specific request for that pathogen as well as *C. difficile* toxin should be made. Viral cultures may need to be considered in immunocompromised patients.

Sigmoidoscopy and colonoscopy

Sigmoidoscopy and biopsy will help establish the presence or absence of colitis and histology may help differentiate between infectious colitis and an initial attack of inflammatory bowel disease. However the two can sometimes be difficult to differentiate on histology alone.

A colonoscopy is usually not needed in the work-up of acute diarrhoea. The presence of bleeding with a normal sigmoidoscopy or the suspicion of ischaemic colitis are situations in which colonoscopy may need to be considered.

THERAPY

Acute diarrhoeal illnesses range from minor self-limited episodes of diarrhoea to devastating illnesses with overwhelming sepsis and profound dehydration. Therapy will need to be tailored depending on the severity of the illness, the nature of the underlying aetiology and the competence of the host's defence mechanism.

Hospitalisation is usually necessary for those with sepsis or severe dehydration, and should be considered for those who have an impaired immune response.

Hydration

Maintenance of adequate hydration is the only treatment necessary for the majority of episodes of acute diarrhoea. In the presence of nausea, this may require the frequent intake of small amounts of fluid orally. Soups and fruit juice will usually supply the sodium, potassium and glucose necessary for adequate fluid absorption. Oral rehydration solutions are available commercially or can be prescribed, and are used for mild-to-moderate dehydration. Oral rehydration solutions play an important role in developing countries where gastrointestinal infections are common and medical facilities are limited. Intravenous fluids are indicated for severe dehydration.

Diet

The tradition of limiting food during intakes of diarrhoea carries the disadvantage of restricting caloric intake during a catabolic event. Restriction of milk and milk products is usually indicated as secondary lactase deficiency may be present. Products containing sorbitol, including some fruit juices, will exacerbate diarrhoea and are best avoided. Anorexia is obviously a factor during diarrhoeal illnesses, but the maintenance of caloric intake should be encouraged.

Antidiarrhoeal agents

Agents such as loperamide and diphenoxylate are widely used for symptomatic relief of diarrhoea. They are usually effective and have few side effects. However, they should be avoided in patients with colitis in view of the potential to cause toxic megacolon. They should also be avoided in young children as they are usually ineffective and may prolong intestinal recovery.

Antibiotics

Antibiotics should be avoided in the routine treatment of acute diarrhoea. They are usually ineffective in reducing the duration of the illnesses and in some cases may prolong excretion of the pathogen. They also have significant side effects and indiscriminate use will increase drug resistance. There are a limited number of situations where antibiotics may be helpful. Table 12.4 outlines the indication for antibiotics and these are discussed in more detail under disease headings.

TABLE 12.4: Indication for antibiotics

- *Shigella* spp.
- *Salmonella* spp.
  - Extraintestinal infections
  - Associated toxicity
  - Predisposed individuals
- *Campylobacter jejuni*—prolonged or severe infection
- *Clostridium difficile* infection
- *Giardia lamblia*
- *Entamoeba histolytica*
- Travellers' diarrhoea—moderate to severe symptoms
- *Yersinia enterocolitica*

CONDITIONS CAUSING FOOD-BORNE ILLNESSES

Food-borne illnesses are caused by the consumption of contaminated food and result in significant worldwide morbidity and mortality. They can be caused by the consumption of bacteria or bacterial toxins, viruses, parasites or chemicals.

Clinical syndromes resulting from such diverse aetiological agents vary, but nausea, vomiting, diarrhoea and abdominal pain are common to most. Neurologic, hepatic and renal syndromes may also occur. The rapid onset of symptoms (within six hours) suggests ingestion of a preformed toxin. A longer incubation period is associated with bacterial or viral agents.

Some of the common causes of food-borne illnesses are discussed below under aetiological headings.

Bacterial food poisoning

Common causes of food-borne illnesses include *Salmonella*, *Campylobacter* and *Escherichia coli*—these are discussed later in this chapter. Other major bacterial causes of food-borne illnesses are discussed below.

Clostridium perfringens

C. perfringens is a common food-borne pathogen with an incubation period of 8–24 hours. The illness usually results from the ingestion of meat or poultry and results in watery diarrhoea and crampy abdominal pain. The symptoms are short-lived and usually last 24 hours. Symptomatic therapy with attention to hydration is usually all that is necessary.

C. perfringens may also cause a severe and often fatal illness—enteritis necroticans or pigbel—which is seen only in under-developed tropical countries. Abdominal pain and bloating, vomiting and diarrhoea with shock occur usually after a feast.

Staphylococcus aureus

Staphyloccocal food poisoning results in profuse vomiting, followed by crampy abdominal pain and diarrhoea. These symptoms result from staphylococcal toxins and occur 1–6 hours after the ingestion of contaminated food. Symptomatic therapy only is necessary with recovery occurring within 24–28 hours, although occasional deaths have been reported.

Bacillus cereus

Food poisoning with *B. cereus* is associated with two distinct syndromes: a vomiting syndrome and a diarrhoeal syndrome. Ingestion of a preformed toxin will result in vomiting similar to that of *S. aureus* lasting about 12 hours. Fried rice has been implicated as the vehicle in the majority of cases. The diarrhoeal illness occurs 6–14 hours after ingestion of contaminated food and results from the production of an enterotoxin. Diarrhoea, crampy abdominal pain and, less commonly, vomiting last for 20–36 hours.

Vibrio parahaemolyticus

V. parahaemolyticus is associated with seafood and causes food poisoning outbreaks after ingestion of shellfish or raw fish. It causes an explosive watery diarrhoea with an incubation period of 12–24 hours. The diarrhoea may be associated with nausea and vomiting and fever occurs in about 25% of patients. Occasionally, a dysenteric syndrome may result with bloody diarrhoea. Symptoms are generally short-lived and require no specific therapy.

Clostridium botulinum

C. botulinum produces a heat-labile neurotoxin and outbreaks of food-borne botulism have been reported from ingesting home preserved foods that have been improperly prepared.

Symptoms usually begin within 12–24 hours and consist of bilateral cranial neuropathy with symmetrical descending paralysis. The diagnosis is made by demonstrating the toxin in serum, stool or food ingested.

Respiratory support may be necessary and an anti-toxin is available, which can prevent further paralysis. Full recovery may take months.

Non-bacterial food-borne illnesses

Heavy metals including zinc, iron, tin, copper and cadmium can cause gastric irritation with abdominal pain, nausea and vomiting. Poisoning usually results from storage of food or beverages in metal containers.

Neurotoxin food-poisoning syndromes can be caused by Scombroid fish, ciguatera fish (see below) shellfish and mushrooms.

Viral (hepatitis A) and parasitic (*Trichinella spiralis* and *Giardia lamblia*) food poisoning are further examples of non-bacterial food-borne illnesses.

Ciguatera fish poisoning

Results from the ingestion of fish containing a neurotoxin, which originates in algae. Symptoms begin within 5 minutes to 30 hours and consist of nausea, vomiting, diarrhoea as well as photophobia, blurred vision and paraesthesia. Bradycardia, heart block and hypotension may also occur. No specific antidote is known.

TRAVELLERS' DIARRHOEA

International travel is now a common event and, of those travelling to developing countries, between 30 and 50% will develop diarrhoea. Symptoms are generally short-lived but carry the potential to disrupt a well planned holiday excursion or business trip. Pre-travel advice should include recommendations for prevention as well as treatment.

Aetiology and transmission

Travellers' diarrhoea is predominantly due to gastrointestinal infective illnesses, with an enteropathogen being documented in up to 80% of cases (Table 12.5). Causes vary considerably with country of destination, but the commonest pathogen isolated in most studies is enterotoxigenic *E. coli*, which accounts for up to 50% of travellers' diarrhoea. In about 20% of cases no pathogen is isolated and this group may represent known pathogens not identified due to insensitive or inadequate culture technique, unknown pathogens or non-infectious causes of diarrhoea, such as stress, alcohol and medications.

Travellers' diarrhoea is acquired through the ingestion of contaminated food or water. Enteropathogens may be found in tap water, ice, dairy products, vegetables, unpeeled fruit and raw shellfish. Contaminated food is the most important cause of travellers' diarrhoea, although waterborne transmission also occurs.

TABLE 12.5: Aetiology of travellers' diarrhoea

Escherichia coli	50%
Shigella spp.	10%
Salmonella spp.	5%
Campylobacter jejuni	3%
Yersinia enterocolitica	2%
Entamoeba histolytica	1%
Giardia lamblia	4%
Cryptosporidium spp.	3%
Viruses	3%
Unknown	19%

Clinical manifestations

The onset of travellers' diarrhoea is usually abrupt, with symptoms beginning within 3–4 days of arrival at the country of destination. Typically, the illness is mild with less than six bowel actions daily and it lasts for 3–4 days in 85% of untreated sufferers. Occasionally, symptoms may be more severe with profuse watery diarrhoea leading to dehydration, or are associated with a high fever and blood in the stool. The presence of blood suggests invasive disease (see conditions causing acute bloody diarrhoea).

Prevention

Diet. The logical approach to prevention is to avoid ingesting enteropathogenic agents. Hence, common advice to travellers is to avoid tap water, raw shellfish, dairy products, uncooked vegetables, unpeeled fruit and eating from street vendors (boil it, cook it, peel it or forget it). Unfortunately, studies examining the efficacy of these recommendations have failed to demonstrate that they significantly reduce the incidence of diarrhoea. This is partly because it is difficult to follow such strict dietary advice when on holidays and partly because enteropathogens can be found in food from five-star hotels, bottled drinks and food too hot to touch. Nevertheless, it remains prudent to avoid foods that obviously carry a higher risk of contamination.

Antibiotics. Antibiotics have been documented to be of value in reducing the incidence of diarrhoea when taken prophylactically. A wide range of antibiotics, including sulfonamides, doxycycline, cotrimoxazole, ciprofloxacin and rifaximin (not available in Australia) have been shown to reduce the attack rate for travellers' diarrhoea by 30–85%. Despite this efficacy, routine prophylaxis cannot be recommended as travellers' diarrhoea is usually self-limited and effective treatment is available. Also, side effects may occur and drug resistance will undoubtedly increase if millions of travellers take antibiotics each year. Exceptions to this rule may include those especially inconvenienced by travellers' diarrhoea or those who are at risk of severe illness, such as those immunocompromised or those with impaired gastric acidity.

Investigations

Mild resolving diarrhoea does not require investigation. The presence of blood in the stool, high fever or severe watery diarrhoea should prompt stool cultures and examination, as noted under investigation of acute diarrhoea.

Treatment

Hydration

The only treatment necessary for the majority of sufferers of travellers' diarrhoea is maintenance of adequate hydration. Proprietary rehydration solutions or fruit juice and soups with added salt will help replace sodium, potassium and fluid losses.

Antibiotics

Antibiotics have been shown to be effective in shortening the length of the illness and should be considered in those with moderate-to-severe symptoms. Norfloxacin, ciprofloxacin, doxycycline, cotrimoxazole and rifaximin (a non-absorbable antibiotic) have all been shown to be effective.

Antidiarrhoeal agents

Agents such as loperamide or diphenoxylate are widely used for symptomatic relief of symptoms, although there is limited evidence available to show that they shorten the course of the illness. In addition, in some settings they may prolong excretion of pathogens and should be avoided in those who have bloody diarrhoea, severe abdominal pain, a high fever, and in children.

Medical advice

Medical advice should be sought in those with bloody diarrhoea, persisting severe symptoms, severe abdominal pain or a high fever not responding to antibiotics.

CONDITIONS CAUSING ACUTE WATERY DIARRHOEA

1. *Giardia lamblia*

Giardia lamblia is a flagellated protozoan. It exists as a trophozoite, the active form, and as a cyst, the inactive form. The trophozoites multiply by binary fission and encyst as they pass down the intestine. The cystic form is shed in the stool and can survive in the environment.

G. *lamblia* has a worldwide distribution and transmission is by way of contaminated water or food when large outbreaks may occur, or by direct person-to-person spread. The latter is common in daycare centres and various institutions.

Clinical manifestations

Ingestion of *G. lamblia* cysts results in a spectrum of symptoms, ranging from asymptomatic cyst passage to an acute diarrhoeal illness or chronic diarrhoea with malabsorption. After an incubation period of 1–2 weeks, a minority of patients will develop a symptomatic infection with prolonged passage of cysts. Those who develop symptoms will report watery diarrhoea with crampy abdominal pain, nausea and excessive flatus. The stools are often malodorous and may develop typical features of malabsorption, becoming greasy, bulky, pale and floating. The symptoms usually settle after 1–3 weeks but prolonged infection with marked weight loss has been reported. Blood and pus are not found in the stool and fever is not a feature of the illness.

Diagnosis

A stool examination for cysts is relatively simple but not very sensitive—even examination of three samples yields a positive diagnosis in only 50–70% of cases. Duodenal aspiration and duodenal mucosal biopsies are accurate in 95% of cases, but are relatively invasive for what is usually a self-limited illness. Immunoassay kits have now been developed which have a sensitivity and specificity range of 90–100%. In practice, a therapeutic trial of metronidazole or tinidazole is more often carried out.

Treatment

Metronidazole or tinidazole remains the treatment of choice and can be administered as a single dose. Albendazole has also been reported to have a high efficacy in children. Treatment failures are uncommon but persisting infection can be treated with repeated courses or prolonged therapy. Treatment of other members of the family may be necessary to prevent person-to-person spread.

2. Cholera

Cholera is a severe diarrhoeal illness due to *Vibrio cholerae*, a Gram-negative bacterium that elaborates an enterotoxin. It is endemic in Asia and Africa, from where pandemics spread around the world. The high mortality rate (which can exceed 50% if untreated) is due to dehydration. Stool output can exceed 1 L per hour and death may result within 2–3 hours of the onset of the illness. There are two major biotypes of cholera: 'classical' and El tor. They cause a similar clinical illness, although the El tor infection tends to be milder.

Pathogenesis

Cholera organisms elaborate an enterotoxin composed of five binding (B) subunits and an active (A1) subunit. The B subunits bind to a specific receptor on the enterocyte surface. The A subunit then becomes internalised into the cell membrane and irreversibly activates adenylate cyclase on the inner cell membrane. This results in a continuing conversion of ATP to cAMP, and raised intracellular levels of cAMP change net absorption of fluids into the small intestine into net excretion. Fluid loss from the small intestine results and diarrhoea occurs when the capacity of the colon to absorb excess fluid is overwhelmed.

'Rice water' stools may result and the purging action of the diarrhoea clears all pigment from the stool which then becomes clear fluid with flecks of mucus.

Clinical features

There is a spectrum of clinical manifestations from asymptomatic carrier state or mild diarrhoea through to massive faecal fluid loss with hypovolaemic shock. Symptoms usually begin with abdominal discomfort leading to cramping abdominal pain. This is followed by diarrhoea that increases rapidly, reaching faecal outputs of 15–20 L per 24 hours in some patients. These large volume rice water stools become isotonic with plasma. Vomiting may also occur compounding severe dehydration. There is a significant mortality associated with untreated cholera infection due to hypovolaemic shock.

Diagnosis

The diagnosis is made by stool culture using appropriate culture media. A presumptive diagnosis may be made by examining stools under dark field or phase microscopy, where Vibrios display a typical 'shooting star' motility.

Treatment

The treatment of cholera involves adequate fluid replacement. The glucose/sodium co-transport system is not affected by the cholera toxin and oral rehydration solutions may be adequate for mild-to-moderate dehydration. Patients with more severe dehydration or persisting vomiting will require intravenous fluids. Hypokalaemia may be severe necessitating oral or intravenous replacement. Bicarbonate is required when acidosis supervenes. Antibiotics are not used for the standard treatment of cholera, but have been shown to reduce fluid losses and marginally reduce the time of excretion of Vibrio organisms.

3. Viral infections

Occurrence and transmission

Viral gastroenteritis has become recognised as a common cause of diarrhoea in adults and children. The rotavirus has been identified as a leading cause of gastroenteritis in young children and the Norwalk virus documented as a cause of epidemics of acute infectious diarrhoea in older children and adults. Other viruses implicated in causing diarrhoea include enteric adenoviruses and astroviruses. However, new viruses almost certainly remain to be discovered, as no viral agent can be identified in up to a third of cases of suspected viral gastroenteritis.

Rotavirus

Rotavirus causes gastroenteritis in children aged between 6 and 24 months and is more likely to occur in winter months. The symptoms of vomiting and watery diarrhoea typically begin after an incubation period of 48–72 hours. The diarrhoea usually lasts 4–8 days, and the combination of diarrhoea and vomiting often leads to dehydration. A milder disease occurs in older children and adults, but most children have been found to develop antibodies to rotavirus by the age of 24 months. Human colostrum and milk contain antibodies to rotavirus and it is known that breastfeeding reduces the incidence of gastroenteritis in children. Transmission is mainly by the oro-faecal route and viruses can be shed in the faeces for up to 21 days.

Rotavirus infection can be diagnosed by an immunoassay using an ELISA test, by polymerase chain reaction technique or by isolation from stool samples.

There are no effective antiviral agents against rotavirus and treatment involves adequate oral or, if needed, intravenous hydration. Vaccines are being developed (one was in use but has been withdrawn).

Norwalk virus

The Norwalk virus is a common cause of epidemics of acute gastroenteritis. Oro-faecal and waterborne spread has been reported and direct person-to-person spread also occurs. The virus typically causes symptoms in older children and adults and is usually mild with diarrhoea, nausea and vomiting occurring after an incubation period of 24–48 hours. Cramping abdominal pain, fever and myalgia may also occur and the symptoms usually last for several days. No effective antiviral agent is available and treatment is symptomatic with fluid replacement as appropriate.

CONDITIONS CAUSING ACUTE BLOODY DIARRHOEA

The differential diagnosis is summarised in Table 12.3.

1. *Shigella*

Occurrence and transmission

Shigella organisms are more common in developing countries with poor sanitation and overcrowding, but *Shigella* infections can also occur in developed countries. There are four major subgroups (*S. boydii*, *S. dysenteriae*, *S. flexneri*, *S. sonnei*), and all are capable of causing dysentery, a term that refers to diarrhoea containing blood and pus. *Shigella* infections occur only in humans and transmission is by the oro-faecal route. The organism is highly contagious and direct person-to-person spread can occur resulting in a high secondary household transmission rate.

Clinical manifestations

Symptoms following ingestion of *Shigella* organisms vary from fever, with or without mild watery diarrhoea, to typical dysentery with diarrhoea containing blood and pus. There is associated cramping abdominal pain, frequently with tenesmus.

Shigellae produce intestinal damage both by direct invasion of the colonic epithelium and by production of an enterotoxin. The capacity to invade colonic cells is essential for virulence and results in a localised severe inflammatory response. The development of oedema, crypt abscesses and ultimately mucosal ulceration gives rise to the typical dysenteric stool.

Complications include rectal prolapse, toxic megacolon and colonic perforation. Extraintestinal symptoms include the haemolytic uraemic syndrome, febrile seizures in young children, reactive arthritis and pneumonia.

Diagnosis

The diagnosis of shigellosis is made by stool culture, and antibiotic sensitivity should be performed at the same time, as drug resistance is common.

A patchy colitis with ulceration may be demonstrated at sigmoidoscopy and biopsies will help exclude inflammatory bowel disease and amoebic colitis.

The differential diagnosis includes other infectious cases of colitis (enteroinvasive *E. coli, C. jejuni, Y. enterocolitica, C. difficile, E. histolytica*) and inflammatory bowel disease.

Treatment

General supportive measures include maintaining hydration and lowering high fever, especially in children. Antidiarrhoeal drugs should be avoided.

Antibiotics are indicated in most patients with *Shigella* infections as they reduce the severity and shorten the duration of the illness. Trimethoprim-sulfamethoxazole and ciprofloxacin are generally effective, but drug resistance is emerging as a significant problem, especially for ampicillin.

2. *Salmonella*

Salmonellae are Gram-negative motile bacilli that can cause a wide clinical spectrum of illness in humans, including gastroenteritis, typhoid fever, bacteraemia and localised infection. An asymptomatic carrier state also occurs.

Serotypes include *Salmonella typhi, S. paratyphi, S. enterica* (previously called *S. choleraesuis)* and *S. enteritidis*. The term non-typhoidal salmonellosis refers to enteric disease caused by infection with salmonellae other than *S. typhi*.

2a. Non-typhoidal salmonellosis

Non-typhoidal salmonellosis is a common cause of food-borne disease around the world, and its incidence has increased in many developed countries. Food-borne epidemics are frequent and transmission from animal products, especially eggs and poultry, are recognised sources of infection. In addition, pets such as turtles and ducklings have been implicated in the spread of salmonellosis. Direct person-to-person spread seems to be uncommon.

The incubation of *S. enteritidis* is short, within the range of 24–48 hours. There is a spectrum of symptoms ranging from mild diarrhoea to severe watery diarrhoea with cramping abdominal pain and fever. Risk factors for severe disease or complications include extremes of age, haemolytic disease, immunocompromised hosts and the presence of prosthetic devices (Table 12.6).

Complications include bacteraemia, osteomyelitis, localised abscesses, meningitis and pneumonia.

Diagnosis

The diagnosis of non-typhoidal salmonellosis relies upon isolation of *Salmonella* organisms from stool or blood culture.

Treatment

Maintenance of hydration with fluid and electrolyte replacement is indicated, as appropriate. The routine use of antibiotics should be avoided, as they do not shorten the average illness and may prolong excretion of the organism. Antibiotics should be reserved for those with severe symptoms or at risk of complications (see Table 12.6). Antimicrobial resistance is an emerging problem. Antibiotics that are effective include quinolones, trimethoprim-sulfamethoxazole and amoxycillin.

TABLE 12.6: Risk factors for severe *Salmonella* infections and complications

- Extremes of age
- Immunosuppression:
  - AIDS
  - Immunosuppressive drugs
  - Congenital and acquired immunodeficiency
  - Transplantation patients
- Malignancies (especially lymphoproliferative disorders)
- Prosthetic devices
- Haemolytic anaemia

2b. Typhoid fever

Typhoid fever is a distinctive clinical syndrome usually associated with *S. typhi* or *S. paratyphi*. The clinical features include a prolonged fever with bacteraemia leading to the stimulation of the reticuloendothelial system and metastatic spread. Multiple organ damage follows, which may include the intestine, but despite the term enteric fever, gastrointestinal symptoms are not prominent, especially early in the syndrome.

Clinical manifestations

The incubation period varies from 1–3 weeks but can range up to 60 days. The illness evolves over a period of four weeks, beginning with a high fever, headache and chills. A bradycardia relative to the fever may occur and the typical 'rose spots' rash is seen during the first week in some patients. Hepatosplenomegaly is common. Intestinal manifestations are not prominent early in the disease and both constipation as well as mild diarrhoea may occur.

The fever is persistent over a period of four weeks with the illness becoming more severe during the second and third week—persistent high fever, delirium and complications from waves of bacteraemia including meningitis, nephritis, osteomyelitis and hepatitis. Diarrhoea may develop at this stage of the disease with haemorrhage or perforation.

Symptoms generally start to abate after the third week but relapses may occur.

Diagnosis

The diagnosis is established by isolating the organism, on either blood or stool culture. Blood cultures are positive in up to 90% of cases during the first week and stool cultures do not usually become positive until the second or third week. Bone marrow culture is positive in over 90% of patients. Serological tests are less reliable and may indicate previous exposure in endemic areas.

Transmission

Transmission of *S. typhi* is usually by water or food contaminated by an individual who either has typhoid fever or is an asymptomatic carrier.

3. *Campylobacter jejuni*

Occurrence and transmission

C. jejuni is a common cause of acute diarrhoeal illnesses, and in many developed countries it is the most common pathogen detected in patients with diarrhoea. It is usually a food-borne illness and sources of infection include contaminated milk, sick pets, occupational exposure to poultry eggs and contaminated water.

Clinical manifestation

After an incubation period of 2–6 days, symptoms begin with the onset of diarrhoea or prodromal features of lassitude, fever, myalgia and headaches. The diarrhoea is initially watery, but may progress to contain blood and mucus. Cramping abdominal pain is common and may be severe.

Diagnosis

The diagnosis is made by stool culture. Special incubating techniques at 42°C with microaerobic conditions are necessary. Sigmoidoscopy may demonstrate colitis in up to 80% of cases, although this finding does not help in making a specific diagnosis.

Treatment

Maintenance of hydration is all that is usually necessary in those patients with a self-limited illness, and in whom symptoms are usually improving at the time of diagnosis. For those with more severe symptoms or who are immunosuppressed, erythromycin is the antibiotic of choice. Quinolones are also effective, although resistance is an emerging problem.

4. *Yersinia enterocolitica*

Occurrence and transmission

Y. enterocolitica has a worldwide distribution and causes a gastrointestinal illness which more commonly affects children and young adults. Transmission is via the oro-faecal route and numerous food and waterborne epidemics have been reported. Direct person-to-person spread has also been documented.

Clinical manifestations

Diarrhoea and abdominal pain are the two dominant symptoms resulting from *Y. enterocolitica* infection, but the clinical manifestations tend to vary according to age. The incidence of bloody diarrhoea in reported series is higher in children and less commonly seen in adults. The illness is self-limited and usually lasts less than two weeks.

In older children and adults, the diarrhoea may be associated with right iliac fossa pain due to an infective ileitis. These symptoms may be clinically indistinguishable from acute appendicitis or Crohn's disease.

Infrequently, a more severe illness may result with enterocolitis, septicaemia and extraintestinal infective complications, such as meningitis or abscesses in bones, joints or sinuses. This is more likely to occur in immunosuppressed individuals or those with iron-overload states (e.g., haemochromatosis or haemolytic diseases) who seem particularly predisposed to infection with *Y. enterocolitica*.

Postinfective sequelae of *Y. enterocolitica* include reactive arthritis, Reiter's syndrome, pericarditis, erythema nodosum, erythema multiforme, glomerulonephritis and thyroiditis.

Diagnosis

The diagnosis is established by culture of the organism, usually in the stool. It may also be cultured from atypical cases at surgery from lymph nodes or from free peritoneal fluid. Serologic tests are also available.

Treatment

The illness is usually self-limited and symptomatic treatment without antibiotics is all that is needed. Antibiotics should be administered to those with septicaemia or extraintestinal abscesses and those predisposed to *Y. enterocolitica* infection. Quinolones, trimethoprim-sulfamethoxazole and tetracyclines are usually effective.

5. *Escherichia coli*

E. coli is a common inhabitant of the gastrointestinal tract in humans, where it may be present either as a commensal or as a pathogen. There are currently five recognisable categories of *E. coli* which cause diarrhoea, each with distinct clinical and epidemiological features: enterotoxigenic *E. coli* (ETEC), enteropathogenic *E. coli* (EPEC), enteroinvasive *E. coli* (EIEC) enterohaemorrhagic *E. coli* (EHEC), and enteroaggregative *E. coli* (EAEC). Further categories may emerge in the future.

Clinical manifestations

Enterotoxigenic *E. coli*. ETEC is a common cause of diarrhoea in children in the developing world and it is also a leading cause of travellers' diarrhoea. Transmission is usually by contaminated food or water, with direct person-to-person spread being uncommon.

ETEC adheres to gut mucosa and produces several enterotoxins, one of which is very similar to the cholera toxin. The clinical syndrome that results consists of watery diarrhoea, cramping abdominal pain and nausea. The illness is usually mild with 5–6 loose stools per day and lasts 3–5 days. Less frequently, a cholera-like illness with profuse watery diarrhoea and dehydration may occur. Natural immunity to ETEC after infection has been documented.

Enteropathogenic *E. coli*. EPEC is a cause of diarrhoea usually in infants and young children. The clinical illness consists of watery diarrhoea, which may occasionally follow a prolonged course. Vomiting, fever and failure to thrive may also occur. It lacks invasive and toxin-producing properties with pathogenicity apparently related to its enteroadhesive properties.

Enteroinvasive *E. coli*. EIEC has the capacity to invade intestinal mucosa causing diarrhoea which often contains blood and mucus. Constitutional symptoms with fever, myalgia and general malaise are common. The illness usually lasts for 3–4 days but may persist for up to two weeks.

Enterohaemorrhagic *E. coli.* EHEC causes haemorrhagic colitis with bloody diarrhoea after an incubation period of 3–4 days. Outbreaks from restaurants and nursing homes have been reported. EHEC does not invade the intestinal mucosa but produces several toxins, one of which is very similar to the *Shigella* toxin.

Complications of infection with EHEC (e.g., subtype 0157:H7) include the haemolytic uraemic syndrome, thrombotic thrombocytopaenic purpura and toxic megacolon. The haemolytic uraemic syndrome occurs most often in children where the incidence ranges from 5–10%. In this syndrome, there is haemolytic anaemia, thrombocytopaenia and fibrin occlusion of small renal vessels that cause renal failure.

Enteroaggregative *E. coli.* Diffusely adhering EAEC produce mild symptoms in some volunteers given this strain of *E. coli*. It may play a more significant role in children and further studies are needed.

Diagnosis

Techniques for the diagnosis of pathogenic *E. coli* are not widely available, except in research laboratories. Patients with bloody diarrhoea should have a sigmoidoscopy or colonoscopy and other infective and non-infective causes of colitis excluded.

Treatment

Mild illness resulting from pathogenic *E. coli* does not require any specific therapy beyond maintenance of hydration. The use of antibiotics in the treatment of enterohaemorrhagic *E. coli* infection remains controversial because of the potential risk that the incidence of haemolytic uraemic syndrome may be increased. The management of travellers' diarrhoea is discussed elsewhere.

6. *Entamoeba histolytica*

Occurrence and transmission

E. histolytica is a protozoan parasite that exists as an invasive trophozoite and as an infective cyst. It resides in the large intestine where asymptomatic colonisation is usual, but it has the potential to become invasive resulting in colitis or spreading to involve the liver and, rarely, other organs.

There is a worldwide distribution of *E. histolytica* with a prevalence ranging from 1% in industrialised nations up to 50% in some developing nations. The cystic form can survive in the environment and is responsible for spread of the disease via the faecal-oral route. Direct person-to-person transmission is usual, but food and waterborne spread can occur. Several other species of amoebae, including *E. dispar*, reside in the lumen of the large intestine and are non-pathogenic but need to be distinguished from *E. histolytica*.

Clinical manifestations

The motile trophozoites live in the lumen of the large intestine where they require either bacteria or tissue substrates for survival. Factors responsible for triggering invasion are incompletely understood, but include the strain of *E. histolytica*, intestinal factors such as the nature of bacteria within the colon, and host resistance. Host factors which increase susceptibility to invasion include extremes of age, malnutrition, pregnancy and immunosuppressive states, including AIDS.

Symptoms following invasion vary from mild diarrhoea through to fulminating amoebic dysentery. A majority of patients develop a diarrhoeal illness lasting 3–4 weeks. The stools frequently contain blood and pus and most attacks resolve spontaneously or with treatment, but chronic amoebiasis or fulminating disease may result. The latter is characterised by a high fever, profuse diarrhoea with bleeding, abdominal pain and tenderness.

Complications of amoebic infection include perforation, strictures, amoeboma and involvement of extraintestinal sites, usually the liver.

A liver abscess may occur during the acute attack or present weeks to months later. It may also complicate asymptomatic infections and be present in patients with no history of preceding diarrhoea. Fever, malaise and right upper quadrant pain are the common manifestations. The onset may be abrupt or insidious.

Diagnosis

The diagnosis of intestinal amoebiasis may be made by identification of the organism in the stool or in colonic biopsies. However, microscopic identification of the organism does not differentiate between pathogenic and non-pathogenic species of *Entamoeba*, which can be done by antigen testing or serology.

The diagnosis of liver abscess depends on imaging and serological tests as amoebae are seldom demonstrated in either intestinal cultures or from abscess aspirate. The indirect haemagglutination assay (IHA) is positive in up to 99% of patients with amoebic liver abscess, although the test may be negative early in the course of the illness.

Treatment

Metronidazole is the drug of choice for intestinal amoebiasis as well as amoebic liver abscess. A prolonged course may be necessary as encysted organisms can survive in the intestine and can be followed by asymptomatic passage of cysts over a long period of time.

ANTIBIOTIC-ASSOCIATED DIARRHOEA AND *C. DIFFICILE* COLITIS

Introduction

Antibiotics can cause diarrhoea through a variety of mechanisms, including an osmotic diarrhoea due to an impairment of colonic fermentation of unabsorbed carbohydrates as well as toxin-producing *Clostridium difficile* infection. Of those infected with *C. difficile*, less than half will develop a diarrhoeal illness.

Occurrence and transmission

C. difficile becomes established in the large bowel, usually after the normal flora of the colon has been changed by antibiotics. Hospital acquisition of infection is common, as the two conditions for colonisation (antibiotic therapy and environmental contamination) often occur together. *C. difficile* forms heat-resistant spores, which act as a source of recurrent infection.

Clinical manifestations

Exposure to *C. difficile* results in a spectrum of illness ranging from asymptomatic carriage to severe pseudomembranous colitis. More than 50% of healthy neonates are asymptomatic carriers and the majority of hospital inpatients exposed to *C. difficile* are asymptomatic.

Those who develop symptoms usually do so during or shortly after antibiotic therapy. The illness begins as diarrhoea with cramping abdominal pain. A low-grade fever may be present together with lower abdominal tenderness. A small proportion of patients progress to colitis, which may become life-threatening, with severe bloody diarrhoea, diffuse abdominal tenderness and abdominal distension. Fulminating colitis with toxic megacolon has been reported.

Diagnosis

The diagnosis is made by demonstrating the specific cytotoxin in the stool. Cytotoxin assay and culture of *C. difficile* must be specifically requested and a careful history of preceding antibiotic usage taken. The toxin is demonstrated by tissue culture assay and is neutralised by a specific *C. difficile* antitoxin.

Sigmoidoscopy or colonoscopy may document the typical raised white plaques of pseudomembranous colitis. Although characteristic, these are uncommon, except in those with more severe symptoms. A diffuse or patchy colitis may be present and biopsy may reveal non-specific colitis or even pseudo-membranous colitis in the absence of plaques. Patchy colitis beyond the reach of the flexible sigmoidoscope has been reported.

Treatment

Antibiotic therapy should be discontinued where possible. If symptoms are severe, or mild symptoms fail to settle spontaneously, then therapy with oral metronidazole or oral vancomycin is indicated. Vancomycin is expensive and should be reserved for very ill patients or those who fail to respond to metronidazole. A relapse of symptoms and infection may occur in 15–20% of patients. On rare occasions, frequent relapses require prolonged treatment.

CRYPTOSPORIDIOSIS

Occurrence and transmission

Cryptosporidium parvum is a protozoan parasite that causes diarrhoea in both normal and immunocompromised populations. Oro-faecal transmission occurs from contaminated water and food and large epidemics have been reported. Direct person-to-person spread is also common. It has been estimated that *C. parvum* is responsible for 5–10% of infectious diarrhoea in developing countries and 1–3% of cases in the developed world.

Clinical manifestations

Profuse watery diarrhoea with abdominal pain and nausea is the usual presentation. Vomiting may occur and a low-grade fever is common. The illness usually abates after 1–2 weeks, although in some individuals voluminous diarrhoea and weight loss may persist.

In immunocompromised individuals, chronic diarrhoea is common and this is usually indolent, but may be devastating with profound fluid loss.

Diagnosis

Cryptosporidium oocysts may be identified in stool samples with appropriate concentration and staining techniques. Organisms can also be demonstrated at the luminal surface by duodenal or colonic biopsies. Enzyme immunoassay kits are available and are highly sensitive and specific.

Treatment

No effective treatment is available. A variety of antibiotics have been trialled with little persistent effect noted. Immune reconstitution in immunocompromised individuals is the most effective treatment available.

DIARRHOEA ASSOCIATED WITH AIDS

Diarrhoea is a common gastrointestinal symptom in AIDS with a frequency ranging from 30–90%, depending on the stage of the illness and environmental factors. The host immunodeficiency results in persisting infection and frequent re-infection. In addition, severe illness with septicaemia and infections with organisms not usually pathogenic are common. Malnutrition may result from associated malabsorption or a chronic diarrhoeal illness with anorexia. The presence of chronic diarrhoea influences quality of life as well as morbidity and mortality.

Aetiology

Potential pathogens involved in AIDS diarrhoea are listed in Table 12.7 and vary with the stage of the illness and degree of immunocompetence of the host. Some patients with AIDS develop diarrhoea without any detectable pathogens and non-infectious causes of diarrhoea, including drugs, pancreatic insufficiency and tumour invasion, may be involved. The AIDS virus itself and small bowel bacterial overgrowth may also be responsible for diarrhoea in some patients.

Diagnosis

Stool samples should be obtained for culture and sensitivity and be examined for cysts, ova and parasites. An assay for *C. difficile* toxin and special acid-fast stains for *Cryptosporidium* should be performed.

If no cause is forthcoming with stool cultures, then sigmoidoscopy or colonoscopy and biopsy may help identify cytomegalovirus and herpes simplex virus. Endoscopic duodenal biopsies for culture, histopathology and electron microscopy may help the diagnosis of *G. lamblia*, cytomegalovirus and *C. parvum*. Multiple pathogens may be present and the identification of one pathogen does not exclude the possibility of other agents causing diarrhoea.

Treatment

Supportive therapy with rehydration and antimotility drugs should be introduced where appropriate. The immune response should be reconstituted where possible, although antiretroviral drugs are not available in many developing countries. Identifying the cause of diarrhoea enables specific therapy to be instituted. Long-term suppressive therapy is often necessary, as a recurrence of infection is common. Subcutaneous octreotide may be useful in patients with refractory diarrhoea.

TABLE 12.7: Pathogens associated with AIDS diarrhoea

Bacterial	Viral	Protozoal
Mycobacterium avium intracellulare (MAI)	Cytomegalovirus	Cryptosporidium parvum
Salmonella spp.	Herpes simplex virus	Giardia lamblia
Shigella spp.	Adenovirus	Isospora belli
Campylobacter jejuni		Entamoeba histolytica
Clostridium difficile		Microsporidium spp.

Further reading

Butzler JP. *Campylobacter*, from obscurity to celebrity. *Clin Microbiol Infect* 2004; 10: 868–76.

Clark B, McKendrick M. A review of viral gastroenteritis. *Curr Opin Infect Dis* 2004; 17: 461–9.

Gore JI, Surawicz C. Severe acute diarrhea. *Gastroenterol Clin North Am* 2003; 32: 1249–67.

Jabbar A, Wright RA. Gastroenteritis and antibiotic-associated diarrhea. *Prim Care* 2003; 30: 63–80, iv.

Reisinger EC, Fritzsche C, Krause R, Krejs GJ. Diarrhea caused by primarily non-gastrointestinal infections. *Nat Clin Pract Gastroenterol Hepatol* 2005; 2: 216–22.

Sentongo TA. The use of oral rehydration solutions in children and adults. *Curr Gastroenterol Rep* 2004; 6: 307–13.

Thom K, Forrest G. Gastrointestinal infections in immunocompromised hosts. *Curr Opin Gastroenterol* 2006; 22: 18–23.

chapter **13**

CHRONIC DIARRHOEA AND FATTY STOOLS

Chronic diarrhoea can be simply defined as the frequent or urgent passage of unformed stool for at least one month. As with acute diarrhoea (Chapter 12), a careful history and physical examination will often help suggest the diagnosis and direct investigations.

HISTORY

Determine what the patient means by diarrhoea. Ask about the frequency and consistency of the stools. Distinguish diarrhoea from rectal urgency alone or faecal incontinence (Chapter 14).

Clues to the cause of the diarrhoea can be obtained from the history and examination (Table 13.1). Small-volume frequent stools suggest large bowel disease and tenesmus (a constant sense of the need to defecate) suggests rectal involvement. Large-volume watery stool is consistent with small bowel disease; while obvious clinical steatorrhoea with pale, bulky, oily stools that float suggests the presence of small bowel or pancreatic disease.

The presence of blood may indicate local anal bleeding or other colonic disease. Bright red blood that is separate from the stool is consistent with an anal or rectal cause, but may occur with more proximal colonic disease. Altered blood, or blood mixed with stool is in keeping with higher colonic bleeding, such as from inflammatory bowel disease or colon cancer (Chapter 9).

Symptoms associated with the diarrhoea may also provide valuable information about the nature of the underlying disease process. Weight loss suggests an organic disorder and may be marked with malabsorption, carcinoma or inflammatory bowel disease. Large joint arthritis or sacroileitis suggests inflammatory bowel disease.

The presence of a skin rash may suggest coeliac disease (e.g., dermatitis herpetiformis) or inflammatory bowel disease (e.g., erythema nodosum or erythema multiforme). Crampy abdominal pain occurs with diarrhoea of any cause, but pain shortly after eating raises the possibility of partial bowel obstruction (e.g., Crohn's disease or bowel cancer). Abdominal pain is also a feature of chronic pancreatitis, associated with malabsorption. Abdominal bloating may occur with most forms of diarrhoea but, in association with alternating diarrhoea and constipation, suggests the presence of the irritable bowel syndrome. The duration of symptoms may also be helpful, as diarrhoea occurring over many years is more in keeping with a benign process.

There may be a correlation between diarrhoea and diet. Milk consumption in lactose-intolerant individuals or in those with a high sorbitol intake (in chewing gum and fruit juices) can cause diarrhoea. Changing to a high-fibre diet may also cause a change in bowel habit with loose stools.

A history of systemic disease may be relevant. Disorders such as diabetes mellitus and hyperthyroidism may be relevant.

A drug history may identify the cause of diarrhoea and a wide variety of medications have been implicated. Antibiotics and antacids are frequent offenders in this category. Alcohol is also a cause of chronic diarrhoea and surreptitious laxative abuse needs to be considered in difficult cases.

A sexual history is important in the evaluation of a chronic diarrhoeal illness, as diarrhoea is a very common symptom in patients with HIV/AIDS. Overseas travel before the onset of diarrhoea may implicate a gastrointestinal infection or, more frequently, a postinfectious irritable bowel syndrome.

The family history should be obtained as inflammatory bowel disease, bowel cancer and coeliac disease have an increased incidence in families.

TABLE 13.1: Clinical features in chronic diarrhoea	
Clinical feature	**Conditions to consider**
Young age	Coeliac disease, inflammatory bowel disease, lactase deficiency, irritable bowel syndrome
Oil droplets in stool	Pancreatic insufficiency
Previous surgery	Bacterial overgrowth, dumping, post vagotomy diarrhoea, ileal resection, short bowel syndrome
Peptic ulcer	Zollinger-Ellison syndrome
Medications	Laxatives, magnesium antacids, antibiotics, lactulose, colchicine
Frequent infections	Immunoglobulin deficiency
Marked weight loss	Thyrotoxicosis, malignancy, malabsorption
Arthritis	Inflammatory bowel disease, Whipple's disease, hypogammaglobulinaemia
Hyperpigmentation	Whipple's disease, Addison's disease, coeliac disease
Fever	HIV, inflammatory bowel disease, lymphoma, Whipple's disease
Flushing	Carcinoid syndrome
Chronic lung disease	Cystic fibrosis
Neuropathy	Diabetes mellitus, vitamin B12 deficiency, amyloidosis
Family history of diarrhoea	Colon cancer, coeliac disease, inflammatory bowel disease
(Based on Talley NJ, Internal Medicine, 2nd edn, MacLennan & Petty, with permission from Elsevier Australia.)	

PHYSICAL EXAMINATION

Evidence of malnutrition and wasting should be sought and the skin examined for rashes, pigmentation and evidence of nutritional deficiency. There may be evidence of iron deficiency (pallor, cheilosis, glossitis and koilonychia) or vitamin B12 deficiency (peripheral neuropathy, glossitis). Protein deficiency may result in peripheral oedema and white nails.

Further clues to the cause of diarrhoea may be obtained from abdominal examination. An abdominal mass or liver secondaries may be identified. A rectal mass may be present on rectal examination or faecal impaction, particularly in elderly patients, may be noted. Perianal disease with fissures, fistulae and abscesses is common in Crohn's disease (Chapter 11).

ASSESSMENT

The history and physical examination will often direct the order and nature of investigations.

Clinical steatorrhoea will initiate tests for malabsorption, and blood in the stool will direct investigations towards the large bowel.

In those in whom the diagnosis is not obvious, a variety of factors will influence the order and extent of investigations, especially the age of the patient and the length of the history. A long history suggests a benign illness, although disorders, such as coeliac disease and Crohn's disease, may not be diagnosed for many years because of subtle symptoms. Conversely, the development of new symptoms in a patient over the age of 40 would raise concern about the possibility of bowel cancer.

A full blood count and erythrocyte sedimentation rate (ESR) is a simple initial blood investigation and may provide information about anaemia due to iron, folate or vitamin B12 deficiency. It may also show an elevated white cell count or ESR suggesting the presence of inflammation. The serum albumin will often be low with chronic inflammatory processes or with malnutrition.

The stool examination may provide information about parasites, such as *Giardia lamblia*, and may also document white blood cells implicating inflammation or infection, or red blood cells in bleeding (e.g., carcinoma). The stool weight provides some evidence of the severity of diarrhoea.

Sigmoidoscopy may establish the presence of inflammation or tumours. A biopsy should always be performed in patients with diarrhoea to exclude microscopic or collagenous colitis. Melanosis coli may be obvious macroscopically and will also be demonstrated on biopsy. A colonoscopy requires a full bowel preparation with sedation, but has the advantage of examining the entire bowel length and often the terminal ileum can be intubated as well. Disorders that may require colonoscopy for diagnosis include bowel cancer, polyps, segmental colitis and terminal ileitis.

Radiological investigations that may aid in the investigation of diarrhoea include a plain abdominal X-ray, small bowel series, barium enema and abdominal CT scan.

If small bowel disease is suspected, a small bowel biopsy (usually performed endoscopically) may provide further information. A disaccharidase assay can be carried out at the same time as a small bowel biopsy.

Further investigations that may be needed if no diagnosis is reached include stool examination for laxatives and blood tests for thyroid function (thyroid-stimulating hormone) and hormone-secreting tumours (e.g., gastrin, vasoactive intestinal polypeptide).

MALABSORPTION

The basic physiological problem the body faces in assimilation of food is the passage of nutrients across the limiting cell membrane of the enterocyte. The problem is solved by breaking food particles down to basic components (digestion) and the insertion of special carrier proteins into the absorptive cells to facilitate absorption. The term malabsorption is generally used to encompass both impaired digestion and defective absorption. A classification of malabsorption is shown in Table 13.2.

Physiology

Understanding malabsorption requires knowledge of the physiology of normal digestion and absorption.

The enterocyte

The small intestine is lined by specialised cells called enterocytes and, like all cells, they are surrounded by a limiting membrane (a lipid bilayer) with the function of preventing loss of cytosol and the entry of unwanted molecules. The purpose of digestion is to break down nutrients into molecules small enough to be absorbed. The lipid bilayer allows diffusion of fats into the cell and is equipped with carriers to enable absorption of sugars and amino acids. Anatomical modifications in the small intestine (valvulae conniventes, villi and microvilli) increase the luminal surface area by approximately 600-fold.

Carbohydrate digestion and absorption

Carbohydrates in western society account for 50% of dietary energy and comprise about 60% starch, 30% sucrose and 10% lactose. Starch is a high molecular weight compound consisting of two polysaccharides: amylose and amylopectin. Amylose is a straight chain polymer of glucose linked by 1,4 glycosidic bonds. Amylopectin is similar, but in addition to the 1,4 linkages there are 1,6 linkages for every 20–30 glucose molecules.

Starch is digested by salivary and pancreatic alpha amylase. An endoenzyme breaks 1,4 linkages. Terminal 1,4 linkages, 1,6 linkages and 1,4 linkages near 1,6 bonds are resistant. Thus, the products of amylase digestion are maltose, maltotriose and alpha limit dextrins (small carbohydrates of four to six molecules containing 1,6 linkages). The brush border enzymes maltase and sucrase isomaltase hydrolyse maltose and maltotriose to glucose. Sucrase and lactase break down sucrose (to glucose) and lactose (to glucose and galactose). Glucose and galactose are actively transported across the enterocyte membrane by a sodium-dependent carrier. Fructose is transported by facilitated diffusion.

Protein assimilation

Protein digestion begins in the stomach with the action of pepsin, which breaks down protein into large polypeptides. These enter the duodenum and are further hydrolysed by pancreatic enzymes. Pancreatic secretion is stimulated by pancreozymin/cholecystokinin from the duodenal mucosal cells. Each pancreatic enzyme is secreted as an inactive precursor, with the initial activation being carried out by enterokinase. This is secreted by the mucosal brush border and converts trypsinogen to trypsin.

Intraluminal digestion of protein occurs by the sequential action of the proteolytic endopeptidases (trypsin, chymotrypsin, elastase) and exopeptidases (carboxypeptidase A and B).

The products of luminal proteolysis are amino acids and small peptides of two to six amino acid residues. Peptidases in the brush border break down these small peptides to amino acids which are actively transported into the enterocyte. Small peptides are also actively transported across the brush border and are broken down to amino acids within the enterocyte by peptides in the cytosol.

Fat assimilation

The various processes involved in fat absorption include the secretion of bile and pancreatic juice, emulsification of fats, enzymatic hydrolysis of triglycerides, soublisation with micelles, uptake by the enterocytes, intracellular reassembly of triglycerides and the release of fats as chylomicrons.

The process begins with bile salts which form micelles and function as detergents, thus solubilising fats. The pancreas secretes bicarbonate, as well as lipase and co-lipase. Bicarbonate raises the pH to 7 or 8 where the lipase is maximally active. Lipase acts on triglycerides cleaving the ester linkages at positions 1 and 3, yielding free fatty acids and monoglycerides. Co-lipase displaces bile salts from triglycerides to enable the lipase to be maximally active.

Enterocytes absorb free fatty acids and monoglycerides and carry fats to the interior surface membrane. Bile salts are finally absorbed in the terminal ileum. Within the enterocyte, monoglycerides are re-esterified to triglycerides and coated with small amounts of protein to form a chylomicron. These pass into the mesenteric lymphatics and enter the blood stream via the thoracic duct.

TABLE 13.2: Classification of malabsorption and examples of causes

1. Lipolytic phase defects

   a) Chronic pancreatitis, pancreatic carcinoma
   b) Cystic fibrosis

2. Micellar phase defects

   a) Bacterial overgrowth
   b) Terminal ileal disease or resection: < 100 cm—bile salt diarrhoea
                                      > 100 cm—steatorrhoea
   c) Extrahepatic biliary obstruction or chronic cholestatic liver disease

3. Mucosal phase defects

   a) Coeliac disease
   b) Tropical sprue
   c) Lymphoma, Whipple's disease, small bowel ischaemia or resection, hypogammaglobulinaemia, amyloidosis, AIDS

4. Delivery phase defects

   a) Intestinal lymphangiectasia
   b) Tumour infiltration of lymphatics

(Based on Talley NJ, Internal Medicine, 2nd edn, MacLennan & Petty, with permission from Elsevier Australia.)

CLINICAL APPROACH TO THE PATIENT WITH MALABSORPTION

Diagnosis in malabsorption requires firstly suspecting its presence, secondly confirming its existence and thirdly demonstrating the cause (Table 13.3).

Suspecting malabsorption

Suspecting the presence of malabsorption may be easy when it is gross, but early symptoms are often subtle and non-specific. The diagnosis is usually considered in patients with marked weight loss and the presence of typical steatorrhoea: pale, bulky, offensive stools that are difficult to flush and may contain oil. Anaemia is common and may be due to malabsorption of vitamin B12, folate or iron. Deficiency of fat-soluble vitamins may cause bruising (vitamin K), tetany and bone pain (vitamin D), or hyperkeratosis of the skin. Night blindness may occur with vitamin A deficiency.

Protein deficiency may result in muscle wasting and oedema from hypoalbuminaemia. Peripheral neuropathy may occur following vitamin B12 deficiency.

Early malabsorptive symptoms are often non-specific and may include minor weight loss, general malaise, loss of energy and a slight change in bowel habit. Presentation with a single-nutrient deficiency (e.g., iron deficiency anaemia) is quite common. Aphthous ulcers, glossitis and cheilosis may also occur. Presentation in children is usually with diarrhoea, irritability and growth failure.

Confirming malabsorption

Faecal fat excretion

The 3-day faecal fat estimation remains the 'gold standard' for malabsorption. A 100 g fat per day diet must be maintained for 3 days prior to and during the stool collection for accurate results. Fat excretion of greater than 7 g per day is considered abnormal.

Qualitative estimation of faecal fat by staining faecal smears with Sudan III is simpler but less sensitive.

Breath tests

The triolein breath test for fat malabsorption involves the ingestion of ^{14}C-labelled triolein and measurement of ^{14}CO$_2$ in the expired air. Its lack of sensitivity has limited its clinical use.

Hydrogen breath tests have been used to measure carbohydrate malabsorption. In the mammalian body, hydrogen is only produced by bacterial action, usually on unabsorbed carbohydrate in the colon. Thus, if a carbohydrate that is normally absorbed in the small intestine is malabsorbed, a breath hydrogen peak will occur about 90 minutes after its ingestion when it first arrives in the colon and is broken down by bacterial action. Similarly small bowel bacterial overgrowth will be detected by an early hydrogen peak. Malabsorption of lactose or a standard rice meal can be detected in this way. Unfortunately, the limited sensitivity and specificity of breath hydrogen tests restrict their usefulness.

TABLE 13.3: Typical test results in malabsorption

Investigation	Coeliac disease	Bacterial overgrowth	Whipple's disease	Terminal ileal disease	Chronic pancreatitis
Stool fat	High-normal	High	High	High	Very high
D-xylose[1]	Low	Low	Low	Normal	Normal
Schilling's test with/without intrinsic factor[2]	Normal (rarely abnormal due to ileal involvement)	Abnormal	Normal	Abnormal	Abnormal (40%)
Folate (serum)	Low (> 50%)	High-normal	Low	Normal	Normal
Small bowel biopsy (proximal)	Flat biopsy (subtotal/total villous atrophy)	Normal	Clubbing and flattening of villi PAS-positive inclusions[4]	Normal	Normal
Small bowel X-ray[3]	Normal (unless lymphoma)	Normal (may find diverticula)	Normal	Abnormal	Normal

1. This is a test of proximal small bowel function. Falsely low values occur in chronic renal failure, dehydration, ascites, hyperthyroidism and in elderly patients.

2. While pernicious anaemia corrects with intrinsic factor, ileal disease does not correct. Bacterial overgrowth corrects with antibiotics and pancreatic insufficiency with pancreatic supplements. False negative results occur with incomplete urinary collections, decreased extracellular volume and renal disease.

3. A small bowel series may be abnormal in severe mucosal disease (e.g., dilatation, flocculation of barium, loss of fine mucosal pattern), but this is not specific. It should be ordered to exclude anatomical abnormalities (e.g., diverticula, Crohn's disease). A wireless capsule endoscopy study may provide additional information in difficult cases, and appears more accurate than a small bowel X-ray.

4. May also occur with *Mycobacterium avium intracellulare* (MAI) in AIDS patients.

PAS = periodic acid-Schiff technique.

(Based on Talley NJ, Internal Medicine, 2nd edn, MacLennan & Petty, with permission from Elsevier Australia.)

D-xylose test

This test measures small bowel mucosal absorption and involves the ingestion of D-xylose and measuring its excretion in the urine. As well as mucosal absorption, bacterial action, renal function and the completeness of urine collection and the action of drugs can influence the result.

Nutritional status

Nutritional status can be determined by the body mass index (BMI), mid-arm circumference and skin-fold thickness. Blood tests that have been used to assess nutritional status include serum albumin, transferrin, serum prealbumin and lymphocyte count. Specific nutrient deficiencies should be sought by serum iron studies, vitamin B12 and folate levels, calcium, international normalised ratio (vitamin K) and vitamin assays (A, D and E). A full blood count may document anaemia, macrocytosis, microcytosis or a mixed picture or even the presence of hyposplenism (seen in coeliac disease).

Finding the cause of malabsorption

History

The list of causes of malabsorption (Table 13.4) is daunting, and a thorough history is essential to target investigations. Common causes of malabsorption include coeliac disease, chronic pancreatitis, small bowel bacterial overgrowth and gastric surgery.

A cause may be obvious from the history if gastric surgery or a small bowel resection has been performed or there is known chronic pancreatitis. Childhood diarrhoea, failure to thrive or anaemia may suggest the possibility of coeliac disease. An associated skin rash of dermatitis herpetiformis (Figure 13.1) or a positive family history may also be clues to the diagnosis of coeliac disease.

Abdominal pain, alcohol excess or a history of passing 'oil' suggests chronic pancreatitis. Abdominal pain may also be a feature of Crohn's disease and there is sometimes a positive family history of inflammatory bowel disease. Intestinal lymphoma and mesenteric ischaemia may also present with abdominal pain.

A careful history may elicit drugs that may result in malabsorption including cholestyramine, neomycin, colchicine and cathartics. The history should also be directed towards identifying systemic disorders that may be associated with malabsorption including AIDS, scleroderma, thyrotoxicosis or diabetes mellitus.

TABLE 13.4: Causes of malabsorption

More common

- Coeliac disease
- Chronic pancreatitis
- Post gastrectomy
- Crohn's disease
- Small bowel resection
- Small intestinal bacterial overgrowth
- Lactase deficiency

Less common

- AIDS (*Mycobacterium avium intracellulare*, AIDS enteropathy)
- Whipple's disease
- Intestinal lymphoma
- Immunoproliferative small intestinal disease (alpha heavy chain disease)
- Radiation enteritis
- Collagenous sprue
- Tropical sprue
- Non-granulomatous ulcerative jejuno-ileitis
- Eosinophilic gastroenteritis
- Amyloidosis
- Zollinger-Ellison syndrome
- Intestinal lymphangiectasia
- Systemic mastocytosis
- Chronic mesenteric ischaemia
- Abetalipoproteinaemia (autosomal recessive)

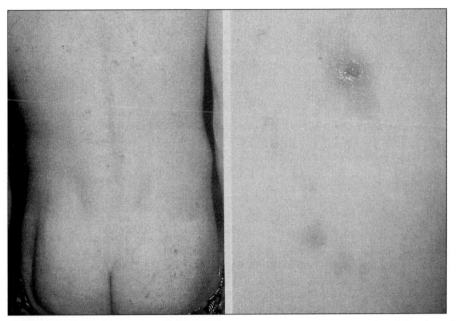

FIGURE 13.1: Dermatitis herpetiformis. Typically, the lesions are grouped and distributed over the scapulae, sacrum and buttocks (left), elbows and knees. Severe pruritus accompanies the disease and results in much excoriation and 'dug-out' skin (right).
(From Misiewicz JJ et al, Slide Atlas of Gastroenterology, with permission.)

Investigations

The nature and order of investigations carried out is dependent on the history. In many instances a cause will be suggested and investigations can be targeted. For example, upper abdominal pain may suggest pancreatitis, directing investigations towards demonstrating pancreatic disease. Crampy lower abdominal pain and diarrhoea would lead investigations towards exclusion of Crohn's disease. Specific investigations are set out below.

Pancreatic disease suspected. A plain abdominal X-ray may show pancreatic calcification, which establishes the diagnosis of chronic pancreatitis. An abdominal CT scan is more sensitive in documenting calcification and may show a dilated pancreatic duct or a pancreatic mass.

Endoscopic retrograde cholangiopancreatography (ERCP) will document changes of chronic pancreatitis with dilated and/or irregular ducts. A magnetic resonance pancreatogram (MRCP) is less invasive and may also document typical pancreatic duct changes.

Direct tube tests such as the secretin stimulation test remain the 'gold standard' for assessment of exocrine function but are seldom used today. They involve placement of a tube into the second part of the duodenum, the administration of secretin or cholecystokinin and the measurement of bicarbonate or enzymes in the aspirated duodenal juice. These tests are expensive to perform, uncomfortable for the patient and may yield false positive results if duodenal collection of juice is inadequate. Alternative non-invasive tests for pancreatic function have been developed and include the bentiromide test, the pancreaolauryl test, the faecal chymotrypsin assay and the faecal elastase assay. None of these tests have achieved sufficient sensitivity or specificity to attract widespread use, but this is a developing area.

In children with malabsorption, a sweat test is required to exclude cystic fibrosis.

Small bowel disease suspected. A small bowel biopsy at upper endoscopy is usually performed in patients with unexplained malabsorption. This may be preceded by serologic tests for coeliac disease (see later). In addition to the diagnosis of coeliac disease (a common cause of malabsorption), rare causes of malabsorption such as lymphangiectasia and Whipple's disease can also be detected. *Giardia lamblia* trophozoites may sometimes be visible on routine histology and a disaccharidase assay can be performed.

Barium studies of the small bowel may define defects that give rise to malabsorption, such as strictures, diverticula or fistulae. Small bowel endoscopy or wireless capsule endoscopy can be useful in difficult cases.

Small bowel bacterial overgrowth can only be reliably detected by measurement of viable counts of bacteria in fasting proximal small intestinal aspirates obtained at upper endoscopy. This requires small intestinal intubation as well as a specialist unit experienced in anaerobic bacterial culture.

A variety of indirect tests have evolved for the diagnosis of small bowel bacterial overgrowth. These include the ^{14}C glycocholate test, which relies upon bacterial deconjugation of bile acid and an increase in $^{14}CO_2$. This test has a high false positive and false negative rate.

The ^{14}C-D-xylose breath test relies upon bacterial metabolism of ^{14}C-D-xylose by bacteria in the proximal small intestine. $^{14}CO_2$ is formed, which is then absorbed and excreted in the breath. Although some reports suggest this test has a high sensitivity and specificity, others have been unable to substantiate this claim. The test's role in the investigation of small intestinal bacterial overgrowth remains unclear.

Other indirect tests, including the lactulose breath test, glucose breath hydrogen test and rice breath hydrogen test, all have unacceptable sensitivity and specificity levels.

Ileal absorptive function can be determined by Schilling's test performed with intrinsic factor in three stages (without intrinsic factor, with intrinsic factor and after a course of treatment), or with a SeHCAT (^{75}Se-labelled homocholic acid taurine) test. Vitamin B12 and bile acids are absorbed in the terminal ileum. The Schilling test is frequently abnormal with and without intrinsic factor in terminal ileal disease. Vitamin B12 absorption in pernicious anaemia corrects with intrinsic factor. SeHCAT is the taurine conjugate of a synthetic bile acid and the test includes measurement of body ^{75}Se retention after administration of ^{75}SeHCAT. Retention of less than 50% after three days suggests bile acid malabsorption.

DISORDERS THAT MAY CAUSE CHRONIC DIARRHOEA OR MALABSORPTION

Coeliac disease (gluten-sensitive enteropathy)

Coeliac disease is a disorder of the small intestine caused by sensitivity to gluten, a protein component of cereals found in wheat, rye, barley, triticale and possibly oats. Exposure to gluten causes small bowel damage characterised by inflammation and villous atrophy.

Aetiology

The current understanding of the aetiology of coeliac disease is that gluten triggers mucosal damage due to an immune response in genetically predisposed individuals. Virtually all those affected are HLA-DQL or DQ8.

Clinical features

Individuals with coeliac disease may present with classical malabsorptive symptoms of steatorrhoea with pale bulky stools, crampy abdominal pain, abdominal distension and weight loss. Growth failure or failure to thrive in children is also common.

In adults, symptoms may be much more subtle with abdominal bloating, occasional diarrhoea or nutrient deficiencies. Other presentations include infertility, miscarriage, mouth ulcers, osteoporosis or unexplained anaemia. With the availability of serologic screening programmes, many individuals have been diagnosed who are asymptomatic. Iron deficiency anaemia is common and combined iron and folate deficiency is typical of coeliac disease. Bruising due to vitamin K deficiency or tetany due to vitamin D deficiency and hypocalcaemia may be the presenting features.

Dermatitis herpetiformis (see Figure 13.1) presents with a pruritic papulovesicular rash on extensor surfaces of the limbs and also on the buttocks. Small bowel changes of coeliac disease are usual, but may be patchy. The condition responds to a gluten-free diet.

Diagnosis

Small bowel biopsy

The diagnosis of coeliac disease is made by documenting the typical mucosal changes (Figure 13.2) on small bowel biopsies, which are usually obtained at endoscopy. Multiple biopsies should be obtained from the second part of the duodenum.

Screening

Serological tests are now available, which are useful for screening in coeliac disease (Table 13.5). Tissue transglutaminase appears to be the target antigen detected by the endomysial antibody assay.

Table 13.5: Serological tests in coeliac disease		
Test	**Sensitivity (%)**	**Specificity (%)**
IgA AGA	75–90	82–95
IgG AGA	69–85	73–90
EMA	85–90	97–100
TGA	93–96	99–100
AGA = antigliadin antibody; EMA = endomysial antibody; TGA = tissue transglutaminase antibody.		

Note that up to 5% of individuals with coeliac disease are IgA deficient and will have false negative screening tests to IgA antigliadin antibody, endomysial antibody and transglutaminase antibodies.

A diagnosis of coeliac disease should not be made on serological tests alone and a small bowel biopsy is always required for confirmation.

Screening tests are useful for those with a low probability of coeliac disease and to monitor the response to a gluten-free diet.

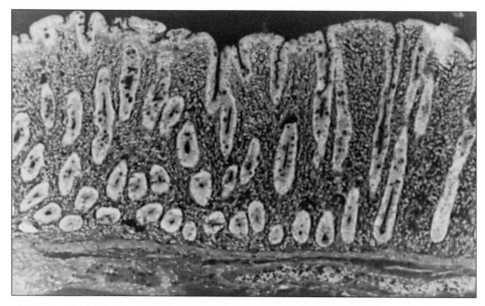

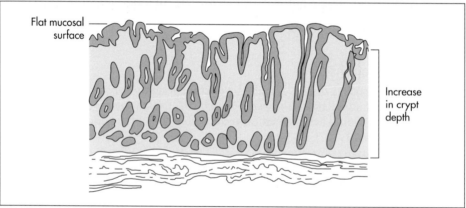

Flat mucosal surface

Increase in crypt depth

FIGURE 13.2: Subtotal villous atrophy showing total absence of villi and a corresponding increase in depth of the crypts, producing an apparently increased mucosal thickness.
(Photomicrograph from and illustration based on Misiewicz JJ et al, Slide Atlas of Gastroenterology, *with permission.)*

Treatment

The treatment of coeliac disease requires a lifelong gluten-free diet and the exclusion of wheat, rye, barley and triticale from the diet. It is not clear whether oats cause disease, but should be avoided as oats are often contaminated with small amounts of gluten from wheat and barley.

Patients should be educated in the importance of maintaining a gluten-free diet and referred to a dietician who is experienced in advice to patients with coeliac disease.

Associations with coeliac disease

Patients with coeliac disease have a greater incidence of a variety of other disorders, including malignant disease and diseases associated with altered immunity. The incidence of malignancy, particularly lymphoma and gastrointestinal malignancies, is significantly increased. This increased risk is reduced or eliminated after maintaining a gluten-free diet for a number of years. Ulcerative jejuno-ileitis and coeliac disease refractory to treatment may both represent early T-cell lymphoma, complicating coeliac disease.

Autoimmune disorders associated with coeliac disease include autoimmune thyroid disease, Type 1 diabetes mellitus, hyposplenism, dermatitis herpetiformis, autoimmune liver disease and infertility.

There are also associations with neurologic disease (ataxia, epilepsy) as well as Down and Turner's syndromes.

Tropical sprue

Tropical sprue is a diarrhoeal disorder characterised by malabsorption occurring in residents of tropical areas. It may also occur in visitors to the tropics who stay for more than four weeks. Current evidence suggests it is caused by small bowel bacterial overgrowth.

The diagnosis is established by demonstrating villous atrophy on small bowel biopsy in an appropriate clinical setting. Other causes of villous atrophy, including coeliac disease, need to be excluded.

Tropical sprue responds to folic acid, which often reverses signs and symptoms of tropical sprue. Antibiotic therapy is also effective, although it often needs to be prolonged and relapses occur.

Whipple's Disease

Whipple's disease is a rare disorder characterised by chronic diarrhoea, abdominal pain, skin pigmentation, arthralgia and low-grade fever, usually in middle-aged men. The small intestine is always involved, but multiple other sites can also be involved including the brain, heart, synovium and kidney. Central nervous system involvement becomes more common with time and may lead to dementia or cranial nerve signs.

Whipple's disease is caused by a bacillus, *Tropheryma whipplei* and can be diagnosed by small bowel biopsy. PAS-positive macrophages can be identified in the small bowel biopsy and the diagnosis can be confirmed by electron microscopy, if necessary.

Treatment with antibiotics has changed the course of the disease resulting in recovery in most patients. Trimethoprim-sulfamethoxazole has replaced tetracycline as the antibiotic of choice due to the high relapse rate with tetracycline. Treatment needs to be prolonged.

Intestinal lymphoma

Both primary (arising from the gastrointestinal tract) and secondary lymphomas can involve the intestine and cause chronic diarrhoea and malabsorption. Primary gastrointestinal lymphomas can be classified into T- or B-cell lymphomas.

Enteropathy-associated T-cell lymphoma (EATL) occurs as a complication of coeliac disease. Symptoms include failure to respond to a gluten-free diet, abdominal pain, diarrhoea with malabsorption and weight loss. EATL can sometimes be the initial presentation of coeliac disease. An abdominal CT scan may reveal a small intestinal mass or lymphadenopathy, and a small bowel biopsy may provide the diagnosis. Laparoscopy is sometimes necessary for confirmation.

Immunoproliferative small intestinal disease is a B-cell lymphoma occurring in Middle Eastern countries and seems to be associated with poor sanitation and small bowel bacterial overgrowth. Chronic diarrhoea, malabsorption and weight loss occurs with advanced disease.

Eosinophilic gastroenteritis

Eosinophilic gastroenteritis is characterised by eosinophilic infiltration of the gut wall, often associated with peripheral blood eosinophilia.

Clinical features

Symptoms and signs of eosinophilic gastroenteritis depend on the layer of the gastrointestinal tract involved, and it is usually classified as predominantly mucosal disease, muscle-layer disease or subserosal disease.

Mucosal disease. This may present with abdominal pain, bloating, nausea and diarrhoea. Symptoms are often non-specific and similar to irritable bowel symptoms.

Muscle-layer disease. The eosinophilic infiltration involves the muscle layer of the gut and often produces obstructive symptoms of the area involved, which may be oesophageal, antral, small bowel or colonic.

Subserosal disease. Subserosal disease results in eosinophilic ascites characterised by a very high eosinophil count.

The diagnosis of eosinophilic gastroenteritis should be considered in patients with peripheral eosinophilia. It is confirmed by demonstrating eosinophilic infiltration on biopsy. The treatment depends on the severity of symptoms, with steroids usually considered for more severe symptoms. Dog hookworm has been implicated as causing cases of ileocolonic disease in Australia and will respond to a course of mebendazole (100 mg twice a day for three days).

Short bowel syndrome

The small intestine has a functional reserve of around 40–50% and when disease or resection exceeds this, diarrhoea and malabsorption results. As well as the extent of resection, the site of resection (jejunum or ileum), the loss of the ileocaecal valve and the loss of the colon will determine the severity of the symptoms.

Aetiology

The short bowel syndrome in adults may follow vascular injury, for example due to mesenteric vascular occlusion or bowel obstruction with strangulation. Multiple bowel resections for Crohn's disease may also cause a short bowel syndrome and small intestinal function may be further compromised by disease in the remaining small bowel. A deliberately induced short bowel syndrome will follow jejuno-ileal bypass for the management of obesity.

If part of the terminal ileum is resected, bile salt malabsorption may result in watery diarrhoea. With more extensive terminal ileal resection (> 100 cm), bile salt loss results in steatorrhoea.

Clinical features

Diarrhoea is the prominent symptom and fluid losses may be massive, especially shortly after resection before adaptation occurs. Malabsorption results from loss of surface area, malabsorption of bile salts, small bowel bacterial overgrowth and gastric hypersecretion of acid with inactivation of pancreatic enzymes. Weight loss, dehydration and nutritional deficiency may follow.

Management

Maintenance of hydration and nutrition is the primary aim in the early phase. Early enteral feeding will encourage intestinal adaptation, but should be introduced slowly. Small frequent feeds will help reduce the osmotic load in the gut. Vitamin and trace element levels should be monitored and replaced as necessary.

Cholestyramine will help control diarrhoea in patients with limited (< 100 cm) terminal ileal resection. Acid suppression with a proton pump inhibitor will help control gastric hypersecretion.

Long-term parenteral nutrition or small bowel transplantation will need to be considered in those patients whose nutritional needs cannot be met by enteral feeding.

Lactose deficiency

This is discussed in Chapter 16.

Small intestinal bacterial overgrowth

The small intestine is usually relatively sterile with bacterial colony counts being less than 10^4/mL of jejunal fluid. This relative sterility is maintained by normal small intestinal motility, gastric acidity, surface mucus and mucosal immunity, including secretory IgA.

Small bowel bacterial overgrowth may lead to mucosal damage and malabsorption of certain nutrients. Patients may be asymptomatic or have abdominal bloating, watery diarrhoea and weight loss.

Multiple mechanisms are responsible for malabsorption, including intestinal mucosal damage with loss of disaccharidases, and bacterial deconjugation of bile salts. Vitamin B12 malabsorption is common due to bacterial utilisation of this vitamin. The production of toxins may be important in certain liver diseases such as cirrhosis and non-alcoholic steatohepatitis.

Causes of small intestinal bacterial overgrowth

Small intestinal bacterial overgrowth usually occurs with conditions causing small intestinal stasis. Those with impaired immunity and the elderly are also susceptible (Table 13.6).

Diagnosis

Small intestinal aspiration and culture remains the 'gold standard' but is technically difficult and requires a unit experienced in the test with appropriate microbiological support. Breath tests include the ^{14}C-glycocholate test and the ^{14}C-D-xylose test, but they are neither very sensitive nor specific.

Treatment

Correction of the underlying cause is ideal (e.g., surgery for strictures) but is usually not possible. Antibiotics remain the mainstay of therapy and often need to be used long term.

TABLE 13.6: Causes of small intestine bacterial overgrowth

- Gastric surgery—Billroth II (see Chapter 5)
- Small bowel diverticula
- Small bowel stricture:
  - Crohn's disease
  - Radiation enteritis
- Impaired small intestinal motility:
  - Scleroderma
  - Diabetes mellitus
  - Chronic intestinal pseudo-obstruction (see Chapter 5)
- Miscellaneous/multifactorial
  - Elderly
  - Immune deficiency syndrome
  - Chronic pancreatitis
  - Cirrhosis

Radiation enteritis

Radiation to the small intestine may result in either acute or chronic damage. Acute injury during radiotherapy is common and results in diarrhoea, abdominal pain and nausea. Mucosal damage is frequently present with inflammatory changes and partial villous atrophy. Chemotherapy may potentiate radiation damage. Symptoms often begin shortly after commencement of radiotherapy and resolve within two weeks of cessation of therapy.

Chronic radiation damage to the small intestine may present months or years after treatment. It is mediated primarily by ischaemic changes induced by arteritis. Symptoms depend on the site of injury and include diarrhoea, malabsorption, weight loss, nausea and bloating as well as abdominal pain. Complications include intestinal obstruction due to strictures and perforation. Incomplete obstruction with strictures may result in bacterial overgrowth with malabsorption.

Treatment

Treatment depends on the nature and site of the underlying damage. Symptomatic treatment for diarrhoea may be necessary. A low-fibre diet helps in the presence of a stricture. Antibiotic therapy is useful when intestinal stasis occurs and surgery may be required for tight strictures. A parenteral diet may be necessary as well as nutritional replacement with malabsorption. Hyperbaric oxygen has been used in this setting.

Protein-losing enteropathy

The passage of plasma protein across the mucosa and loss into the gut may occur with inflamed or ulcerated mucosa (e.g., inflammatory bowel disease, Ménétrier's disease), abnormal cell structure (e.g., coeliac disease) or increased lymphatic pressure (e.g., carcinoma, lymphoma, intestinal lymphangiectasia). Patients present with oedema and features of the underlying disease. Protein loss may be identified in the stool by measuring stool alpha-1 antitrypsin levels or by the use of intravenously administered radio-labelled macromolecules such as indium-111.

Treatment

Management involves treatment of the underlying condition where possible. A low-fat, high-protein diet supplemented with a medium-chain triglyceride may be beneficial together with replacement of fat-soluble vitamins, minerals and trace metals as necessary.

Endocrine diseases

Steatorrhoea may occur in:

- diabetes mellitus due to intestinal stasis causing small bowel bacterial overgrowth or exocrine pancreatic insufficiency, or because of co-existing coeliac disease;
- hyperthyroidism (from rapid intestinal transport);
- the Zollinger-Ellison syndrome (see Chapter 5);
- carcinoid syndrome (usually diarrhoea rather than steatorrhoea plus cutaneous flushing);
- adrenal insufficiency (rare); or
- hypoparathyroidism (rare).

INFLAMMATORY BOWEL DISEASE

The occurrence of colitis has been recognised for many centuries. Initially all cases were considered infective until ulcerative colitis was described over 100 years ago. Terminal ileitis was described by Crohn and co-workers in 1932 and these two disorders are collectively termed inflammatory bowel disease. A clear distinction between the two cannot always be made, particularly at presentation, and up to 10% can be classified only as 'indeterminate colitis'.

Although these two disorders share many features, there are significant differences in the course of the illness and in management and it is important to determine the type of disease if possible.

Ulcerative Colitis

Ulcerative colitis has a prevalence of 40–80/100,000 of the population. It is more common in developed countries and frequently begins in young adults, but may occur at any age.

Aetiology

The aetiology of ulcerative colitis remains unknown. Both host and environmental factors may play a role. It has been postulated that an abnormal immune response to microbes produces inflammation. Alternatively, bacteria may elicit a normal inflammatory response by penetrating a defective mucosal barrier. There is a positive family history of inflammatory bowel disease in up to 20% of cases, and animal models have demonstrated an important role for microbes in the development of colitis. Cigarette smoking lowers the risk of developing ulcerative colitis. Non-steroidal anti-inflammatory drugs can aggravate underlying inflammatory bowel disease.

Pathology

Ulcerative colitis involves only the colon, and usually the inflammation is limited to the mucosa and crypts.

It may involve only the rectum (proctitis) or spread proximally to involve the sigmoid colon, the descending colon (left-sided colitis) or the whole colon (pancolitis). In those who present with proctitis or left-sided disease, proximal spread to involve all of the colon occurs in only 10%, and usually early in the course of the disease.

Distinguishing features in the pathology of ulcerative and Crohn's disease are outlined in Table 13.7.

TABLE 13.7: Pathological features in inflammatory bowel disease

Ulcerative colitis	Crohn's disease
Distribution	
• Colon only • Always continuous	• Colon and/or small intestine • May be discontinuous
Macroscopic appearance	
• Granular mucosa • Superficial ulcers • Pseudopolyps • Exudate of blood and pus	• Aphthoid ulcers • Deep serpiginous ulcers • Strictures
Microscopic appearance	
• Mucosal inflammation • Crypt damage[1]	• Transmural inflammation • Granulomas ($< 15\%$)[2]

1. Preservation of crypt architecture suggests acute self-limited colitis.
2. Granulomas may occur in tuberculosis, schistosomiasis and syphilis.

TABLE 13.8: Common symptoms in inflammatory bowel disease

Ulcerative colitis

- Diarrhoea
- Rectal bleeding and mucus
- Abdominal pain
- Constitutional symptoms: fever, weight loss, anorexia

Crohn's disease

- Abdominal pain
- Diarrhoea
- Rectal bleeding and mucus
- Constitutional symptoms: anorexia, weight loss, fever, lassitude
- Growth retardation (children)

Clinical features

The symptoms of ulcerative colitis depend on the degree of inflammatory changes and the extent of involvement (Table 13.8). When only the rectum is involved, patients may present with rectal bleeding and tenesmus. Diarrhoea is common but occasionally this group can present with constipation.

With more extensive disease, diarrhoea is usual and is associated with blood and mucus. Abdominal pain is common and is often eased by defecation. In severe disease, usually more than six bloody stools per day are passed. Constitutional features occur with more severe attacks, including anorexia, fever, weight loss, tachycardia, dehydration and anaemia. Features suggesting more severe colitis are outlined in Table 13.9.

TABLE 13.9: Clinical classification of ulcerative colitis			
	No. of bowel movements	Bleeding	Other symptoms
Mild[1]	< 4	Minimal	No toxic symptoms
Moderate	4–6	Moderate	Low-grade fever, malaise
Severe[2]	> 6	Severe	High fever, tachycardia

1. Most have proctosigmoiditis—10% progress to more extensive disease.
2. Most have pancolitis—may progress to toxic megacolon.

Both local and extraintestinal complications may be associated with ulcerative colitis (Table 13.10). The colon may dilate in severe attacks (toxic megacolon); this is a precursor to colonic perforation. It occurs when extensive colonic ulceration exposes the muscle layer of the colon, which then becomes atonic. In those patients with features of severe colitis, it is essential to carry out regular abdominal X-ray examinations to detect toxic megacolon.

Haemorrhage usually occurs as persisting bleeding in proportion to the severity of the diarrhoea. Occasionally massive haemorrhage can occur, although this is more common in Crohn's disease.

Extraintestinal manifestations which may occur in ulcerative colitis are listed in Table 13.10. Some are related to disease activity but others pursue an independent course. The latter group may precede active colitis or may occur after the cure of disease by total colectomy.

As with symptoms, signs in ulcerative colitis depend on the extent and severity of the attack and the presence or absence of complications.

With a mild attack the patient may look well and have only mild abdominal tenderness. With more severe colitis there may be associated pallor and a tachycardia associated with a low-grade fever, and abdominal tenderness may be more pronounced.

Diagnosis

The diagnosis of ulcerative colitis is based on typical clinical features, confirmation of colitis and exclusion of other causes of colonic inflammation.

Stool culture and microscopy. Stool microscopy may document red cells in those without macroscopic bleeding. The occurrence of white cells is evidence of inflammation or infection.

Infection must be excluded. Stool culture may demonstrate a pathogen known to cause colitis (e.g., *Shigella, Yersinia, Campylobacter, Entamoeba*, enterohaemorrhagic *E. coli*), although a negative stool culture does not automatically exclude infection. *Clostridium difficile* culture and toxin should be specifically requested in those where appropriate (e.g., recent hospitalisation or recent antibiotics).

TABLE 13.10: Complications of inflammatory bowel disease

Local complications
- Toxic megacolon
- Perforation
- Haemorrhage
- Carcinoma
- Stricture
- Abscess
- Fistula (Crohn's disease)

Extraintestinal complications
- Joints
  - Large joint arthritis[1]
  - Sacroileitis/ankylosing spondylitis (HLA-B27 positive)
- Mucocutaneous
  - Aphthous ulcers[1]
  - Erythema nodosum[1]
  - Pyoderma gangrenosum[1]
- Ocular
  - Conjunctivitis/episcleritis[1]
  - Uveitis/iritis[1]
- Hepatobiliary
  - Fatty infiltration[1]
  - Sclerosing cholangitis
  - Chronic hepatitis
  - Cholangiocarcinoma
  - Micronodular cirrhosis (ulcerative colitis)
  - Gallstones (Crohn's disease)
  - Granulomatous hepatitis (Crohn's disease)
  - Amyloid (Crohn's disease)
- Haematological
  - Iron deficiency (blood loss)[1]
  - Folate deficiency (poor intake; sulfasalazine)
  - B12 deficiency (Crohn's disease; terminal ileal disease; bacterial overgrowth)
  - Haemolytic anaemia (autoimmune; medication use)
  - Thrombosis (dehydration; bed rest; increased platelets; increased II, VIII levels)[1]
- Other
  - Renal stones (oxalate in Crohn's disease)
  - Renal disease (amyloid in Crohn's disease; hydronephrosis or hydroureter)
  - Growth retardation

---

1. Related to disease activity.

Haematology and biochemistry. The full blood count may be normal in mild colitis; with more severe attacks, the white cell count and ESR or C-reactive protein are often elevated. Anaemia with falling haemoglobin and serum albumin levels are features of more severe colitis. Abnormal liver function tests may indicate an extraintestinal manifestation such as sclerosing cholangitis.

Sigmoidoscopy and biopsy. All patients with ulcerative colitis have rectal involvement and a rectal biopsy should be performed if colitis is suspected. Histopathology may show colitis with 'chronic changes' such as crypt damage indicating inflammatory bowel disease. These chronic changes are absent in infectious colitis, but are not always present in patients with inflammatory bowel disease.

Colonoscopy. Colonoscopy is helpful in the differential diagnosis of colitis, and is useful in determining the extent of disease. The terminal ileum can usually be intubated to assess whether inflammation or ulceration is present.

Colonoscopy is also used for surveillance of carcinoma and assessment of strictures and polyps.

There is little to gain from carrying out a full colonoscopy in patients with severe active colitis, as there is a significant risk of perforation. The severity of colitis is best assessed by clinical features rather than colonoscopy.

Radiology. A plain abdominal X-ray will demonstrate toxic dilatation or perforation in patients with fulminating colitis (Figure 13.3).

Barium enema studies are rarely used now because of the wide availability of colonoscopy. A barium enema can provide information on the extent of disease (but often underestimates the extent of disease compared with colonoscopic evaluation) and the assessment of strictures (Figure 13.4).

Treatment

The treatment of ulcerative colitis will depend upon the extent and severity of disease. A different approach is taken to treat an acute attack and maintaining remission. Medical therapy is summarised in Table 13.11.

TABLE 13.11: Medical therapy in inflammatory bowel disease

General measures
- Correct anaemia and dehydration
- Emotional support
- Nutritional support
- Dietary advice

Symptomatic measures (for incomplete responders to first-line therapy but not in acutely ill cases)
- Antidiarrhoeal agents (e.g. loperamide, bile salt sequestering agents)
- Antispasmodic drugs

Specific drug therapy
- 5-amino salicylates: sulfasalazine, olsalazine, mesalazine
- Corticosteroids, budesonide
- Azathioprine
- 6-mercaptopurine
- Methotrexate (Crohn's disease)
- Cyclosporin (salvage therapy in fulminant colitis)
- Antibiotics (e.g., ciprofloxacin, clarithromycin, metronidazole)
- Infliximab (and other anti-TNF antibodies) (Crohn's disease)

Drugs being evaluated
- Probiotics
- Mycophenolate mofetil (ulcerative colitis)
- Monoclonal antibodies against alpha-4 integrin (e.g., natalizumab) and anti-interleukin 12 antibody (Crohn's disease)
- Thalidomide (Crohn's disease)
- MAP-kinase inhibitors (Crohn's disease)

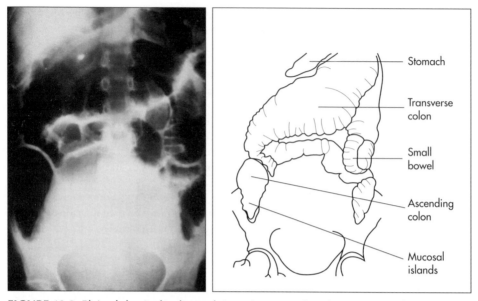

FIGURE 13.3: Plain abdominal radiograph in toxic megacolon showing a grossly dilated transverse colon with mucosal islands in the ascending colon. Concomitant distension of the small bowel is associated with very active colitis.

(Radiograph from and illustration based on Misiewicz JJ et al, Slide Atlas of Gastroenterology, with permission.)

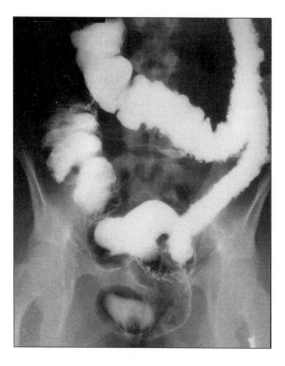

FIGURE 13.4: Left-sided colitis on barium enema.

General measures. Emotional support is important, especially at initial diagnosis and during relapses. Self-help groups in inflammatory bowel disease can provide additional support. Nutritional support is also important and anaemia, iron deficiency and malnutrition should be corrected.

5-amino salicylates. 5-amino salicylates are effective in the treatment of active colitis and in reducing relapses, but local release at the inflamed site is essential.

Sulfasalazine was the first drug used in this group. It consists of a 5-aminosalicylic acid (5-ASA) molecule linked by an azo bond to sulfapyridine. The azo bond is split by bacteria in the large intestine releasing 5-ASA, which is the active molecule. The sulfapyridine acts as a carrier preventing the release and absorption of 5-ASA until it reaches the colon.

Side effects occur in up to 20% of patients taking sulfasalazine and most are due to the sulfonamide component (Table 13.12).

TABLE 13.12: Side effects of sulfasalazine[1]

Dose related—slow acetylators

- Nausea, vomiting, anorexia (most common)
- Headache
- Diarrhoea
- Macrocytosis (folate deficiency)
- Haemolysis (Heinz body)
- Proteinuria, haematuria

Non-dose related

- Skin rash (and Stevens-Johnson syndrome)
- Agranulocytosis, aplastic anaemia
- Reversible male infertility (oligospermia, dysspermia)
- Hepatitis
- Pancreatitis
- Fibrosing alveolitis
- Vasculitis, lupus

---

1. Start at one 500 mg tablet, twice daily on the first day after meals, then increase by two tablets every second day until the patient is taking the full amount (typically, 1 g four times a day in acute disease; and 1 g twice a day for prophylaxis). Usually efficacious within 2–4 weeks (in 40–80% of patients). A blood count and urinalysis should be performed before starting therapy and then regularly during the first 3 months of treatment, and thereafter every 6 months. Supplement with folate, 1 mg/day orally. The drug may also be of specific benefit for the arthropathy in ankylosing spondylitis associated with inflammatory bowel disease.

This has led to the development of new drugs including olsalazine and mesalazine.

Olsalazine consists of two 5-ASA molecules bonded together. It has been shown to be effective in the treatment of active colitis and in maintaining remission. It is devoid of the sulfonamide side effects, but may induce diarrhoea in up to 8% of patients.

Mesalazine consists of 5-ASA protected by an acrylic coating which dissolves at pH 7. This releases 5-ASA in the terminal ileum and colon. This has advantages in patients with terminal ileal (Crohn's) disease, but at the expense of an increased absorption of 5-ASA. Thus, caution should be exercised when using mesalazine in patients with renal disease.

5-amino salicylates are available in suppository and enema form, which is the preferred mode of administration for those with proctitis or left-sided disease. Oral 5-ASA should be used for more extensive colitis.

Corticosteroids. Corticosteroids are effective in the treatment of ulcerative colitis and may be administered topically, orally or parenterally. Topical preparations (suppositories, liquid enemas and foam) are useful for disease limited to the rectum or left side of the colon. Topical steroids have the advantage of limited absorption and minimal side effects.

Oral corticosteroids are used for moderate to severe cases of ulcerative colitis, or milder cases which fail to respond to salicylates. They are generally administered at a high dose initially (e.g., 40–60 mg of prednisolone) until there is a clinical response, and then tapered down by 5–10 mg weekly until 20 mg is reached, then by 2.5 mg weekly.

Budesonide is an alternative oral corticosteroid that may have reduced steroid side effects because of its high first pass metabolism in the liver.

In severe or fulminating attacks of ulcerative colitis patients should be hospitalised and intravenous corticosteroids administered (e.g., hydrocortisone, 300 mg/day by continuous infusion). Regular abdominal X-ray examination for toxic megacolon is mandatory in these circumstances. Failure to demonstrate improvement in 7–10 days may be an indication for colectomy. In specialised centres, intravenous cyclosporin may be considered.

The side effects of corticosteroids can be limited if high dose treatment is restricted to a period of several weeks. Patient with hypertension, diabetes mellitus, cardiac disease or a psychiatric history should be carefully monitored.

Azathioprine, 6-mercaptopurine and cyclosporin. Azathioprine is generally reserved for those who fail to respond to corticosteroids or for a steroid sparing effect in those who require long-term high-dose corticosteroids. Mercaptopurine (6-MP) may be useful in unresponsive colitis, but its onset of action, as with azathioprine, is from 2–6 months.

TABLE 13.13: Azathioprine and 6-mercaptopurine (6-MP)—side effects

- Allergy (high fever, rash, arthritis) (2%)
- Nausea, vomiting, anorexia (1%)
- Bone marrow suppression (leucopaenia, infections)[1] (1%)
- Pancreatitis (1%)
- Abnormal liver function tests (transaminases increase)[1]
- Cholestatic jaundice (rare: may progress despite stopping drug)
- Malignancy (rare)
- Male infertility (reversible depression of spermatogenesis)

1. Dose-related side effects—reduce the dose.

The dose-dependent toxicity of azathioprine and 6-MP (bone marrow suppression, hepatic dysfunction) is related to the metabolite thiopurine–s–methyltransferase (TPMT) (Table 13.13). Deficiency or low activity of TPMT occurs in 10%; testing is done in some centres to detect TMPT activity and, if absent, the patient does not receive azathioprine or 6-MP. Azathioprine is traditionally started at 50 mg per day and gradually increased to a maximum of 2.5 mg/kg. Close monitoring is essential in view of the potential side effects of bone marrow suppression and a full blood count should be performed weekly initially and then monthly.

Cyclosporin given intravenously in high dose as a continuous infusion is of use in severe ulcerative colitis resistant to steroids. Some patients respond to this treatment, but severe side effects and relapse of disease remain a problem. Side effects include renal (hypertension, acute renal failure), neurological (seizures, tremor), infections (*Pneumocystis carinii* prophylaxis is recommended), cancer (skin, lymphoproliferative) and gingival hyperplasia. Blood levels of drug should be monitored and cholesterol checked (low cholesterol predisposes to seizures on the drug). If the patient with fulminant colitis fails to respond in 7–10 days, surgery is indicated. A possible alternative to cyclosporin in this setting is infliximab, but more data are needed.

Preventing relapse. 5-ASA compounds have been shown to be useful in reducing the rate of relapse and should be continued long term. Azathioprine is also effective in reducing the relapse rate.

Complications

Both local and extraintestinal complications may occur in ulcerative colitis (see Table 13.10). As indicated, some of these complications are related to disease activity but others are independent of disease status and may begin before the onset of colitis or develop after colectomy.

Toxic megacolon is the most feared complication of severe ulcerative colitis because it is a precursor of perforation and is associated with a high mortality. It should be suspected in patients with severe colitis who develop increasing abdominal pain with fever. It can be detected on plain abdominal X-ray and is defined as dilation of the colon in excess of 6 cm. In addition to intravenous steroids, the patient should be kept nil by mouth and given antibiotics. Lack of improvement within 72 hours is an indication for colectomy.

Massive bleeding may occur in ulcerative colitis, but is more common in Crohn's disease.

Surgery

In contrast to Crohn's disease, only a minority of patients with ulcerative colitis require surgery during the course of their disease. During acute disease surgery may be necessary for fulminating colitis not responsive to medical therapy, toxic megacolon, perforation or massive haemorrhage. Indications in chronic disease include disabling chronic symptoms and carcinoma or carcinoma risk (severe dysplasia) (Table 13.14).

Colon carcinoma. This is a complication of long-standing ulcerative colitis where disease extends beyond the splenic flexure. It may be multicentric. The risk begins 8–10 years after the onset of pancolitis, and approximately 0.5–1% of patients per annum will develop colon cancer. Screening is recommended although the cost effectiveness of regular surveillance with colonoscopy and biopsy is controversial and the yield is low. Currently, colonoscopy every year with multiple biopsies (2–4 at 10 cm intervals) is recommended after 8 years in those with extensive colitis, and after 15 years in those with left-sided colitis above the rectosigmoid junction. If high grade dysplasia is detected, or if dysplasia (high or low-grade) is found with a lesion or mass at colonoscopy (dysplasia associated lesion of the mucosa or DALM) then colectomy is indicated. Pathological interpretation of the presence of dysplasia may be controversial, and active colitis can make biopsies misleading.

Proctocolectomy is the original standard procedure but a permanent ileostomy is required. An ileo-anal anastomosis after proctocolectomy is an alternative; a reservoir is constructed from ileal loops to form a pouch. Pouchitis occurs in up to 50% of cases and frequent bowel movements are usual after the procedure.

TABLE 13.14: Indications for surgery in inflammatory bowel disease

Ulcerative colitis

- Failed medical therapy (fulminant colitis)
- Toxic megacolon
- Perforation
- Massive haemorrhage
- Chronic disabling symptoms
- Carcinoma or high risk of carcinoma

Crohn's disease

- Acute colitis—same as ulcerative colitis
- Chronic disabling symptoms
- Bowel obstruction
- Fistulae
- Abscesses
- Perforation
- Perianal complications
- Growth retardation (children)

Crohn's disease

Aetiology

The current evidence suggests that Crohn's disease is due to either an abnormal immune response to an environmental antigen, such as bacteria, or abnormal exposure of the immune system to that antigen due to an excessively permeable mucosal barrier. An inflammatory bowel disease gene has been reported (IBD1, that encodes a protein NOD2 (also called CARD15) that may regulate intestinal epithelial cell immunity). Mutations in this gene result in an increased susceptibility to Crohn's disease (ileal and fibrostenosing disease) in some populations. Smoking increases the risk of Crohn's disease two-fold.

Clinical features

Symptoms and signs in Crohn's disease vary according to the site of involvement and the degree of activity. Small bowel disease may result in abdominal pain after meals, diarrhoea and weight loss. Terminal ileal disease may also present with fever or right iliac fossa pain that is indistinguishable from acute appendicitis. With large bowel involvement, diarrhoea and rectal bleeding is common (see Table 13.8).

Symptoms in Crohn's disease may begin insidiously and the diagnosis is often delayed. Systemic features are common (fever, lassitude and weight loss) and perianal disease (fissure, fistulae, abscesses) is a frequent early clue to the diagnosis (Chapter 11).

The physical examination may reveal an abdominal mass or localised tenderness, especially in the right iliac fossa. There may be evidence of weight loss or anaemia and perianal involvement may be noted (Chapter 11). Growth retardation may be observed in children and can be the presenting complaint.

Extraintestinal manifestations occur as with ulcerative colitis (see Table 13.10; Figure 13.5).

Investigations

Stool culture and examination. Exclusion of infective causes of diarrhoea and bleeding is important at initial presentation (Chapter 12). A *Clostridium difficile* toxin assay should be included where appropriate (e.g., recent hospitalisation or antibiotics). Cytomegalovirus virus infection can also complicate inflammatory bowel disease and cause a relapse of symptoms, especially in those on immunosuppressants. Infective causes should be considered during relapses if there is a high level of suspicion, such as with watery diarrhoea without bleeding, or if there is a high risk of infection (e.g., after an overseas trip).

Blood screen. Abnormalities of the full blood count are common in Crohn's disease, including anaemia due to iron deficiency, or folate or vitamin B12 deficiency, an elevated white cell count, elevated platelets and a high ESR or C-reactive protein.

Serum albumin levels may be low if there is associated nutritional deficiency. Abnormal liver function test results due to extraintestinal complications or drug therapy may be present.

Antibody testing. Anti-*Saccharomyces cerevisiae* antibody (ASCA) positivity and antineutrophil cytoplasmic antibody (p-ANCA) negativity suggests Crohn's disease. However, these tests lack sufficient accuracy alone for diagnosis.

Sigmoidoscopy/colonoscopy. Colonoscopy is usually the investigation of choice for the diagnosis of Crohn's disease. Changes may be patchy and involve both the colon and terminal ileum or the terminal ileum only. Changes may be subtle with scattered aphthous ulcers or dramatic with deep serpiginous ulcers and spontaneous bleeding. Diffuse colitis resembling ulcerative colitis may also be seen. Biopsies may show non-specific colitis or sometimes granulomas typical of Crohn's disease.

Radiology. A plain abdominal X-ray is the initial investigation in patients with a suspected bowel obstruction. A barium enema may show features typical of Crohn's disease with skip areas, deep ulcers and strictures. It is used less frequently now that colonoscopy is widely available, but remains the best investigation to detect fistulae. Small bowel radiology may document Crohn's disease involving the terminal ileum or elsewhere in the small bowel (Figure 13.6). Abdominal CT scanning may be helpful in the diagnosis of an abscess complicating Crohn's disease or local inflammatory changes around the small or large bowel. A small bowel wireless capsule study may be considered in difficult diagnostic cases but may become obstructed in a strictured small bowel segment requiring surgical removal.

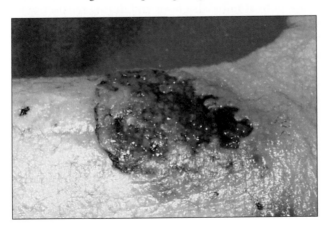

FIGURE 13.5: Pyoderma gangrenosum on the lower leg.

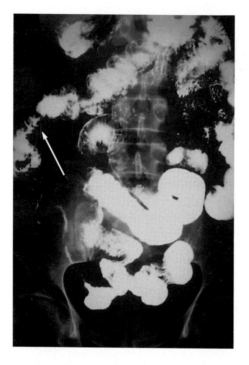

FIGURE 13.6: Terminal ileal disease due to Crohn's disease (string sign)

Radionuclide scanning. This technique involves labelling the patient's white cell counts with indium and injecting them intravenously. The white cells accumulate in areas of inflammation. The test is non-specific but may provide additional evidence of Crohn's disease.

Treatment

The treatment of Crohn's disease depends on the site of involvement and the severity of the disease. Medical therapy is summarised in Table 13.11.

General measures. Correction of anaemia, malnutrition or dehydration may be necessary and hospital admission is indicated for severe disease. Advise the patient to stop smoking.

Emotional support is important both at initial diagnosis and during relapses. Self-help groups may provide a valuable role here.

A low-fibre diet may help reduce symptoms in those patients with significant small bowel disease. Vitamin and mineral supplements including iron, folate and vitamin B12 may be necessary.

5-amino salicylates. Sulfasalazine is effective in the treatment of active colonic Crohn's disease, but its role in small bowel Crohn's disease is less clear as there is little release of 5-ASA into the small bowel. It has significant side effects mainly related to the sulfapyridine moiety (see Table 13.12).

Mesalazine, a coated salicylate which is released in the terminal ileum and colon, is more effective treatment for active terminal ileal disease.

Olsalazine can be used for active colitis but may cause diarrhoea in some patients.

5-ASA drugs have only a modest benefit in preventing relapse of Crohn's disease in remission.

Corticosteroids. Corticosteroids are effective in the treatment of both active small and large bowel disease. As with ulcerative colitis, they are usually started at high doses (e.g., 40–60 mg of prednisolone), and tapered gradually according to the response. Intravenous administration is preferred for more severely ill patients. Budesonide has also been shown to be effective in the treatment of active ileal Crohn's disease. Steroids are not useful for preventing relapse.

Antibiotics. Oral metronidazole is useful for complicated perianal disease. Long-term use is precluded by side effects, such as peripheral neuropathy, which may be irreversible. Other antibiotics that have been trialled for the treatment of ileal Crohn's disease as well as perianal disease include ciprofloxacin, clarithromycin and the cephalosporins.

Immunosuppressive agents. Azathioprine and 6-mercaptopurine are generally used in patients who are resistant to corticosteroids or for their steroid-sparing effect in those who require high-dose steroids. Their onset of action is slow (from 2–6 months) and bone marrow suppression and liver toxicity is a potential side effect (Table 13.13). At the usual dose (2 mg/kg/day) adverse events are uncommon, but careful monitoring with a full blood count monthly is mandatory.

Methotrexate may be useful in patients with unresponsive Crohn's disease, especially those with associated arthropathy. Hepatic toxicity and bone marrow suppression are significant complications.

Elemental diet. An elemental diet has been shown to be effective in several studies in the treatment of active Crohn's disease. However, compliance is a problem and even motivated patients have difficulty in continuing with the unpalatable diet for more than a week or so. Total parenteral nutrition is an alternative way of allowing bowel rest in patients who are ill and hospitalised or who are malnourished.

Infliximab. Infliximab is a mouse–human chimeric antibody to tumour necrosis factor alpha. It was initially introduced for the treatment of fistulae in Crohn's disease but is now also used for active ileal and colonic Crohn's disease. It has a high response rate for severe Crohn's disease and fistulae, but relapses may start within two months. Some advocate long-term treatment every two months, but the long-term side effects are not yet clear and severe complications, mostly related to immune suppression, have been reported.

Preventing relapse. The 5-ASA drugs do not reduce relapse of disease. Immunomodulating agents such as azathioprine are useful for preventing relapse. Repeated infusions of infliximab are used in some centres to maintain remission.

Surgery

Up to 80% of patients with long-term Crohn's disease will require surgery at some stage during their disease (see Table 13.14). Surgery will not prevent recurrence of the disease, but may relieve symptoms for a long period. Colonoscopic studies suggest that, after resection, approximately 70% have evidence of recurrent disease (often asymptomatic) within a year; re-operation for small bowel and colonic disease at 15 years is about 70% and 40%, respectively.

However, because recurrence is usual, it is important to avoid extensive small bowel resection. With multiple strictures or previous small bowel resection, a conservative approach such as stricturoplasty may relieve symptoms. The risk of colon and small bowel cancer is slightly increased in Crohn's disease, but surveillance is not recommended.

Surgery is also indicated for complications such as abscesses or fistulae (Table 13.14).

Inflammatory bowel disease in pregnancy

Ulcerative colitis and Crohn's disease do not have any effect on fertility or increase the incidence of fetal malformation, but spontaneous abortions and prematurity are increased if disease is active. Prognosis is not affected by pregnancy but Crohn's disease may flare up postpartum. Similarly, neither sulfasalazine or corticosteroids increase the risk of congenital abnormalities and can be continued during pregnancy. Azathioprine can also be continued during pregnancy without major risk to fetus or mother.

COLLAGENOUS AND MICROSCOPIC COLITIS

Collagenous colitis is a diarrhoeal disorder characterised by thickening of the subepithelial collagen plate in the colon. Intraepithelial lymphocytes are also often increased. In microscopic colitis, there is no increased collagen.

A typical syndrome of watery diarrhoea results usually in middle-aged to elderly women. At colonoscopy the macroscopic appearance is often normal and biopsies are necessary to establish the diagnosis.

Symptoms may improve with sulfasalazine or corticosteroids but, often, symptomatic therapy with loperamide or diphenoxylate is all that is necessary.

Further reading

Akobeng A, Gardener E. Oral 5-aminosalicylic acid for maintenance of medically-induced remission in Crohn's disease. *Cochrane Database Syst Rev* 2005; (1): CD003715.

Alaedini A, Green PH. Narrative review: celiac disease: understanding a complex autoimmune disorder. *Ann Intern Med* 2005; 142: 289–98.

Camilleri M. Chronic diarrhea: a review on pathophysiology and management for the clinical gastroenterologist. *Clin Gastroenterol Hepatol* 2004; 2: 198–206.

Dubinsky MC. Azathioprine, 6-mercaptopurine in inflammatory bowel disease pharmacology, efficacy, and safety. *Clin Gastroenterol Hepatol* 2004; 2: 731–43.

Duggan JM. Coeliac disease: the great imitator. *Med J Aust* 2004; 180: 524–6.

Fujioka K. Follow-up of nutritional and metabolic problems after bariatric surgery. *Diabetes Care* 2005; 28: 481–4.

Headstrom PD, Surawicz CM. Chronic diarrhea. *Clin Gastroentrol Hepatol* 2005; 3: 734–7.

Keuchel M, Hagenmuller F. Video capsule endoscopy in the work-up of abdominal pain. *Gastrointest Endosc Clin N Am* 2004; 14: 195–205.

Kornbluth A, Sachar DB, Practice Parameters Committee of the American College of Gastroenterology. Ulcerative colitis practice guidelines in adults (updates): American College of Gastroenterology, Practice Parameters Committee. *Am J Gastroenterol* 2004; 99: 1371–85.

Kucik CJ, Martin GL, Sortor BV. Common intestinal parasites. *Am Fam Physician* 2004; 69: 1161–8.

Mahnel R, Marth T. Progress, problems, and perspectives in diagnosis and treatment of Whipple's disease. *Clin Exp Med* 2004; 4: 39–43.

Panaccione R, Sandborn WJ. Medical therapy of Crohn disease. *Curr Opin Gastroenterol* 2004; 20: 351–9.

Pardi DS. Microscopic colitis: an update. *Inflamm Bowel Dis* 2004; 10: 860–70.

Schiller LR. Chronic diarrhea. *Gastroenterology* 2004; 127: 287–93.

Travis SP, Strange EF, Lemann M *et al.* European evidence based consensus on the diagnosis and management of Crohn's disease: current management. *Gut* 2006; 55 Suppl 1: i16–35.

chapter 14

LEAKAGE OF STOOL (INCONTINENCE)

INTRODUCTION

Faecal incontinence is a common condition, with 10% of the adult population being affected. When the condition is chronic, it can cause restriction of lifestyle or even social isolation. In many cases, it is the factor resulting in an elderly person requiring entry into a nursing home. It has been estimated that only one-fifth of people with incontinence consult their doctor about the problem—the remainder fail to do so, citing as their reason embarrassment or the belief that no treatment is available. A recent Commonwealth Government analysis has shown that treatment of incontinence in Australia stands at several hundred million dollars annually and places a significant financial burden on the community. It is therefore vital to understand the condition, and improve treatment as well as methods of prevention.

DEFINITIONS

Continence is defined as the ability to control the onset of rectal evacuation. Minor incontinence refers to mucus discharge or incontinence of liquid or solid stool less than once per week. Major incontinence is loss of liquid or solid stool more than once a week, or sufficiently frequently to be causing social embarrassment for the patient. A more objective numerical continence scoring system, taking into account the exact frequency and nature of incontinence, is now commonly used in specialist centres and a simplified version is helpful for routine clinical assessment (Table 14.1). It is important to focus on the exact nature of the incontinence as described above in order to decide whether the condition warrants full investigation and treatment.

TABLE 14.1: Simplified Wexner scoring system for faecal incontinence (0–20): 0 = normal continence, 20 = severe incontinence

	Never	< 1/month	< 1/week	< 1/day	> 1/day
Leakage of solid stool	0	1	2	3	4
Leakage of liquid stool	0	1	2	3	4
Flatus	0	1	2	3	4
Pad used	0	1	2	3	4
Lifestyle changed	0	1	2	3	4

HISTORY

The causes of faecal incontinence are summarised in Table 14.2. A good history will often lead the clinician to the diagnosis of the cause. The physical examination and targeted investigations will determine whether the sphincter is normal, and will identify the likely pathology in most cases. The three most common causes of faecal incontinence requiring surgical treatment are rectal prolapse, sphincter trauma and neurogenic incontinence. These conditions account for the majority of patients who suffer severe long-standing symptoms.

The essential historical features that need to be established in these patients are:

- Is the incontinence for solids, liquids or gas? Determine whether complaints of incontinence reflect only perianal soiling by mucus. Mucus seepage occurs with local anal conditions such as anal mucosal prolapse and haemorrhoids.

- Is it passive incontinence, where there is involuntary seepage of stool without awareness? Passive incontinence occurs with internal sphincter weakness.

- What is the frequency, duration and time course (variable, constant or progressive) of the incontinence?

- Is urgency present—is the patient able to defer defecation for a reasonable time? Urgency and incontinence often occurs when the sphincter is normal, such as in proctitis, rectal cancer, or with diarrhoea. With diarrhoea, incontinence results from rapid transit of stool through the lower colon. It may be preceded by lower abdominal crampy pain and occasional perianal pain prior to the incontinent event. Alternatively, urgency may be an expression of the lack of normal rectal capacitance such as can occur with proctitis, when the rectum acts only as a conduit rather than a capacitance organ.

- Does the incontinence date from a particular medical event, e.g., perianal surgery or a difficult vaginal delivery? Perianal trauma may not present with incontinence immediately after the event, but rather many years later. Thus, the anal sphincter mechanism can compensate for a badly damaged sphincter due to anal surgery (e.g., for fistula), an unsatisfactorily repaired episiotomy or third-degree tear, or prolonged stretching of the pudendal and sacral nerves during second-stage vaginal delivery.

- Are there any other symptoms of anal or rectal disease?

TABLE 14.2: Causes of faecal incontinence

Normal sphincter

- Diarrhoea
- Anorectal conditions:
  - Rectal carcinoma
  - Inflammatory bowel disease
  - Haemorrhoids
  - Mucosal prolapse
  - Fissure-in-ano
  - Abnormal rectal sensation

Abnormal sphincter

- Congenital abnormalities
- Anal sepsis
- Neurological conditions
- Rectal prolapse
- Sphincter trauma
- Neurogenic (idiopathic) incontinence

EXAMINATION

Examine the patient in the left lateral position with the hips flexed to allow the examiner good access to the perineum and anal region. Inspect the area for soiling, and for excoriation of the perianal skin as evidence of chronic irritation secondary to incontinence. Look for any external prolapse at the anus (Table 14.3). Also look for an asymmetrical sphincter secondary to trauma and perianal scarring.

Digital anorectal examination is carried out next and the resting tone (produced by the internal sphincter) is noted. Estimate the functional length of the anal canal in centimetres. The strength of the pelvic floor muscles is estimated by posterior pressure on the examining finger. External sphincter strength is assessed by asking the patient to contract the sphincter and, thereafter, to cough. A shortened, weak sphincter (caused by poor contraction of the puborectalis muscle) is found in neurogenic incontinence. A weak sphincter of normal length is caused by a sphincter defect due to trauma. The sphincter is examined circumferentially between the thumb and index finger and a defect may be palpable.

The rectal mucosa is then examined circumferentially for a tumour; this should not be done at the beginning of the examination since discomfort from deep pelvic examination may impair subsequent ability of the patient to cooperate with contraction and relaxation of the sphincter.

The patient is next asked to bear down while the examiner looks for rectal prolapse. Palpate the ischial tuberosities and assess the plane of the perineum in relation to the position of an imaginary line drawn between the tuberosities. If the perineum descends below this line when the patient is asked to bear down, then this is evidence for abnormal descent associated with neurogenic weakness of the pelvic floor muscles. If rectal prolapse is suspected but not demonstrated in this position, the examination should be repeated with the patient squatting over a paper towel or sitting on a commode. Internal prolapse can sometimes be demonstrated by digital rectal examination. An internal prolapse where the intussusception does not pass the anal sphincter can be detected by digital examination while the patient is bearing down.

If there is a history suggestive of a neurological condition, then a full neurological examination should be carried out.

TABLE 14.3: Causes of external prolapse at the anus

Anal canal
- Haemorrhoids
- Anal mucosal prolapse
- Fibroepithelial polyp

Rectum
- Rectal mucosal prolapse
- Full-thickness rectal prolapse
- Polyp
  - Juvenile polyp (haematoma)
  - Adenoma

Colon
- Intussusception of pedunculated adenoma

Proctoscopy and sigmoidoscopy

At proctoscopy, anal mucosal prolapse and haemorrhoids can be diagnosed. Sigmoidoscopy is essential to exclude rectal pathology including proctitis and rectal tumours (Chapter 20). The patient at the end of the examination is asked to strain down on the sigmoidoscope as an internal (occult) rectal prolapse can sometimes be diagnosed in this way.

PHYSIOLOGICAL ANORECTAL EXAMINATION

Before considering physiological investigation of anal incontinence it is important to consider the physiology of continence. Continence is maintained by a complex process that has both sensory and motor components.

Physiology of continence

Normal continence depends on an interaction of the following factors.

1. Anal sphincter

The anal canal is surrounded by a muscular tube that produces a high-pressure zone exceeding the pressure in the rectum. The sphincter contains two layers (Figure 14.1): an inner layer of involuntary smooth muscle (internal sphincter) and an outer layer of skeletal muscle (external sphincter). The internal sphincter is a distal continuation of the circular muscle of the rectum and is in a state of constant contraction, maintained by a process of intrinsic muscle stimulation. Relaxation of the muscle occurs during defecation, mediated by a local neural reflex within the wall of the anorectum in response to distension of the rectum by the faecal bolus, as well as by extrinsic autonomic control via the presacral sympathetic nerves. The external sphincter is under voluntary control but also contracts involuntarily in response to an increase in intra-abdominal pressure via a spinal reflex through the anterior horns of the S2–S4 spinal segments.

The puborectalis muscle lies immediately above the external sphincter and forms a muscular sling behind the anus (Figure 14.2). It supports the anus and maintains the anorectal angle, and contributes to the high-pressure zone.

2. Anal cushions

There are three anal cushions in the 3, 7 and 11 o'clock positions formed from expansions of the submucosa of the anal canal. The cushions are compressed when the sphincter pressure is high, but expand at other times and lie in apposition to each other, thereby assisting continence.

3. Sensory mechanism

The anal mucosa contains an abundance of sensory nerve endings. Spontaneous relaxation of the upper part of the internal sphincter occurs intermittently to allow the anal mucosa to 'sample' the contents of the rectum (the sampling reflex). This allows us to normally distinguish flatus from stool in the rectum.

4. Stool consistency

The nature of the stool in the rectum has an important impact on continence, a fact often overlooked.

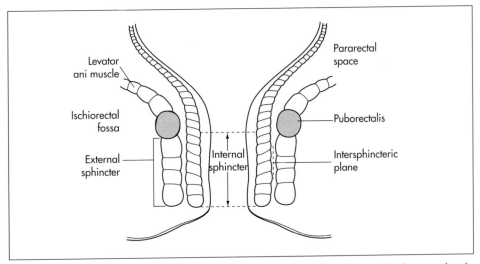

FIGURE 14.1: Anal sphincter. The internal sphincter is continuous above with the muscle of the rectum. The external sphincter lies below the puborectalis and levator ani muscles.
(Based on Parks et al, 1976; 63(1): 1–12, John Wiley & Sons Ltd, with permission.)

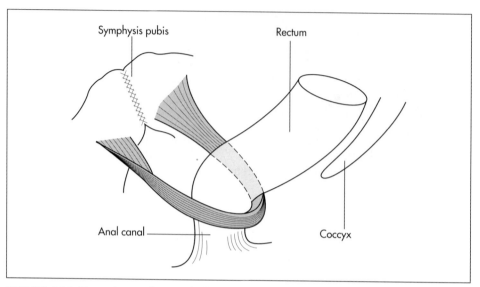

FIGURE 14.2: The puborectalis muscle forms a sling behind the junction of the anus and rectum.

(Based on Anderson, Grants Atlas, *1978, with permission from the publisher.)*

5. Rectal compliance

The rectum is a storage organ and its wall must be compliant in order to fulfil this reservoir function. Diseases affecting the rectal wall may make it less compliant and impair continence.

Diagnostic tests

Anorectal manometry

Pressure in the anus and rectum is measured using a small plastic catheter placed inside the anal canal and connected to a pressure transducer and recording apparatus. The pressure at rest reflects the strength of the internal sphincter, and pressure during voluntary contraction of the muscles is a measure of the external sphincter strength (Figure 14.3). Relaxation of the internal sphincter is tested by inflating a balloon in the rectum while recording anal pressure. Manometry is a very useful test because it defines which muscle is affected in a patient with sphincter weakness. It also demonstrates that sphincter function is normal in a patient whose incontinence is due to diarrhoea or excessive colonic propulsion, or due to a local anal condition such as haemorrhoids and, hence, confirms that sphincter weakness is not the cause of the incontinence.

Electrophysiology

Nerve conduction studies. In patients with suspected neurogenic incontinence the function of the pudendal nerves is tested. *Motor conduction* is measured by transrectal stimulation of the nerves, using a fine disposable electrode mounted on the gloved index finger. The left and right pudendal nerves are stimulated at the point that each passes around the ischial spine and the conduction time to the external anal sphincter is recorded (Figure 14.4). Stretch-induced damage to the nerves caused by difficult vaginal delivery or chronic excessive straining at stool is reflected in slowing of

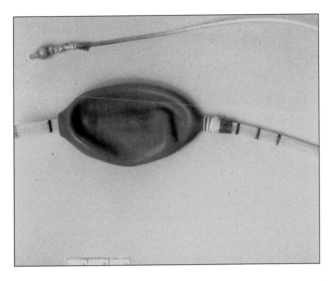

FIGURE 14.3A: Anorectal manometry. Recording catheter microballoon (above), and multi-channel catheter for recording simultaneously at several levels, and with a balloon near the tip for distension of the rectum (below).

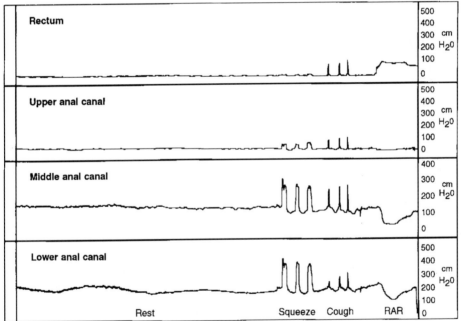

FIGURE 14.3B: Anorectal manometry. Manometry recording—pressures recorded simultaneously at three levels in the anal canal and one site in the rectum. Pressure at rest reflects the internal sphincter; increase above the resting pressure is produced by a squeeze or cough, due to the external sphincter contraction. The rectoanal reflex (RAR) shows relaxation of the internal sphincter (seen as a fall in pressure in the anal recording) due to distension of the rectum with a balloon (seen as a rise in pressure in the rectum).

conduction in the nerves due to axonal degeneration. Sensory conduction is measured by delivering a small current to the anal mucosa. The current is increased in fractions of a milliamp until a slight painless tapping feeling is reported by the patient, and the threshold of stimulation is measured. With pudendal nerve damage there is loss of sensation, reflected as an increased threshold of stimulation.

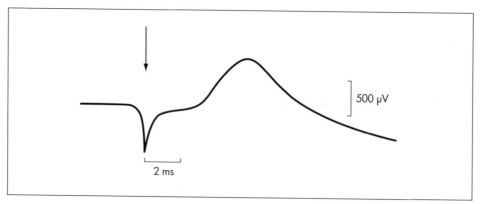

500 μV

2 ms

FIGURE 14.4: Recording of pudendal motor latency. The arrow indicates the onset of the stimulus delivered to the pudendal nerve; there is then a delay (2 ms) due to the conduction time along the nerve (pudendal latency), followed by contraction of the external sphincter shown by a rise and fall in the trace. Damage to the pudendal nerve results in an increase in pudendal latency.

Electromyography. This is carried out using a fine needle electrode inserted into the external sphincter muscle. Muscle contraction is amplified and displayed as spikes of electrical activity. Normal muscle activity can be clearly distinguished from non-functional scar tissue, allowing the site and extent of a sphincter defect to be clearly defined (Figure 14.5).

Ultrasound

Endoanal ultrasound has become a valuable tool to study anal function. It is very accurate in identifying a defect in the internal or external sphincter (Figure 14.6). Much of the information previously sought from electromyography can now be obtained from endoanal ultrasound, which is non-invasive.

Proctography

Barium studies of the anorectum are used to test the ability of the anal sphincter to maintain continence. Semi-solid barium paste of similar consistency to soft stool is instilled into the rectum. Lateral X-ray examination is made of the rectum and anus while the patient coughs, moves and during a Valsalva manoeuvre, and the amount of leakage is assessed (Figure 14.7). This examination is used to confirm the diagnosis of neurogenic incontinence.

Computerised tomography

CT scans of the pelvis or lumbosacral spinal cord are useful if a spinal cord lesion is suspected.

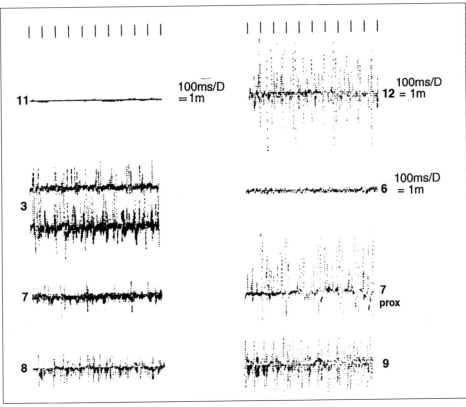

FIGURE 14.5: Electromyography of the external sphincter showing normal muscle activity at 3, 7, 8, 9, and 12 o'clock, and loss of activity at 6 and 11 o'clock due to sphincter damage.

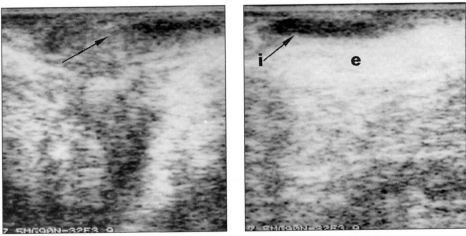

FIGURE 14.6: Anal ultrasound in a patient with faecal incontinence showing the longitudinal view of the anal canal. Normal muscle at 9 o'clock (right); internal anal sphincter (i) seen as a black band, external anal sphincter (e) seen as a dense white band. Damaged sphincter muscle at 12 o'clock (left), showing loss of internal and external sphincter bands (arrow).

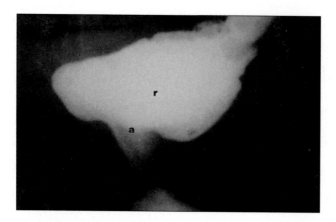

FIGURE 14.7: Proctography. Lateral X-ray film of the rectum (r) and anal canal (a) showing leakage of barium during coughing in a patient with neurogenic incontinence.

CONDITIONS CAUSING INCONTINENCE WITH A NORMAL SPHINCTER

Diarrhoea

Aetiology

Diarrhoea, either acute or chronic, may overcome the ability of the normal sphincter to resist the forceful passage of liquid stool. High pressures generated in the colon may exceed the maximum pressure of the anal sphincter, and incontinence is then inevitable. Incontinence may even occur when stool consistency and frequency are normal, due to sudden excessive colonic propulsion.

Clinical features

In patients with diarrhoea, incontinence is sometimes preceded by crampy lower abdominal pain or a sudden urgent call to stool. Other clinical features are discussed in Chapters 12 and 13.

Treatment

When there is a colonic cause for incontinence, simple antidiarrhoeal medication may produce a very dramatic improvement in some patients. Chronic diarrhoea should be investigated with fresh stool specimens sent for microscopy and culture, and sigmoidoscopy or colonoscopy. Special tests for malabsorption or more rare causes of diarrhoea (see Chapter 13) will be indicated in some cases.

Once secondary causes have been excluded, diarrhoea should be treated with a small *regular* prophylactic dose of loperamide, usually one 2 mg tablet taken daily in the morning. The aim of treatment is to suppress colonic activity sufficiently to produce slight firmness of the stool. There is no benefit gained from taking this medication after a loose stool is passed. Loperamide also has the added benefit of producing direct contraction of the internal sphincter muscle and, hence, raising resting anal pressure in some patients.

Anorectal conditions

Anal mucosal prolapse and prolapsing haemorrhoids can result in incontinence. Prolapse is caused by straining at stool. Most commonly the anterior mucosa is affected, but circumferential prolapse may also occur. Anal fissure may produce a keyhole deformity near the anal verge as a result of chronic fibrosis through which seepage of mucus and stool may occur.

In older patients with a short history of incontinence, conditions to consider include rectal cancer (Chapter 20), inflammatory bowel disease (Chapter 13) and ischaemic proctitis (Chapter 4).

In a small number of patients there is loss of rectal sensation so that there is reduced awareness of faeces in the rectum with resulting overflow incontinence. The cause for this sensory loss is unknown.

Treatment

With a normal sphincter, treatment, if successful, will result in the return of normal continence. Rectal cancer presenting with incontinence is treated by surgery according to conventional principles (Chapter 20). Prolapsing haemorrhoids and anal mucosal prolapse causing incontinence usually require rubber band ligation (Chapter 11). Occasionally when the prolapse is large, surgical excision is required. Anal fissure causing incontinence is always a deep chronic fissure, which should be treated surgically by lateral sphincterotomy. Abnormalities in rectal sensation may respond to loperamide because of the constipating effect of the drug.

CONDITIONS CAUSING INCONTINENCE WITH AN ABNORMAL SPHINCTER

Congenital abnormalities

There are two basic forms of anorectal abnormalities. Low defects affect only the lower anal canal and are usually easily corrected in infancy, with normal continence resulting. High defects affect the anal sphincter, pelvic floor muscles and, in some cases, also the urogenital tract, and surgery may be accompanied by varying degrees of incontinence in later life. Many of these patients require a permanent colostomy, although recent developments in sphincter reconstruction allow this to be avoided in some cases.

Anal sepsis

Perianal sepsis may be severe enough to result in sphincter destruction and incontinence (Chapter 11). Complex anal fistulae with longstanding sepsis, or hidradenitis suppurativa (infection in perianal apocrine glands) are the most common causes.

Neurological conditions

Faecal incontinence due to a neurological cause is not commonly encountered. Nevertheless, this diagnosis is an important one to consider because localised conditions such as spinal cord or pelvic tumours may be amenable to surgery or radiotherapy. Neurological conditions causing incontinence may be supranuclear or infranuclear, depending on their relation to the Onuf's nucleus.

Supranuclear lesions. The cerebral control of sphincter function is located in the orbitofrontal cortex and conditions affecting this area, such as dementias, are particularly liable to present with incontinence. Upper motor neurone lesions also result from multiple sclerosis, multifocal atherosclerotic vascular disease, or spinal trauma above the S2 level. Some disorders, especially motor neurone disease, are accompanied by widespread muscle wasting but relative preservation of the sphincter muscles because of sparing of the motor neurones in the Onuf nucleus.

Infranuclear lesions. Lower motor neurone lesions cause denervation of the sphincter muscles and hence incontinence. This results from damage to the sacral nerve roots in the pelvis or within the cauda equina. Cauda equina disease results from sacral spondylosis, disc prolapse, trauma, or intraspinal neoplasms. Pelvic lesions include tumours, either primary presacral tumours or recurrent carcinoma after excision of the rectum.

Treatment

There is no effective curative treatment for most supranuclear lesions, including multiple sclerosis, and most dementias. Localised spinal conditions such as disc prolapse or tumours may be amenable to surgical treatment.

Rectal prolapse

Rectal prolapse is a circumferential intussusception of the rectum, which passes through the anal sphincter and beyond the anal verge to the exterior (Figure 14.8). It occurs in females in 90% of cases. In over two-thirds of patients there is associated neurogenic weakness of the anal sphincter (see neurogenic incontinence), but unlike patients with neurogenic incontinence, where almost all are multiparous women, almost half the women with rectal prolapse are nulliparous.

Aetiology

Rectal prolapse is a primary intussusception of the bowel. Constipation and impaired rectal evacuation leading to straining at stool are sometimes present and may contribute to the development of prolapse. Trauma during childbirth is probably not a

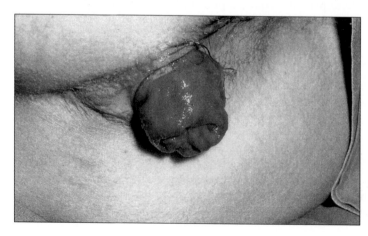

FIGURE 14.8: Rectal prolapse.

significant contributing factor as many women with prolapse are nulliparous. Almost all cases of prolapse in children are due to constipation and straining.

Clinical features

The condition is most common over the age of 50 years, and a smaller number of patients are in the 20–50-year age group. It occasionally occurs in children.

Most elderly patients complain of a prolapse during defecation, which either reduces spontaneously or must be manually reduced. Sometimes the prolapse occurs spontaneously when the subject walks about. The prolapse is accompanied by mucus discharge.

There are two distinct forms of rectal prolapse:

1. In two-thirds of cases there is associated marked neurogenic weakness of the anal sphincter and faecal incontinence is present; and

2. In one-third of cases the anal sphincter is normal—there is mucus discharge, but incontinence usually does not develop.

Treatment

Rectal prolapse in children is usually due to constipation and straining and should be treated conservatively with dietary measures (Chapter 10).

In adults, if the prolapse is small, reduces spontaneously and is not accompanied by incontinence, then it can be treated conservatively. With mild symptoms or a patient with poor functional status, conservative treatment including encouragement to avoid straining at stool and treatment of constipation with bulk-forming agents (e.g., psyllium, sterculia) might be all that are indicated.

If the prolapse is more severe then surgery is needed. There are many operative procedures used in the treatment of rectal prolapse, indicating that no procedure produces an entirely satisfactory result. There are two approaches that can be used: an abdominal procedure or a perineal procedure. With an abdominal operation there is a low long-term incidence of recurrent prolapse and also a 75% chance of curing the incontinence, but this is achieved with the risks and morbidity that accompany a major abdominal operation. This is particularly relevant in very elderly patients with prolapse. Perineal procedures are associated with very little pain or other morbidity, but carry a higher incidence of recurrent prolapse. Incontinence is cured less frequently by these procedures than by an abdominal procedure. The choice of a particular procedure in a patient therefore needs to take into account such factors as the age and general medical status of the patient, the expected remaining lifespan, and the severity and nature of the symptoms. For example, a young patient with prolapse and severe incontinence would be well suited to abdominal rectopexy; an elderly, frail patient with a large prolapse and less severe incontinence would be treated with a perineal procedure.

Abdominal procedures. Abdominal rectopexy involves mobilising the rectum out of the pelvis, and then securing it to the sacrum with sutures to prevent prolapse. This procedure can now be done using laparoscopic techniques, avoiding a formal laparotomy.

Perineal procedures. Anal encirclement procedures involve placing a stainless steel wire or nylon suture subcutaneously around the anal canal after reducing the prolapse. Although still used today in some centres for high-risk patients, it really has no place at all because the wire inevitably fails to control the prolapse (being too loose), or ulcerates through the skin, or is too tight, resulting in constipation.

The Delorme procedure involves excision of the mucosa over the prolapsing section of rectum and then plication of the underlying rectal wall. Reported recurrence rates range from 5–30%.

Perineal rectosigmoidectomy involves excision of the entire prolapsing section of rectum and sigmoid, with anastomosis of the colon to the anus. In principle this is a very sound procedure, but the reported recurrence rates are as high as with the Delorme procedure. The high rates found in some series are probably because of incomplete removal of the prolapsing bowel, and in those centres where a more complete excision is practised, recurrence rates as low as 5% are found. Since there is minimal blood loss with the procedure and virtually no morbidity, this is a very good option for elderly patients.

Sphincter trauma

Aetiology

Direct trauma to the sphincter is most commonly due to an obstetric tear, or damage resulting from surgery for anal fistula. Other less common causes are impalement on a sharp object, pelvic fracture, stab wound or gunshot wound.

Obstetric injuries are the most common cause of sphincter trauma. In North America and some parts of Europe where midline episiotomy is practised routinely, division of the anal sphincter and imperfect repair may cause a sphincter defect; while in Australia, the UK and most of Europe, lateral episiotomy is made and third-degree perineal tears are the cause. Recent studies of the anal sphincter using the technique of intra-anal ultrasound have identified injuries to the anterior sphincter in a much higher proportion of cases than is recognised clinically, and in some of these cases of occult sphincter injury, incontinence will develop in later life.

Surgery for anal fistula is the most common iatrogenic cause of incontinence. Laying open of a fistula which has not been recognised as suprasphincteric or extrasphincteric will result in incontinence. However, these fistulae are rare, and more commonly incontinence results from treatment of a trans-sphincteric fistula which crosses more than 50% of the external sphincter muscle.

Impalement injuries generally result from falling astride a sharp object, such as a fence, and can result in severe damage. Secondary infection may occur if adequate surgical debridement is not performed, resulting in further tissue loss. There may be an associated injury to the rectum above the sphincter. Pelvic fractures may produce widespread disruption of the anal sphincter and can present a particularly difficult problem for surgical repair.

There are several iatrogenic injuries apart from those resulting from fistula surgery. These injuries are due to poor surgical technique and should be completely avoidable. Minor incontinence after haemorrhoidectomy is well recognised and occurs in up to 10% of cases in some series, usually due to damage to the internal sphincter or lower part of the external sphincter during the haemorrhoidectomy, but in some cases, anal dilatation carried out at the time of haemorrhoidectomy may be the cause of the incontinence. Lateral sphincterotomy for anal fissure should only include the lower part of the internal sphincter—if the external sphincter is divided, then incontinence will result. Anal dilatation has been advocated for haemorrhoids and anal fissure. Although this procedure is an effective treatment for these conditions by disrupting the internal sphincter spasm, it is a frequent cause of incontinence, particularly in multiparous women, and should be completely avoided.

Clinical features

A damaged sphincter may be recognised by a visible keyhole defect externally or a palpable defect on physical examination. The defect is best assessed prior to surgical intervention with endoanal ultrasound.

Treatment

Repair of the damaged sphincter ranges from a relatively simple procedure when the sphincter has been cleanly divided, to a very complex procedure when the sphincter has been widely disrupted with accompanying sepsis and tissue necrosis. Preoperative establishment of the precise extent of the scar tissue greatly facilitates planning of the procedure and accurate repair. In most cases, a covering stoma is not required, and the use of a stoma is restricted to three situations: underlying Crohn's disease; repeat sphincter repair; or with a very extensive injury. The principles of surgery are to expose the injured area, excise the scar tissue, and create an overlapping repair using healthy muscle on either side of the scar.

The results of sphincter repair are very satisfactory. Almost 70% of patients will achieve continence and up to half of the remaining patients will be partially improved, although the results do deteriorate over time. In those cases where there is no improvement and severe incontinence persists, the two available alternatives are a permanent colostomy or reconstruction of a new sphincter mechanism. Complete sphincter reconstruction involves the procedure called stimulated graciloplasty, in which the gracilis muscle in the thigh is detached from its insertion on the tibia and tunnelled around the anus to construct a neo-sphincter. Since the gracilis is a conventional fast-twitch skeletal muscle that fatigues quickly, it must be stimulated using an implanted subcutaneous pacemaker which converts it to a fatigue-resistant slow-twitch muscle by continuous low-frequency stimulation, eventually allowing it to remain continuously contracted.

Neurogenic incontinence

Aetiology

A global weakness of the anal sphincter and pelvic floor muscles is a common cause of severe incontinence requiring surgery. This condition was previously known as 'idiopathic incontinence', but new methods of investigation have shown that the sphincter weakness is due to an injury to the distal part of the nerve supply to the anal sphincter and pelvic floor muscles.

The nerve supply to the external anal sphincter is via the pudendal nerve (arising from S2–S4 sacral segments). The puborectalis and levator ani (pubococcygeus) muscles are supplied by direct branches from the sacral nerve plexus (S3, S4) (Figure 14.9). During vaginal delivery there is marked descent of the pelvic floor with stretching of the pudendal and sacral nerves, and a temporary reversible nerve injury occurs in some cases. Somatic nerves can normally withstand a stretch injury of up to 12% of their length and it has been calculated that stretching of 20% may occur during vaginal delivery. In the majority of cases, the neuropraxia resolves over a six-week period, but a permanent injury remains in others. This may not result in muscle weakness immediately, but as the pelvic floor muscles age, particularly after menopause, then a cumulative weakness develops leading to incontinence.

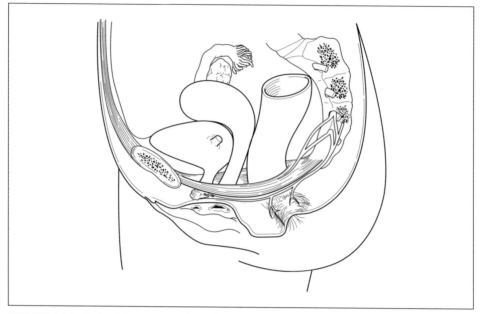

FIGURE 14.9: Pudendal nerve supply to the external anal sphincter; sacral nerves to the puborectalis muscle.
(Based on Henry and Swash, 1985, with permission from the publisher.)

Factors shown to be associated with nerve damage are prolonged second stage of labour, forceps delivery, and high infant birth weight. In addition to vaginal delivery, chronic straining at stool due to constipation has a similar effect by causing a repeated stretch injury to the pelvic nerves. Women who have a combination of multiple vaginal deliveries and chronic constipation are, therefore, particularly likely to develop neurogenic incontinence.

It can be seen that since direct sphincter trauma and neurogenic muscle weakness are both associated with difficult vaginal delivery, these two conditions may co-exist in some women. Recognition of this dual pathology has important implications for surgical treatment in many cases.

Clinical features

On examination, the sphincter is found to be shortened and gaping, and voluntary squeeze is found to be reduced to absent. The puborectalis sling is lax and there is loss of posterior support of the anus. Anorectal manometry and electrophysiology will confirm the abnormalities.

Treatment

Initial treatment is with biofeedback, where the patient is taught to contract the external sphincter muscle more effectively by showing the patient sphincter pressure measurements during physiotherapy exercises. If this is not successful then the pelvic floor muscle can be stimulated by inserting electrodes into the S2, S3 sacral foramina and stimulating the nerves to the pelvis using an implanted subcutaneous stimulator (sacral neuromodulation). This has been shown to have a high success rate in properly selected patients. Surgical treatment of this condition involves plicating the left and right limbs of the puborectalis muscle posterior to the external sphincter (postanal repair). This has the effect of increasing the functional length of the anal sphincter and improving the efficacy of the puborectalis. This operation does not reverse the denervation process and merely realigns the weakened muscles to create a high-pressure sphincter zone. Over 50% of patients achieve satisfactory restoration of continence. In selected patients in whom the procedure fails and severe incontinence persists, the gracilis neosphincter can then be considered as a final surgical option.

Further reading

Bartram Cl, Sultan AH. Anal endosonography in faecal incontinence. *Gut* 1995; 37: 4–6.

Bharucha AE, Zinsmeister AR, Locke GR *et al.* Prevalence and burden of fecal incontinence: a population-based study in women. *Gastroenterology* 2005; 129: 42–9.

Cook TA, Mortensen NJ. Management of faecal incontinence following obstetric injury. *Br J Surg* 1998; 88: 293–9.

Kamm MA. Obstetric damage and faecal incontinence. *Lancet* 1994; 344: 730–3.

Keighley MRB, Williams NS. Faecal incontinence. In: Keighley MRB, Williams NS (eds), *Surgery of the Anus, Rectum and Colon*, 2nd edn. London: WB Saunders, 1999.

Madoff RD, Parker SC, Varma MG, Lowry AC. Faecal incontinence in adults. *Lancet* 2004; 364: 621–32.

Mander BJ, Wexner ML, Williams NS *et al.* Preliminary results of a multicentre trial of the electrically stimulated gracilis neoanal sphincter. *Br J Surg* 1999; 86: 1543–8.

Matzel KE, Kamm MA, Stosser M *et al.* Sacral spinal nerve stimulation for faecal incontinence: multicentre study. *Lancet* 2004; 363: 1270–6.

Norton C, Chelvanayagam S, Wilson-Barnett J *et al.* Randomized controlled trial of biofeedback for fecal incontinence. *Gastroenterology* 2003; 125: 1320–9.

Sultan AH, Kamm MA, Hudson CN *et al.* Anal-sphincter disruption during vaginal delivery. *N Engl J Med* 1993; 329: 1905–11.

chapter 15

LOSS OF APPETITE AND LOSS OF WEIGHT

INTRODUCTION

Body weight is normally constant despite changes in energy expenditure. The energy value of food is a measure of its capacity to produce heat and is expressed in terms of kcal/g. The energy value of carbohydrates (4.1 kcal/g), proteins (5.6 kcal/g), and fats (9.4 kcal/g) differ significantly. A body mass index (BMI) below 18.5 is considered underweight. BMI (kg/m^2) is calculated by the weight (in kilograms) divided by the square of the height (in metres).

Anorexia refers to a loss of appetite. Appetite is a desire or inclination to satisfy one's natural need for food. This is different from hunger, which is an uneasy or painful sensation caused by lack of food. Hunger may persist despite loss of appetite. Satiety is a sensation of satisfaction experienced after adequate intake of food.

Weight loss is defined as a state when the caloric output (from the basal metabolic rate and voluntary activities) exceeds the input. Weight loss that equals or exceeds 5% of body weight (or 4.5 kg) over a 6-month period is arbitrarily defined as clinically significant. Most individuals can sustain a loss of 5–10% of their body weight without any significant health consequences. In a hospital or institutional setting, patients who have lost weight have increased morbidity and mortality, particularly elderly patients and cancer patients. Those who have lost ≥ 5 kg in the preceding six months also have an increased postoperative morbidity and mortality.

PATHOPHYSIOLOGY OF ANOREXIA AND WEIGHT LOSS

Anorexia

Food intake is regulated by complex central and peripheral mechanisms. The central mechanisms act via the hypothalamus. There are two hypothalamic centres:

- The hunger or feeding centre—situated in the lateral hypothalamus;
- The satiety centre—situated in the ventromedial hypothalamus.

Gastric distension, intestinal hormones (e.g., cholecystokinin, enterostatin, peptide YY, and glucagon), leptin (from fat cells), insulinaemia, glucosaemia, aminoacidaemia and vagal stimulation induce satiety. Ghrelin (from the stomach and duodenum) and neuropeptide Y stimulate increased food intake. Destruction of the feeding centre can result in failure of the person to eat, leading to starvation and death. Conversely, injury to the satiety centre can lead to hyperphagia (exaggerated appetite) and obesity.

Anorexia alone is not a symptom of diagnostic value and can occur in many gut and systemic diseases (Table 15.1). Anorexia should be differentiated from 'sitophobia', which is a term used to describe a fear of food because of subsequent abdominal pain. Sitophobia can occur with chronic mesenteric vascular insufficiency (abdominal angina) or small intestinal Crohn's disease with partial obstruction. Anorexia should also be distinguished from early satiation (a feeling of fullness after eating a small amount such that a normal meal cannot be finished), such as occurs after a partial gastrectomy and in functional dyspepsia.

Weight loss

Involuntary weight loss is a common manifestation of a variety of disease processes (see Table 15.2). Although the precise pathophysiologic mechanisms inducing weight loss are unclear, multiple factors have been implicated.

TABLE 15.1: Selected causes of anorexia

Gastrointestinal tract/liver	- Gastric outlet obstruction or small bowel obstruction
	- Gastric cancer
	- Hepatic metastases
	- Acute viral hepatitis
Metabolic	- Addison's disease
	- Hypopituitarism
	- Hyperparathyroidism
Functional	- Extremely unpleasant sight/smell
Systemic	- Chronic pain
	- Renal failure
	- Severe congestive heart failure
	- Respiratory failure
Psychiatric	- Depression
	- Anorexia nervosa
Medications	- Digoxin
	- Narcotic analgesics
	- Diuretics
	- Antihypertensives
	- Chemotherapeutic agents
	- Amphetamines
Miscellaneous	- Excessive smoking
	- Excessive alcohol intake
	- Oral cavity disease
	- Thiamine deficiency
	- Early pregnancy
	- Hypogeusia or dysgeusia

Cancer patients may be unable to eat or may not feel like eating (secondary to treatment or depression). Failure to down-regulate energy expenditure in the face of decreased caloric intake can lead to energy imbalance, which may be one of the main mechanisms of weight loss in some cancers. Increased caloric utilisation by tumour tissue may also be a factor, although increases in resting energy expenditure have not been shown to occur in all patients with tumours. In the acquired immune deficiency syndrome (AIDS), poor oral intake, malabsorption, tumour development and repeated infections coupled with a relatively high resting energy expenditure may all have a role. In elderly people, preferential oxidation of fatty acids and an increase in anaerobic glucose metabolism result in inefficient expenditure or wastage of adenosine triphosphate (ATP).

At a molecular level, various mediators may be important in promoting loss of weight. Tumour necrosis factor (TNF) is a cytokine produced from activated lymphocytes and macrophages in cancer patients or in patients with emphysema or severe heart failure; in animal studies it gives rise to anorexia and weight loss. Pentoxifylline, an inhibitor of TNF, can reverse the above effects in animal studies. Interleukin 1 (IL-1-beta and IL-6) are potent anorexic cytokines, increasing resting energy expenditure and promoting skeletal wasting.

Although reductions occur from both adipose tissue and muscle (lean mass) in weight loss, the extent from each source can differ. Obese people lose less lean mass than those who are not obese. In uncomplicated starvation, fat tissue is selectively depleted to spare muscle proteins. However in patients with AIDS or cancer, weight loss occurs predominantly from the muscle compartment.

CLINICAL APPROACH TO A PATIENT WITH ANOREXIA AND WEIGHT LOSS

The differential diagnosis is large (Tables 15.1 and 15.2), but investigations should be directed by the history and physical examination.

History

Determine whether the problem is acute or chronic and when it began. Enquire about any loosening of the patient's clothes or changes in belt size. Also ask whether weight loss is ongoing. Previous records or photographs may be helpful for comparison. There are rare situations in which patients claim to have lost weight without having done so.

Next, determine the patient's appetite and eating habits. About one-third of patients with involuntary weight loss plus anorexia have a cancer; up to a quarter have no cause uncovered by tests. Weight loss does not always accompany anorexia. Patients may actually have weight loss with an increase in appetite in malabsorption, hyperthyroidism, uncontrolled diabetes mellitus, phaeochromocytoma or occasionally with lymphoma or leukaemia.

Ask about the number of meals per day and their composition, and usual daily physical activity.

Ask about other gastrointestinal symptoms. For example, recurrent vomiting may indicate bowel obstruction, while dysphagia may suggest oesophageal cancer. The occurrence of diarrhoea immediately after eating can occur in patients with a high intestinal fistula or malabsorption.

Ask whether the patient is afraid to eat because eating precipitates pain or other gastrointestinal symptoms. Abdominal pain that usually occurs after eating suggests peptic ulcer disease, chronic pancreatitis or chronic mesenteric ischaemia (abdominal angina). Pain after eating may also occur in patients with the irritable bowel syndrome or functional dyspepsia, but the relationship is not constant (Chapters 5 and 6).

In elderly patients, poor dentition is a common but often overlooked problem. Oral disease resulting from conditions such as vitamin deficiencies, candidiasis or gingivitis can affect mastication. Ask about alterations in taste (dysgeusia), which may make food seem unpalatable. Zinc deficiency may sometimes be responsible for dysgeusia (Chapter 3).

A detailed current drug history is important. Various medications can cause anorexia and associated nausea and vomiting, which may lead to subsequent weight loss, including digoxin (especially in toxic doses), amphetamines, chemotherapeutic agents and narcotic analgesics. It is important to look up the side effects of drugs being taken if you are unsure.

TABLE 15.2: Selected causes of weight loss

Medical conditions	Examples
• Malignancy	Carcinoma of the pancreas, stomach, oesophagus, colon, liver, lung, breast, kidney
• Gastrointestinal and liver disease	Malabsorptive states, inflammatory bowel disease, secondary to dysphagia, pancreatitis, hepatitis
• Cardiovascular disease	End-stage heart failure
• Respiratory disease	End-stage respiratory failure
• Renal disease	Uraemia
• Endocrine disease	Hyperthyroidism (and hypothyroidism-induced anorexia in elderly patients), hyperparathyroidism, diabetes mellitus, panhypopituitarism, Addison's disease, phaeochromocytoma
• Connective tissue disease	Scleroderma, rheumatoid arthritis
• Infections	HIV, tuberculosis, pyogenic abscess, infective endocarditis, atypical *Mycobacterium*, systemic fungal infections
• Neurological disease	Stroke, dementia, Parkinson's disease
• Drugs	Amphetamines, cocaine, opiates, serotonin reuptake inhibitors

Psychiatric
- Depression
- Anorexia nervosa
- Bulimia nervosa
- Alcoholism
- Neuroleptic-withdrawal   Cachexia

Miscellaneous
- Oral disorders   Ill-fitting dentures, candidiasis, gingivitis
- Hyperemesis gravidarum

Ask about previous medical conditions (e.g., pulmonary tuberculosis, renal disease, previous cancer, cardiac disease) and past surgery. Post-gastrectomy syndromes can cause malabsorption (Chapter 5). Prior abdominal surgery can lead to chronic incomplete intestinal obstruction.

Cigarette smoking and alcohol use may be important (e.g., due to the associations with lung and other cancers and cirrhosis, respectively). The patient's involvement in high-risk behaviour may be relevant (e.g., acquisition of HIV infection).

Ask about social isolation and symptoms of depression (including depressed mood, apathy, insomnia, fatigue, feelings of worthlessness, diminished ability to think and suicidal ideation). Depression, not malignancy, is the most common cause of weight loss in elderly patients and institutionalised patients, and is often missed. It may not always present in its 'typical' form. Ask about body image and self-induced vomiting; anorexia nervosa and bulimia nervosa are important causes of weight loss in young people.

Physical examination

Weigh the patient and measure the patient's height. Milder degrees of weight loss can exist with little or no wasting. In severe weight loss, muscle wasting will usually be obvious.

Look for features of vitamin and mineral deficiencies (Table 15.3). Glossitis, cheilosis or perioral dermatitis can result from deficiency of vitamins such as riboflavin, pyridoxine or niacin, whereas peripheral neuropathy or ataxia can occur due to lack of thiamine or vitamin B12.

Next, conduct a careful gastrointestinal examination. For instance, in a patient with weight loss and jaundice (Chapter 21), a pancreatic cancer with biliary obstruction may be the explanation. If stigmata of chronic liver disease are present and abdominal examination reveals a liver mass with or without a bruit, cirrhosis with development of a hepatoma should be considered. Large abdominal masses can occasionally compress the stomach or small bowel inducing anorexia (Chapter 17).

Look for clues on the general examination. Although usually not pathognomonic, they can help direct investigations of a particular organ system. For instance, clubbing may suggest the presence of co-existing chronic lung infection or cancer, whereas lymphadenopathy could point towards a possible lymphoma, metastatic cancer or chronic infection. In a febrile patient, the presence of a newly detected murmur may suggest a diagnosis of infective endocarditis, whereas localised bony tenderness could occur in osteomyelitis or with bone metastases.

Investigations

The diagnostic work-up needs to be directed towards defining the extent of malnutrition and detecting the underlying cause of weight loss.

1. Tests to estimate nutritional status

Nutritional assessment helps to identify patients who are more likely to develop complications from their malnutrition and, hence, likely to benefit from supportive nutritional therapy. Assessment can be either clinical or based on laboratory tests and measurements.

Calculate the BMI. Other anthropometric measurements include triceps skin-fold thickness and mid-arm muscle circumference to assess the fat reserve and the muscle mass of the body, respectively. These quantitative measurements are useful for follow-up of nutritional status.

The subjective global assessment (SGA) is based on the history and clinical findings. The degree of recent weight loss, dietary alterations, and the level of physical activity is gauged from the history. Examination subjectively assesses the amount of fat reserve, muscle mass and oedema. Patients are then classified into one of three groups; well nourished, moderate (or suspected) malnutrition, and severe malnutrition.

Laboratory tests that detect decreases in serum albumin or lymphocyte count ($< 1.5 \times 10^9$/L (< 1500/mm^3)) are crude but helpful estimates of nutritional status. Estimation of proteins with a shorter half-life, such as transferrin or prealbumin, should be undertaken if enteral or parenteral nutrition is being considered. Vitamin levels (e.g., fat-soluble vitamins A, D and K) need to be checked in patients with suspected severe malabsorption (e.g., pancreatic insufficiency). The prognostic nutritional index (PNI) predicts the likelihood of developing postoperative complications in patients undergoing gastrointestinal surgery. The PNI is based on a simple linear equation incorporating measurements of serum proteins (albumin and transferrin concentration), subcutaneous fat (triceps skin fold), and immunologic function (delayed skin hypersensitivity).

To determine adequate protein intake, nitrogen balance can be assessed by estimating the protein intake and urinary urea nitrogen excretion. To assess adequate caloric intake, energy expenditure can be calculated using the Harris Benedict equation, if weight, height and age are known. To determine lean body mass and total body fat, body composition can be simply measured using bioelectrical impedance.

TABLE 15.3: Clinical findings associated with vitamin and mineral deficiencies

Findings on physical examination	Associated vitamin deficiencies
Mucocutaneous	
• Dermatitis/cheilosis/glossitis	Riboflavin (B2), pyridoxine (B6), niacin
• Bleeding/swollen gums	Vitamin C
• Petechiae/ecchymoses	Vitamin C and K
• Perifollicular haemorrhages/keratitis	Vitamin C
• Rash (face/body: pustular, bullous, vesicular, seborrhoeic, acneiform), skin ulcers, alopecia	Zinc
Neurological	
• Peripheral neuropathy	Thiamine/vitamin B12, chromium, vitamin E
• Dementia/confusion	Thiamine/niacin, zinc, manganese
• Night blindness	Vitamin A
• Ophthalmoplegia	Thiamine
Haematological	
• Pallor (anaemia)	Vitamin B12/folic acid, iron, copper
Miscellaneous	
• Dysgeusia	Zinc
• Fractures	Vitamin D
• Loosening of teeth, periosteal haemorrhages	Vitamin C
• Cardiac failure/cardiomyopathy	Thiamine, selenium
• Hypothyroidism	Iodine

2. Tests aimed at detecting the cause

Diagnostic tests can be arbitrarily classified into those of a screening nature and those that target specific abnormalities detected by the history, physical examination or initial screening test results (Table 15.4). The tests are most successful in finding the cause when they are directed by the history and examination findings.

TABLE 15.4: Investigations for weight loss and examples of diseases to consider	
Diagnostic test	**Examples of diseases screened**
Bedside tests	
• Urine analysis	Renal cell cancer
Laboratory tests	
Routine	
• Full blood count and iron studies	Iron deficiency anaemia from gastrointestinal blood loss
• Folate/B12	Macrocytic anaemia in bacterial overgrowth
• Electrolytes	Renal failure, Addison's disease
• Liver function tests (LFT)	Chronic liver disease
• Calcium/phosphate	Hyperparathyroidism, bony metastases
• Erythrocyte sedimentation rate (ESR) or C-reactive protein (CRP)	Autoimmune disease, inflammatory bowel disease, malignancy
Specific	
• Anti-nuclear antigen (ANA)	Autoimmune disease, e.g., systemic lupus, scleroderma
• Rheumatoid factor	Rheumatoid arthritis
• Thyroid function tests (TFT)	Hyper/hypothyroidism
• Tumour markers	(See Table 15.5)
Imaging tests	
• Chest X-ray	Lung cancer, tuberculosis
• Barium studies of small bowel	Crohn's disease
• CT scan	Empyema, lung/ovarian/liver cancers
Invasive tests	
• Gastroscopy, colonoscopy	Peptic ulcer, oesophagus/stomach/colon cancers
• Endoscopic retrograde cholangiopancreatography (ERCP)/ magnetic resonance cholangiopancreatography (MRCP)	Pancreatic cancer, cholangiocarcinoma, ampullary tumour
• Laparoscopy, laparotomy	Crohn's disease, internal malignancies
• Fine needle aspiration (FNA)	Liver/breast/thyroid/lymph node cancers

Routine tests. These are inexpensive, and may help to identify the basic nature of the problem. A full blood count can detect evidence of iron deficiency anaemia, which may suggest blood loss from a gastrointestinal tract cancer. A high erythrocyte sedimentation rate (ESR) or C-reactive protein (CRP) may suggest inflammation or malignancy. Electrolyte and creatinine tests can identify uraemia as a cause of anorexia.

Liver function tests can be helpful (e.g., elevated transaminase levels in hepatitis, obstructive jaundice due to pancreatic cancer or hypoalbuminaemia in malignancy). A serum calcium test may detect hypercalcaemia caused by a malignancy. A bedside urine analysis may detect proteinuria (e.g., nephrotic syndrome) or haematuria. In the absence of infection or stones, persistent haematuria may indicate renal cancer. A positive result of a stool occult blood test may indicate colorectal neoplasia or inflammatory bowel disease, but this test has low sensitivity and specificity and is less often done (Chapter 9). If malabsorption is suspected, then an appropriate work-up should be done (Chapter 13). A thyroid-stimulating hormone test will detect hyperthyroidism and fasting blood sugar level test, diabetes mellitus. Tumour markers may occasionally help point towards a correct diagnosis in difficult cases but are of most use in following response to treatment (Table 15.5).

Imaging tests. A chest X-ray examination is relatively inexpensive and an adjunct to the clinical examination. It is mandatory in the presence of pulmonary symptoms (e.g., to detect pulmonary tuberculosis or primary lung cancer) or if routine tests are unhelpful. A silent mass lesion, infiltrative process or lymphadenopathy may be detected on the chest X-ray film.

TABLE 15.5: Causes of elevated levels of tumour markers

Carcinoembryonic antigen (CEA)
- Colonic cancer (higher levels if the tumour is more differentiated or is extensive, or has spread to the liver)
- Lung or breast cancer; seminoma
- Cigarette smokers
- Cirrhosis, inflammatory bowel disease, rectal polyps, pancreatitis
- Advanced age

Alpha fetoprotein
- Hepatocellular cancer: very high titres or a rising titre is strongly suggestive, but > 10% of patients do not have an elevated level
- Hepatic regeneration e.g., cirrhosis, alcoholic or viral hepatitis
- Cancer of the stomach, colon, pancreas or lung
- Teratocarcinoma or embryonal cell carcinoma (testis, ovary, extragonadal)
- Pregnancy
- Ataxia telangiectasia
- Normal variant

Prostate-specific antigen
- Prostate carcinoma (localised disease)
- Prostatic hyperplasia
- Prostatitis
- Prostatitic infarction

Cancer-associated antigen (CA-19-9)[1]
- Pancreatic carcinoma (80% with advanced, well-differentiated cancer have an elevated level)
- Other gastrointestinal cancers: colon, stomach, bile duct
- Acute or chronic pancreatitis
- Chronic liver disease
- Biliary tract disease

---

1. Patients who cannot synthesise Lewis blood group antigens (~5% of the population) do not produce CA-19-9 antigen.

CT scans of the chest and abdomen provide excellent anatomical definition and objective assessment which is not operator dependent. They are extremely useful for defining mediastinal and retroperitoneal pathologies. Mediastinal widening seen on chest X-ray films in small cell lung cancer, lymphoma or thymoma can be delineated further with a chest CT scan. Similarly, metastatic lymph notes in the mesentery or in the retroperitoneum, or organomegaly detected on clinical examination can be accurately defined by an abdominal CT scan. Although CT should be reserved for localising a suspected lesion, this test is increasingly used for screening when no diagnosis is forthcoming. Ultrasound examination can provide valuable information about biliary anatomy or pelvic pathology (Chapter 17). Mammography should be done in women if breast cancer is a consideration.

Invasive tests. Gastroscopy and colonoscopy have replaced barium examination as the gold standard for visualising the upper and lower gastrointestinal tract. In patients with altered bowel habits or microcytic anaemia thought to be due to chronic gastrointestinal blood loss, endoscopy is the procedure of choice for detection of underlying pathology (e.g., gastric or colorectal cancer). Barium examinations still have a role to play in screening the small bowel (e.g., Crohn's disease). Fine needle aspirations (FNA) are useful for pathological confirmation of suspected lesions in organs such as the liver.

3. Test yield

Testing will reveal an organic cause for weight loss in 75% of cases. The most common causes are depression and cancer. In one-quarter of patients, despite detailed examination and exhaustive tests, the aetiology remains elusive. In such cases, it is prudent to adopt a wait-and-see approach since the diagnosis may become obvious within the next 6 to 12 months.

MANAGEMENT OF PATIENTS WITH WEIGHT LOSS

Identification and treatment of the underlying medical or psychiatric cause remains the cornerstone of management. It is also important to provide patient support and education; cancer is a feared diagnosis and late stage cancer even more so. Revision of dentures may be required in older patients. Treatment of infection or review and cessation of unnecessary medication may be all that is required in individual cases. Chemotherapy for malignancy may help to alleviate anorexia and cachexia secondary to cancer. Adequate pancreatic enzyme supplements should be prescribed for patients with pancreatic insufficiency. Optimal control of underlying colitis as well as improvement in nutritional status are required in patients with inflammatory bowel disease.

Occasionally, it may be useful to admit a patient to hospital for medical and nursing supervision in order to observe the individual's eating habits closely. Self-induced vomiting in bulimic patients, surreptitious laxative abuse in patients with difficult to diagnose 'diarrhoea' or food faddism, and avoidance of food in anorexic patients may only then become obvious.

Empiric therapy has a place in stimulating appetite and increasing weight in patients with end-stage cancer and AIDS. Cyproheptadine, a serotonin antagonist, has been extensively used in both adults and children and may be of benefit in a few cases. Corticosteroids have an established role in stimulating appetite and improving the sense of well-being in patients with malignancies. However, steroids have side effects and do not usually result in non-fluid weight gain (e.g., increased muscle bulk). Megesterol is a synthetic progestin that is an antiemetic with an appetite stimulating effect. It is helpful in increasing oral food intake and non-fluid weight gain in patients with AIDS. This medication is usually well tolerated but is expensive.

NUTRITIONAL SUPPORT

In patients who cannot or will not eat, nutrition can be provided by enteral or parenteral feeding. Malnourished patients who cannot maintain an adequate intake, especially those already with a significant negative nitrogen balance, require nutritional support. Although it is possible to adequately replenish nutrition with total parenteral nutrition (TPN), the associated higher costs, increased medical and nursing needs and complications make the enteral route the preferred choice in all circumstances. Enteral nutrition also has a beneficial effect on intestinal cells, providing the necessary fuel (e.g., glutamine, volatile fatty acids) for promoting intestinal integrity. A specific indication for enteral feeding is to establish early small bowel adaptation following massive resection. Hence, the enteral route is physiological and allows greater flexibility: *if the gut works, use it.*

Enteral feeding

Enteral feeding is achieved by means of feeding tubes placed either transnasally or percutaneously with the distal end lying in the stomach or the small intestine. Feeding via a nasogastric tube, which can be placed easily at the bedside, is the preferred route for short-term enteral feeding. However, on account of local irritation, it is often inadvertently or deliberately removed by patients. The mode of nutrient delivery can either be continuous (constant rate over 24 hours) or intermittent (boluses of 300–400 mL over 5–10 minutes, every few hours). The entire feeding can be done over 12–16 hours during the night allowing freedom during the day.

Nasoduodenal/jejunal tubes have the added advantage of bypassing the stomach, thereby overcoming problems related to delayed gastric emptying. It is also useful when avoiding pancreatic stimulation is required, for example in patients recovering from severe acute pancreatitis. Placement of a nasoenteric tube beyond the pylorus may require pharmacological assistance (e.g., intravenous metoclopramide or erythromycin) or endoscopic/fluoroscopic assistance (e.g., over the wire placement). With nasoduodenal/jejunal tubes, continuous feeding is usually required to avoid diarrhoea and discomfort from small bowel distension.

Percutaneous enteric gastrostomy (PEG) tubes, placed via an upper endoscopy, are well tolerated. They are indicated for long-term enteric feeding in patients unable to eat long term, such as those with a defective swallowing apparatus from neurological disease (e.g., stroke, advanced Parkinson's disease or motor neurone disease) or occasionally with oesophageal disease (e.g., advanced oesophageal carcinoma). A PEG is relatively contraindicated in patients with a previous gastrectomy and may be difficult in a patient with a midline abdominal scar from other surgery. The procedure-related mortality is approximately 1%; major procedure complications occur in 3% (e.g., perforation of a viscus, sepsis or haemorrhage) and minor procedure complications in 15% (e.g., local infection post procedure, tube dislodgment, blockage, gastrointestinal bleeding, epistaxis and nasal mucosal ulceration). Operative placement (surgical jejunostomy) is considered only when other methods are not possible or complications supervene.

Diarrhoea is a common complication of enteral feeding. Causes include high osmotic load, sorbitol-based compounds, and use of antibiotics leading to altered bacterial flora. Decreasing the osmolality and infusion rate, avoiding sorbitol or magnesium-based compounds, increasing dietary intake of lactobacillus, stopping antibiotic therapy, or regularly using diphenoxylate or loperamide may be helpful in individual cases.

Another specific problem associated with nasogastric or nasoenteric feeding is gastro-oesophageal reflux. Aspiration is also an important complication. Patients with symptomatic aspiration (e.g., aspiration pneumonia) may benefit from elevation of the head end of the bed during and post feeding, and the avoidance of bolus feeding. If aspiration occurs with a PEG despite the incorporation of the above regimen, a revision to jejunostomy tube feeding should be considered. Placement of the tube beyond the pylorus reduces, but does not overcome, this complication. The main indications for use of jejunostomy feeding over gastrostomy include tracheal aspiration, gastroparesis and a partial or total gastrectomy.

Total parenteral nutrition

While the enteral route is always preferable, total parenteral nutrition (TPN) is required when anatomical or physiological abnormalities of the gut preclude enteral feeding. In clinical practice, the most common indications are protracted periods of non-functioning bowel (e.g., major abdominal sepsis). Short gut syndrome occurs infrequently, but requires long-term TPN. Preoperative TPN is of no benefit in healthy patients or even those with mild-to-moderate malnutrition. Indications for TPN are summarised in Table 15.6.

TPN formulae contain a mixture of proteins (4.5–10% amino acids), carbohydrates (25–70% dextrose), fat (lipid emulsions), electrolytes, vitamins and trace elements. The daily protein requirement is around 1.5–2.0 g/kg/day. Glucose is the main energy substrate used, providing approximately 50% of daily calorie requirement. Lipids can be infused 2–3 times per week (500 mL; 10% lipids) as a source of essential fatty acids, or infused daily as a calorie source delivering about 40% of the patient's non-nitrogen calorie requirement. The latter form of infusion minimises catabolism of endogenous proteins and provides an alternative source of calories. It also avoids the metabolic complications that may result from the usage of a higher concentration of glucose (e.g., hepatic steatosis and hyperglycaemia). The usual requirement for sodium is 1–2 mmol/kg/day and potassium is 1 mmol/kg/day. Electrolyte requirements are guided by serum concentrations. Diarrhoea, vomiting or high output fistulae necessitate additional supplementation. Multivitamins and trace elements are usually provided in standard amounts on a daily to weekly basis. Additional care must be exercised in patients with specific organ failure (e.g., hepatic or renal failure).

Complications related to TPN can be either local (i.e., related to insertion and maintenance of the central venous catheter) or systemic (i.e., related to the infusion itself). In patients receiving TPN, local defence barriers may break down, allowing bacterial colonisation and systemic seeding. Strict asepsis and insertion by experienced personnel, followed by patient education in the care of the line, should minimise local complications. Long (pic) lines placed through, for example, the brachial vein to just above the right atrium can be left in place up to a year before needing replacement. As metabolic derangements are frequent, close monitoring by a dedicated TPN team is preferable. The complications are summarised in Table 15.7.

TABLE 15.6: Indications for total parenteral nutrition

- Postoperative (bowel surgery, protracted recovery)
- Severe inflammatory bowel disease (complicated ulcerative colitis, severe Crohn's disease with malabsorption)
- Acute radiation enteritis or chemotherapy enteritis
- Enterocutaneous fistula involving the small bowel
- Short gut syndrome
- Preoperative (severely malnourished patients only when enteral nutrition is not possible)

TABLE 15.7: Complications of total parenteral nutrition

Local (central vein catheter)

- Pneumothorax/haemothorax
- Venous thrombosis
- Air embolus
- Local infection and septicaemia
- Thrombophlebitis

Systemic

- Hyper/hypoglycaemia
- Electrolyte disturbances
- Azotaemia and hyperosmolarity
- Liver dysfunction (hepatocellular or cholestatic) and fatty liver (Chapter 21)
- Acalculous cholecystitis
- Cholelithiasis (long-term therapy)
- Vitamin or mineral deficiency (rare)
- Metabolic bone disease (rare)

DISEASES ASSOCIATED WITH WEIGHT LOSS

Some common gastrointestinal cancers, and anorexia and bulimia nervosa are discussed here. Other diseases are covered elsewhere (e.g., malabsorption: Chapter 13).

Adenocarcinoma of the pancreas

Adenocarcinomas arising from ductal cells constitute 90% of all cases of pancreatic cancer. Islet cell tumours, acinar cell tumours, and cystadenocarcinomas account for most of the remaining 10% of cases (see Chapter 23). The incidence appears to be on the increase, with carcinoma of the pancreas being the second most common gastrointestinal malignancy (after colon cancer).

Pathogenesis

The exact aetiopathogenesis is unclear. It is rare before age 45, and is more common in men and people of African descent. Increasing age (> 60 years) appears to be a factor. Smoking, diabetes mellitus, chronic pancreatitis (especially the rare hereditary pancreatitis) (Chapter 5), some familial cancer syndromes (e.g., Peutz-Jeghers syndrome), *Helicobacter pylori*, obesity and increased dietary fat are also risk factors. There is no convincing evidence that coffee intake is a causal factor. Mutations of CDKN2A, *p53* and K-ras gene have been identified.

Clinical features

It usually manifests in elderly persons and, unfortunately, often at an advanced stage. The initial symptoms and signs can be non-specific, but anorexia, weight loss and upper abdominal pain are common features.

Pain occurs in 75% of patients and weight loss is present in almost all patients. The pain is usually an epigastric dull ache, which may radiate through to the back. Weight loss is primarily due to anorexia, although malabsorption may also contribute. Gastric outlet obstruction with vomiting may occur. With the exception of jaundice, other symptoms are often insidious and delay diagnosis.

Jaundice due to biliary obstruction is found in the majority of patients with cancer of the pancreatic head. Pruritus is often associated. The gall bladder is usually enlarged in patients with cancer of the pancreatic head but is impalpable in more than 50% (Courvoisier's law: if the gall bladder is enlarged and the patient is jaundiced, the cause is unlikely to be gallstones) (Figure 15.1). Migratory thrombophlebitis (Trousseau's sign), venous thrombosis, acute pancreatitis and new onset diabetes mellitus are uncommon presentations of carcinoma of the pancreas. Upper gastrointestinal haemorrhage can rarely result from direct invasion of stomach or duodenum, or from varices due to compression of the portal venous system or involvement of the splenic vein.

Diagnosis

The diagnosis is initially suggested by demonstrating a mass in the pancreas or by dilated bile ducts. On ultrasound scan, this is characteristically hypoechoic. On CT

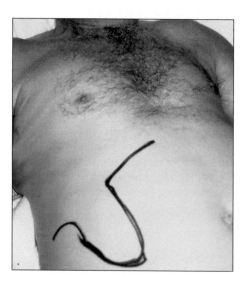

FIGURE 15.1: Enlarged, palpable gall bladder in a patient with carcinoma of the head of the pancreas.

scan, the mass is usually of reduced density compared with the rest of the pancreas. If the tumour is in the head of the pancreas, it commonly produces dilatation of the common bile duct and the main pancreatic duct (double-duct sign). Lymphatic metastases may be apparent as masses in the porta hepatis. Liver metastases may also be apparent. MRI offers no advantage over CT. Helical CT combined with intravenous contrast (CT angiograph) helps evaluate for resectability.

Endoscopic ultrasound (EUS) is useful to make a tissue diagnosis of a small tumour and to assess resectability. While tissue diagnosis can be achieved by CT or ultrasound-guided needle biopsy it has the disadvantage that the tumour might seed the needle track and this track will not be excised by subsequent surgery. This is not the case for an EUS guided biopsy. If the tumour is obviously unresectable (e.g., obvious vascular involvement or metastases) then the issue of seeding the track is irrelevant. If there is no definite mass lesion on CT or ultrasound scan and the patient is jaundiced, endoscopic retrograde cholangiopancreatography (ERCP) provides strong presumptive evidence when there is a long extrinsic compression of the common bile duct; the pancreatic duct may also be compressed (Chapter 23). A tissue diagnosis at ERCP is possible for ampullary carcinoma by biopsy and for cholangiocarcinoma by brush cytology. Magnetic resonance cholangiopancreatography (MRCP) is an alternative to define the anatomy non-invasively. If the mass appears resectable after all imaging, many surgeons will operate without a preoperative tissue diagnosis.

Histological diagnosis is mandatory for confirmation of the tumour and to rule out focal pancreatitis, autoimmune pancreatitis or other neoplasms, such as lymphoma, islet cell tumours and cystadenocarcinoma, where the prognosis and therapeutic options are significantly different (Chapter 23).

The cancer-associated antigen (CA-19-9) is often elevated in advanced disease.

Occasionally, a small (< 2 cm) tumour is demonstrated without evidence of lymphatic or liver metastases in a patient who is young and fit enough to be considered for a major pancreatic resection. Further evaluation is warranted to show that the tumour is resectable and that there are no metastases that have failed to be demonstrated by CT and ultrasound scan. A contrast-enhanced helical CT scan with thin cuts may detect small liver metastases, or encasement of the gastroduodenal artery or superior mesenteric vein or portal vein, demonstrating that the tumour is not resectable. Laparoscopy may demonstrate small peritoneal or liver metastases.

Treatment

Curative surgical resection (e.g., pancreaticoduodenectomy, i.e., a 'Whipple' resection) is the only effective treatment for the disease. Operative mortality in experienced hands is low (2–5%). Unfortunately, fewer than 15–20% of all tumours are resectable at the time of diagnosis. The 5-year survival rate after curative operation is below 30% for node-negative and 10% for node-positive patients. Even in patients who eventually have tumour recurrence, the survival is prolonged three- to four-fold (to a median of 17–20 months) compared with patients not undergoing resection. Untreated non-metastatic pancreatic cancer has a median survival of about 8–12 months (and 3–6 months if there are metastases). Adjuvant chemotherapy alone after resection may improve survival.

The major aim of palliative therapy should be relief of jaundice. This can usually be achieved by endoscopic insertion of a biliary stent. This is attractive because it avoids an operation. If the patient seems likely to survive for more than six months, an expanding metal stent (internal diameter 10 mm) can be used rather than conventional 3 mm plastic stent, which tends to block with sludge and needs changing every three months. Surgical biliary bypass (choledochojejunostomy) is rarely performed these days except in patients operated on with curative intent who are found at operation to be unresectable. In that circumstance a gastroenterostomy can be performed at the same time. Otherwise the 10% of patients who develop gastric outlet obstruction will usually be palliated with an expanding metal uncovered duodenal stent. Chemotherapy and radiotherapy have not been shown to be very effective, increasing median survival by only a few months in locally advanced cancer.

In those with hereditary pancreatitis, screening for pancreatic cancer is recommended from age 35. Similarly, those with a family history of pancreatic cancer can be offered screening 10 years before the age at which the cancer was diagnosed. Spiral CT and EUS are recommended in these cases but the tests are not very sensitive in this setting.

Carcinoma of the oesophagus

Squamous cell carcinoma and adenocarcinoma account for more than 90% of all cases of oesophageal tumour. Smoking, excess alcohol and ingestion of nitrites and fungal toxins have been causally linked to the development of squamous cell carcinoma. Achalasia, Plummer-Vinson syndrome (cervical and oesophageal web and iron deficiency anaemia) and previous lye ingestion may also increase the risk.

Adenocarcinomas arise from the distal oesophagus in metaplastic segments of columnar epithelium (Barrett's oesophagus). The incidence of adenocarcinoma of the distal oesophagus has risen six-fold in the past 20 years. Gastro-oesophageal reflux disease and obesity are risk factors.

Clinical features

Weight loss and progressive dysphagia for solids are the initial symptoms in most patients. Dysphagia progresses later on to include semisolids and liquids. Progressive dysphagia is, therefore, always an alarm symptom and mandates appropriate investigation (see Chapter 2). Unfortunately, however, diagnosis at this stage often indicates incurable disease.

Diagnosis

Endoscopy helps to delineate the nature and the extent of the lesion, and biopsies will usually confirm the diagnosis. The tumour spreads initially through the wall of the oesophagus and then via lymphatics to adjacent lymph nodes. Once the diagnosis is confirmed histologically, tumour extent is ascertained by a CT scan of the chest and upper abdomen and subsequently by PET (positron emission tomography) scanning. PET whole-body scanning is more sensitive for distant metastases than CT, detecting bony as well as liver and lung metastases and also metastases in totally unexpected positions. EUS is being used increasingly for additional regional staging. Thus, it is possible to assess how far through the oesophageal wall the tumour has penetrated and whether enlarged local perioesophageal lymph nodes have been infiltrated by the tumour. Nodal involvement is more reliably ascertained by fine needle aspiration biopsy of one or more of those nodes.

Treatment

Apart from early oesophageal cancers (e.g., those detected during Barrett's screening (see Chapter 1) that are treated by curative surgery), the prognosis is generally poor (the 5-year survival rate is about 5% for all patients, but as high as 20% for patients selected for surgical resection). Nevertheless, surgery offers the only hope of cure and as long as the tumour can be resected with clear margins, this achieves the best palliation. Preoperative chemoradiotherapy has been shown to improve the disease-free interval and possibly survival. Unfortunately, many patients are too old or frail to tolerate this approach. In those unsuitable for surgery by a specialist oesophageal surgeon, palliation of dysphagia can be achieved by placement of an expandable metal stent. Palliative chemotherapy and radiotherapy have limited roles.

Gastric carcinoma

There has been a significant decline in the incidence of gastric carcinoma in many Western countries, yet overall, it remains one of the most common causes of cancer-related deaths in the world. The incidence is highest in Japan, followed by China, South America and countries in Eastern Europe. It is rare under the age of 40.

Pathology

Adenocarcinoma accounts for the majority (> 90%) of gastric carcinomas (Figure 15.2). Lymphomas and leiomyosarcomas account for most of the remainder. Adenocarcinomas can be further classified histologically into intestinal and diffuse types. The intestinal type is characterised by cohesive neoplastic cells, which form gland-like structures and are frequently polypoid. The diffuse cancers lack cohesion, are usually ulcerative and develop throughout the stomach. Adenocarcinomas are also staged into early and advanced cancers. In early cancers, the depth of invasion is limited to the submucosa; if detected early, gastric cancer is potentially curable with resection.

Aetiology

Chronic atrophic gastritis, which begins as a multifocal process, can progress in those predisposed to intestinal metaplasia and dysplasia. This sequence can ultimately lead to cancer. *H. pylori* is classified as a Class I carcinogen by the World Health Organization, it causes chronic atrophic gastritis and is linked to gastric adenocarcinomas, mucosa-associated lymphoid tissue (MALT) lymphoma and B-cell lymphoma. Patients with *H. pylori* infection have a higher risk (three- to six-fold) of developing non-cardia gastric adenocarcinoma. Other risk factors for gastric cancer are listed in Table 15.8. Changes in multiple oncogenes and tumour suppressor genes (e.g., *MCC*, *APC* and *DDC*) have been identified in gastric cancer.

Clinical features

Gastric cancer in its early stages is asymptomatic and is diagnosed either incidentally or through a screening programme. With symptomatic presentation, advanced disease is often already present. The major symptoms are upper abdominal pain and weight loss. Anorexia and nausea also occur in about one-third of patients. Lesions around the cardia can present with dysphagia as the predominant symptom.

Typically gastric carcinomas spread to local lymph nodes and /or the liver.

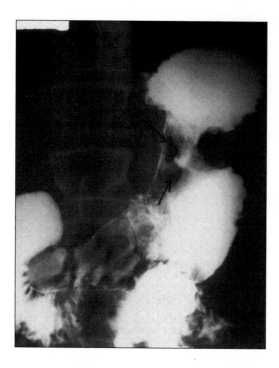

FIGURE 15.2: Gastric adenocarcinoma of the stomach.

Diagnosis

Gastroscopy with biopsy is the standard method for diagnosing gastric cancer. To increase the accuracy, multiple biopsies (> 5) are recommended. All gastric ulcers should be biopsied to rule out the presence of neoplasm.

The tumour is staged prior to surgery firstly by CT scanning looking for lymph node metastases, liver metastases and ascites, then by laparoscopy to detect smaller liver and peritoneal metastases. PET is also used as an adjunct, as it is in assessment of oesophageal tumours.

TABLE 15.8: Risk factors for gastric adenocarcinoma

Genetic factors

- Blood group A
- Family history
- Hereditary non-polyposis colon cancer syndrome

Environmental factors

- Low socioeconomic status
- Decreased consumption of fresh fruits and vegetables, and vitamin C
- Increased consumption of salted or smoked foods

Precursor conditions

- *H. pylori* gastritis
- Pernicious anaemia (autoimmune chronic atrophic gastritis)
- Ménétrier's disease
- Gastric polyps (usually adenomatous, occasionally hyperplastic)
- Previous partial gastrectomy

Treatment

Curative. Complete surgical resection of the tumour (and adjacent lymph nodes) is the only chance for a cure. In distally located tumours, the distal stomach is removed. For proximally located tumours, the whole stomach and sometimes the distal oesophagus are removed. Adjuvant chemoradiotherapy has recently been shown to be beneficial.

Palliative. Surgery may also afford a means of palliation in patients with gastric outlet obstruction or significant gastrointestinal bleeding. Combination chemotherapy can be used to palliate some non-surgical candidates with advanced gastric cancers. However, the medial survival with combination chemotherapy is only 6–10 months, and is toxic.

Prognosis

The most important determinant of prognosis is stage. In early gastric cancer, the incidence of lymph node involvement is about 10%, and the 5-year survival is about 75%. On the other hand, advanced gastric cancer (with serosal involvement) will have spread to lymph nodes in about 70% of cases and has a dismal 5-year survival rate of 5%.

Anorexia and bulimia nervosa

Anorexia nervosa

While usually affecting young women, it can also affect men. It is characterised by a distortion of body image. The disorder has been increasing over the last few decades with a prevalence in Western society of approximately 3%. It has been noted that patients with anorexia, over time, may exhibit symptoms of bulimia.

Clinical features

Young females in the pubertal age group are at the greatest risk. Amenorrhoea is usually present. A history of food fads, food avoidance, excessive use of purgatives or diuretics and self-induced vomiting is common. Mental irritability, depression or agitation can co-exist. These patients typically manifest an extreme loss of fat and muscle bulk, leading to gaunt faces, atrophic breasts and loss of body contour. Hypotension, hypothermia and bradycardia may also be evident. Lanugo (soft down-like hair), dry skin and brittle nails are common.

Pathogenesis

Distorted body image is a central abnormality; even extremely thin and emaciated patients consider themselves to be overweight, inducing them to self-starvation. There exists an association between anorexia and major depressive illnesses, as well as obsessive compulsive behaviour, personality disorders and substance abuse. There is a tendency for these patients to be high achievers and perfectionists.

Complications

The medical complications arise from starvation. Hypokalaemia, hypochloraemia and metabolic alkalosis are typical (Table 15.9). Cardiac complications are the most frequent cause of death in these patients. Prolongation of the QT interval is thought to predict the onset of serious cardiac arrhythmias. As glucose metabolism and insulin secretion are disturbed, hypoglycaemia is common and potentially lethal. Osteopenia from oestrogen deficiency is common and can lead to debilitating fractures.

Treatment

A multidisciplinary approach is required. Outpatient therapy is increasingly employed. Intense cognitive therapy and psychotherapy are the mainstays of treatment. Oral feeding is usually commenced in small amounts but occasionally parenteral nutrition may be needed in dire circumstances. Patients may resort to vomiting, purging, or surreptitious disposal of food or medications. Hospitalisation and a supervised feeding program is needed in patients with moderate to severe disease (i.e., body weight below 75% of ideal weight). Such patients mostly require prolonged hospital admission (average: 60–90 days) to achieve full nutritional rehabilitation. Malnourished patients are less responsive to tricyclic antidepressants and more likely to develop side effects, especially arrhythmias and hypotension; they should only be used when depression is not improving despite weight gain. Fluoxetine (a selective serotonin reuptake inhibitor) is also useful for reducing relapse. Antipsychotics may have a role in some patients.

Approximately 20% of patients have a relapse and 10–20% die as a result of cardiac arrhythmias, opportunistic infections, suicide or starvation. An equal number remain chronically ill. Prognosis is worst in those with later onset of disease.

Bulimia nervosa

Bulimia nervosa is the most common eating disorder. Self-induced vomiting follows excessive gorging. Women outnumber men up to 20:1. For diagnosis, a minimum of two bulimic episodes per week for three months is required, with regular purging behaviour, such as self-induced vomiting or the use of laxatives and diuretics. Unlike anorexic patients who are cachectic, these patients have fluctuations in body weight due to alternately bingeing and fasting. Gastro-oesophageal reflux and Mallory-Weiss tears can occur. Abuse of laxatives or diuretics is common.

Clinical features

Bulimic patients have a tendency to hide their illness. Body weight is usually near normal and only about 50% of patients have amenorrhoea. The following signs may sometimes be present:

- Russel's sign: repeated mechanical trauma to the skin over the dorsum of fingers and metacarpophalangeal joints, leading to erosions and callused knuckles due to self-induced vomiting;
- Painless swelling of salivary glands (sialadenosis); and
- Dental caries and erosion of enamel caused by high acid content in vomit.

Treatment

As with anorexia nervosa, a similar multidisciplinary approach is necessary. Pharmacotherapy has a greater role to play and often higher doses of medications are required. Fluoxetine (up to 60 mg/day) has been best studied but only one-third of patients go into remission. A combination of an antidepressant plus cognitive behavioural therapy appears to be better (up to 50% remission). Individuals who have milder symptoms at the commencement of treatment tend to have a better prognosis than those individuals who are disabled and functioning poorly at the start of treatment. Additionally, other indicators of poor prognosis include premorbid personality disturbance, low self-esteem, impulsiveness and persistent body image dissatisfaction.

TABLE 15.9: Laboratory findings that may occur in patients with anorexia nervosa	
Endocrine investigations	Low gonadotrophin (FSH and LH) levels
	Low oestrogen and testosterone levels
	Sick euthyroid state
	Increased cortisol level
Metabolic investigations	Hypokalaemia, hypomagnesaemia
	Hypocalcaemia, hypophosphataemia
	Hypoglycaemia
	Pre-renal azotaemia
Haematological investigations	Anaemia, pancytopaenia
	Low plasma protein levels

Further reading

Alibhai SM, Greenwood C, Payette H. An approach to the management of unintentional weight loss in elderly people. *CMAJ* 2005; 172: 773–80.

Bouras EP, Lange SM, Scolapio JR. Rational approach to patients with unintentional weight loss. *Mayo Clin Proc* 2001; 76: 923–9.

Brugge WR, Lauwers GY, Sahani D *et al*. Cystic neoplasms of the pancreas. *N Engl J Med* 2004; 351: 1218–26.

Fairburn CG, Harrison PJ. Eating disorders. *Lancet* 2003; 361: 407–16.

Hernandez JL, Matorras P, Riancho JA, Gonzalez-Macias J. Involuntary weight loss without specific symptoms: a clinical prediction score for malignant neoplasm. *QJM* 2003; 96: 649–55.

Hustinx R. PET imaging in assessing gastrointestinal tumors. *Radiol Clin North Am* 2004; 42: 1123–39.

Jankowski JA, Anderson M. Review article: management of oesophageal adenocarcinoma—control of acid, bile and inflammation in intervention strategies for Barrett's oesophagus. *Aliment Pharmacol Ther* 2004; 20 Suppl 5: 71–80.

Lagergren J, Bergstrom R, Lindgren A, Nyren O. Symptomatic gastroesophageal reflux as a risk factor for esophageal adenocarcinoma. *N Engl J Med* 1999; 340: 825–31.

Penman ID, Henry E. Advanced esophageal cancer. *Gastrointest Endosc Clin N Am* 2005; 15: 101–16.

Powers PS, Santana C. Available pharmacological treatments for anorexia nervosa. *Expert Opin Pharmacother* 2004; 5: 2287–92.

Walsh BT, Klein DA. Eating disorders. *Int Rev Psychiatry* 2003; 15: 205–16.

Acknowledgement

Much of the material in this chapter was originally written by Dr S Nandurker and his been adapted for the new edition.

chapter 16

FOOD 'ALLERGY' AND INTOLERANCE

INTRODUCTION

Many individuals presenting with gastrointestinal symptoms—particularly abdominal pain, diarrhoea and abdominal distension—complain of food-induced symptoms and believe that they are 'allergic to food' (Table 16.1). In some of these individuals, there is food intolerance secondary to an underlying disease such as lactose malabsorption. However, the majority have a functional gastrointestinal disorder, in whom the mechanism of the perceived food intolerance is obscure. Only a minority of the food-intolerant individuals will subsequently be found to be truly reacting adversely to components of the food they eat and rarely will this reaction be of an immunological (allergic) nature.

HISTORY AND PHYSICAL EXAMINATION

Determine the pattern of gastrointestinal symptoms and their relationship to meals. Ask if it is always the same food groups that cause symptoms (Table 16.2). In true food allergy, which is rare, only one or a few foods (e.g., eggs, nuts, seafood) cause problems. Milk products may cause excess bloating and diarrhoea in lactose intolerance. In the functional gastrointestinal disorders, symptoms after meals are very common, but no consistent food can be blamed, and symptoms in between meals also are frequent. Ask about the specific symptoms of the irritable bowel syndrome (Chapter 6).

A history of systemic symptoms is vital. Ask specifically about swelling or itching a few minutes after food (which may occur in true allergy). Determine if skin rashes or aphthous ulcers have been experienced. Any history of systemic anaphylaxis after food and atopy is important.

A physical examination is generally unhelpful, unless the patient is currently experiencing symptoms. Angioedema, urticaria, or signs of asthma may occasionally be detected.

TABLE 16.1: Types of adverse reactions to foods	
Reaction type	**Example**
• No established adverse food	Functional gastrointestinal disorders reaction (most common)
• Metabolic disorder	Lactase deficiency causing lactose intolerance
• Psychological effects	Food aversion
• Pharmacological effects	Caffeine, metabisulfite
• Fermentation or microbiological effects	Unabsorbed residues acted on by bowel flora
• Allergy (rare)	Specific immunological reactions to food proteins e.g., egg, milk, nuts, seafood Coeliac disease Eosinophilic oesophagitis, eosinophilic gastroenteritis

PATHOPHYSIOLOGY OF FOOD REACTIONS

Individuals may react to the nutrients in food, such as protein, carbohydrate, fat, vitamins or minerals. True allergic reactions of the immediate hypersensitivity type are rare. In these circumstances, the offending agent is a specific food, such as eggs, nuts, milk or seafood. Food reactions may also be due to a specific enzyme deficiency state. In lactase deficiency, for example, an individual is unable to absorb lactose from dairy products resulting in gastrointestinal tract symptoms including diarrhoea and bloating. A more common form of reaction occurs as part of a generalised pharmacological response to biologically active food chemicals. These may be naturally occurring, be added as preservatives or food additives, or be the result of metabolism during the process of digestion or absorption.

The normal process of protein digestion is complex (Chapter 13). It is initiated in the stomach by pepsin with preferential hydrolysis of peptide bonds at the amino side of aromatic amino acids. Within the small intestine, it is continued by the action of pancreatic exopeptidases including trypsin, chymotrypsin and elastase. Other pancreatic exopeptidases—carboxypeptidase A and B—simultaneously continue this process. As a result, within the lumen of the small bowel, a large number of small peptides, especially di-, tri- and tetra-peptides can cross the healthy intestinal mucosa. With altered intestinal motility or permeability, which occurs with some functional and organic gastrointestinal diseases, a larger number of intact peptides and proteins can be absorbed.

Many small peptides, including dipeptides, have a wide range of biological and pharmacological activities, including neuroactivity. The intestine and the nervous system contain numerous peptide and opioid receptors whose physiological functions may be relevant in the pathophysiology of food-induced reactions.

The particular foods and beverages likely to cause gastrointestinal reactions include milk products (in lactase deficiency), cereal grains, nuts and fruit (particularly citrus fruit). Specific chemicals such as monosodium glutamate (a widely used flavour

---

TABLE 16.2: Foods likely to cause gastrointestinal intolerance

- Cereal grains, e.g., wheat
- Dairy products, e.g., milk
- Fruit, e.g., citrus fruit
- Vegetables, e.g., onions
- Miscellaneous: coffee, eggs, chocolate, nuts, preservatives

---

enhancer), metabisulfite (a food preservative which may be added to food, but which also occurs naturally, particularly in foods such as oranges or orange juice) and food dyes (such as tartrazine) may also be a problem. Only a small minority of individuals will be intolerant of one food alone.

Table 16.1 is an overview of some of the mechanisms of adverse reactions to food. This chapter deals predominantly with adverse reactions to food which are believed to be allergic (of the immunological type) or due to pharmacological effects.

Some specific disorders in which the mechanism may be partly immunological can present as food intolerance. These include gluten-sensitive enteropathy (coeliac disease), cow's-milk-sensitive enteropathy and eosinophilic gastroenteritis, which are discussed in Chapter 13.

ALLERGIC REACTIONS TO FOOD (FOOD ALLERGY)

Food reactions due to Type I hypersensitivity are very uncommon causes of adverse reactions to food (Table 16.3). Here, mast cells degranulate and release mediators when antibodies are cross-linked by the relevant antigen.

These reactions can usually be easily diagnosed by a carefully taken history. Patients tend to be children (but this can occur in adults) with an atopic background. The foods that are the offending antigens are relatively few in number. They include eggs, nuts, milk and seafood. The reaction usually starts with local swelling, itching and burning around the mouth and pharynx. This occurs on most occasions within a few minutes of food ingestion. This reaction may be followed by nausea, vomiting, abdominal cramps and diarrhoea. Systemic anaphylaxis is rare but when it occurs, is often dramatic. In severe reactions, urticaria, angioedema, rhinorrhoea and asthma may also be noted.

The diagnosis can be supported by a positive result on a skin-prick test and a positive RAST (radioallergosorbent test) result to the relevant food, and elevated serum IgE levels. There is a tendency for these reactions to be modified or disappear with age. Whether delayed immunological reactions to food occur is controversial.

In interpreting RAST results, the technical details of the test are crucial. Relevant antigens must be coupled to solid-phase support material. There should be negative control serum samples included to reflect non-specific IgE binding, and there should also be positive control serum samples to confirm that relevant antigens have been coupled to a solid-phase support. A positive RAST result does not necessarily indicate that the reaction to that allergen is of clinical significance. False positive results can occur to cereal grains in individuals who have unrelated inhalant allergies. The RAST inhibition provides a tool to confirm the specificity of IgE antibody.

Treatment involves dietary elimination of the one or two specific foods that precipitate such a reaction.

TABLE 16.3: Characteristics of food allergy—immunologically based

- Rare
- Occurs mainly in childhood with atopic background
- Restricted to a limited number of foods, e.g., eggs, fish, nuts, milk
- Onset is immediate
- Accompanied by local reactions around mouth
- Usually has positive skin-prick tests and RAST results

PHARMACOLOGICALLY-RELATED ADVERSE FOOD REACTIONS

In many individuals, reactions to food are often delayed from between one hour and up to 48 hours after ingestion. It is likely that reactions occur to more than one food, and reactions to each constituent may exhibit a dose–response relationship with a triggering threshold that depends partly on recent intake. Thus, an individual food does not necessarily produce the same reaction on each occasion (Table 16.4). This can result in a delay in diagnosis.

When they involve the gut, the symptoms of pharmacological food reactions can mimic the irritable bowel syndrome. The major symptoms are believed to include nausea, vomiting, recurrent abdominal pain, diarrhoea and bloating. These individuals may also have an atopic background. Commonly, other systems are involved such as the skin, the respiratory tract or the central nervous system. However, this is a controversial syndrome and its prevalence is not well documented.

A carefully taken history will often reveal a history of skin rashes, particularly urticaria, in the past and frequently in childhood. Recurrent aphthous ulceration is infrequent but is characteristically found in salicylate-sensitive individuals. Respiratory symptoms are common, mainly involving the upper respiratory tract. Nasal congestion, excessive mucus production, recurrent sore throats or sinusitis are common. In some individuals, precipitation of asthma occurs with these same foods.

Neurological symptoms are commonly present and are sometimes bizarre including headaches (often migrainous), general lethargy and myalgia. Patients often describe the sensation of feeling 'drugged' or 'hung-over'. Testing may reveal impairment in memory and concentration, confusion, depression, dizziness, paraesthesia, sweating, palpitations and flushing. These patients are often labelled as having recurrent bouts of gastroenteritis or a psychiatric disorder.

Physical examination may be helpful in excluding other disorders but there are no specific signs to support a diagnosis of pharmacologically-related food-induced reactions. Appropriate investigation may need to be performed to exclude other relevant diseases, particularly lactose intolerance, coeliac disease and inflammatory bowel disease. The positive features in the history that would indicate a functional gastrointestinal disorder such as the irritable bowel syndrome should be sought (Chapter 6).

These reactions cannot be diagnosed accurately by any available skin or blood test. Many tests have claimed to be diagnostic of food reactions, including food allergy. These include cytotoxic food testing, provocative subcutaneous testing, sublingual testing, examination of the hair and Vega testing. As yet there is no definite evidence to recommend any of these forms of testing; the American Academy of Allergy has stated that they are of unproven validity and recommends that their use be limited to well-designed clinical trials. These tests have a high frequency of both false positives and false negatives, and are not recommended.

The responsible chemicals are best identified by systematic elimination diets and oral challenge. Since each component compound is often present in many foods and each patient is usually sensitive to several compounds, the elimination diet must be comprehensive. Challenges should be spaced by at least 48 hours to allow for delayed reactions, and any response to a challenge should be followed by a pause of at least three symptom-free days because patients often experience a temporary refractory period during which they are unresponsive to that particular food.

When designing an elimination diet for individuals with potential food-induced problems, it is usually wise to remove cereals, dairy products, citrus fruits, beverages and food additives. A standard exclusion diet should avoid these but be nutritionally adequate and contain meat (often lamb), fruits (particularly pears) and vegetables.

If the individuals are not considered improved after two weeks on an exclusion diet, as a general rule symptoms in these patients are not due to food intolerance and it is likely that they have a functional gastrointestinal disorder.

Thus, diagnosis can be confirmed by the use of an elimination diet to determine whether symptoms remit and re-emerge on subsequent challenge with suspected foodstuffs versus a placebo (preferably double-blind). This means of diagnosis is time-consuming and difficult. Compliance by poorly motivated patients is low. However, the results are dramatic and sustained in some individuals when long-term dietary modifications, based on the results of individual oral provocation results, are undertaken.

TABLE 16.4: Characteristics of adverse reactions to food—pharmacologically based

- Occurs in children and adults
- Can occur with many food items
- Onset is commonly delayed (up to 48 hours)
- Often associated with respiratory and/or neurological symptoms
- No confirmatory laboratory tests
- Requires use of an elimination diet and challenge to support diagnosis

---

LACTASE DEFICIENCY

Lactase is a brush border enzyme which splits the milk sugar, lactose, into glucose and galactose. Absence of the enzyme results in osmotic diarrhoea due to the presence of unabsorbed lactose in the small bowel and colon (Table 16.5). In the colon, lactose is converted to hydrogen and short chain fatty acids by the bacterial flora.

There are three forms of lactase deficiency. Congenital lactase deficiency is present from birth and is very rare. Acquired lactase deficiency occurs in most non-milk-drinking populations around the world and develops in late childhood. Secondary lactase deficiency occurs in situations where small bowel mucosal damage occurs, e.g., after gastroenteritis and with coeliac disease.

There are two main theories put forward to explain acquired lactase deficiency. Lactase persistence is an autosomal dominant trait. The genetic theory postulates that with the onset of dairying about 12,000 years ago, those adults able to absorb lactose enjoyed a selective survival advantage. If those adults who were able to absorb lactose produced on average 1% more surviving children in each of the 400 generations to now, it would account for the current distribution of lactase deficiency. The alternative theory postulates that continued milk drinking induces the enzyme lactase. Lactase non-persistence is associated with the CC genotype of the DNA variant-13910 T/C.

Clinical features

Adults with lactase deficiency may not have any symptoms unless they ingest a significant amount of lactose. Many lactase-deficient adults can tolerate up to 10–14 g of lactose (200–300 mL of milk) without any symptoms. Typical clinical features in those who ingest more lactose include diarrhoea, crampy abdominal pain, abdominal distension and borborygmi.

Lactose intolerance in infants after gastroenteritis, for example, may have more serious implications where lactose is a major component of their diet. Persistent diarrhoea with failure to thrive may follow.

TABLE 16.5: Lactase deficiency

- Majority of adult non-Caucasians have primary brush-border lactase deficiency
- Milk products in lactase-deficient patients can cause diarrhoea, bloating, pain and flatus
- Tolerance of milk products is very variable in lactase-deficient individuals but small amounts of lactose are usually tolerated
- May co-exist with the irritable bowel syndrome which can typically cause pain, diarrhoea and bloating
- Lactase deficiency can occur secondarily to small intestinal diseases (e.g., gastroenteritis, coeliac disease, bacterial overgrowth)
- Relief of symptoms on a two-week lactose-free diet is suggestive of lactase deficiency (versus irritable bowel syndrome)

Diagnosis

Lactase deficiency can be determined directly by measuring lactase in small bowel biopsy specimens. Indirect tests include the lactose breath hydrogen test and the lactose tolerance test (Chapter 7). In the lactose H_2 breath test, 2 g/kg (maximum 25 g) of lactose is ingested and breath H_2 sampled for three hours; a rise in H_2 over 20 parts per million (from bacterial breakdown of non-digested lactose) suggests lactose intolerance. False negatives occur in some normal people who are not H_2 producers (1%) or after antibiotics. The lactose tolerance test involves measuring blood glucose after a lactose load, having first established that glucose tolerance is normal (sensitivity 75%, specificity 96%, with false negatives occurring with bacterial overgrowth, diabetes mellitus and slow gastric emptying). In practice, a trial of withdrawal of milk and milk products is often instituted and a presumptive diagnosis made if symptoms resolve.

Treatment

Treatment consists of reducing milk and dairy products until the symptoms resolve. This does not necessarily mean eliminating all dairy products, which are a rich source of calcium. Many types of cheese contain very little lactose and can be well tolerated. Most patients with lactose intolerance can tolerate 240 mL of 2% fat milk daily; spreading out the lactose load throughout the day remains wise. Commercial lactase preparation (yeast or bacterial beta-galactosidases) are of variable value in reducing symptoms. An adequate calcium intake (500 mg/day) should be recommended. Some people who suffer troublesome symptoms obtain excellent symptom relief and are able to maintain adequate calcium intake by substituting soy-based, calcium-enriched milk products for cow's milk.

Further reading

Bischoff S, Crowe SE. Gastrointestinal food allergy: new insights into pathophysiology and clinical perspectives. *Gastroenterology* 2005; 128: 1089–113.

David TJ. Adverse reactions and intolerance to foods. *Br Med Bull* 2000; 56: 34–50.

Hogenauer C, Hammer HF, Mellitzer K *et al.* Evaluation of a new DNA test compared with the lactose hydrogen breath test for the diagnosis of lactase non-persistence. *Eur J Gastroenterol Hepatol* 2005; 17: 371–6.

Lea R, Whorwell PJ. The role of food intolerance in irritable bowel syndrome. *Gastroenterol Clin North Am* 2005; 34: 247–55.

Nowak-Wegrzyn A, Sampson HA. Adverse reactions to foods. *Med Clin North Am* 2006; 90: 97–127.

Pimentel M, Kong Y, Park S. Breath testing to evaluate lactose intolerance in irritable bowel syndrome correlates with lactulose testing and may not reflect true lactose malabsorption. *Am J Gastroenterol* 2003; 98: 2700–4.

Sampson HA, Sicherer SH, Birnbaum AH. AGA technical review on the evaluation of food allergy in gastrointestinal disorders. American Gastroenterological Association. *Gastroenterology* 2001; 120: 1026–40.

chapter 17

ASYMPTOMATIC PALPABLE ABDOMINAL MASSES

This chapter is included to give guidelines and assistance to the clinician in the following situations:

- An unexpected finding of an asymptomatic abdominal mass during the course of a routine clinical examination of an asymptomatic patient.
  In this case, the finding of the mass is the presenting feature of the disease. An example of this situation is, during a routine health check, finding a right iliac fossa mass due to an asymptomatic carcinoma of the caecum;

- A finding of an asymptomatic abdominal mass during evaluation of a patient who presents with distant but related pathology.
  An example of this situation is asymptomatic hepatomegaly due to metastatic breast carcinoma. Here the pathologies are clearly related. The clinician, having already made a provisional diagnosis of breast carcinoma on the basis of the presenting symptoms and signs, was in this case looking for evidence of metastasis from the primary carcinoma;

- An unexpected finding of an asymptomatic abdominal mass in a patient who presents with an unrelated disease process.
  An example is the finding of a renal mass due to asymptomatic hydronephrosis during physical examination in a patient with decreasing visual acuity due to cataracts. In this situation the patient has two unrelated pathologies. This can be a particularly difficult clinical situation because it may require considerable clinical maturity to realise that there are two pathologies and that they are indeed unrelated. It is appropriate in the first instance to try to relate all of the clinical features to the presenting symptoms;

- A patient who has found an abdominal mass.
  This is an unusual situation. It usually occurs with masses of the abdominal wall and occasionally with large intra-abdominal masses; or

- An unexpected abdominal mass demonstrated on an abdominal scan that was performed for some other reason.
  The organ of origin is often already identified and indeed the pathological process may be apparent. The clinician will then go back to the patient in an effort to ascertain whether there are any symptoms attributable to the mass and whether signs of the mass and its sequelae can be elicited.

Other chapters in this book are orientated to evaluation of abdominal masses presenting with symptoms. Assessment of generalised abdominal distension and lumps in the groin are covered in Chapters 18 and 19, respectively.

EXAMINATION OF THE ABDOMEN

As a routine, this examination is performed from the right hand side of the bed with the patient supine. The environment needs to be quiet, warm and private. The presence of a friend or relative may help the patient relax. The examination must be gentle. Discomfort results in a protective contraction of the abdominal muscles. If an abdominal mass is palpated, it is reasonable to go back to its evaluation in the standard sequence (inspection, palpation, percussion and auscultation), to ensure that no important features have been overlooked.

Abdominal masses may be visible, palpable and audible.

Visible. A mass may occasionally be visible as a generalised distension of the abdominal wall or as a localised deformity of abdominal wall contour. Masses within the anterior abdominal wall may be visible and palpable when quite small. Visible intra-abdominal masses usually imply large lesions and are most easily seen in elderly, thin patients, e.g., a visible right iliac fossa mass caused by a caecal carcinoma.

Palpable. Though the majority of abdominal masses cannot be seen on abdominal inspection, some can be detected by palpation. The information gained on palpation can do much to narrow the diagnostic possibilities.

Audible. A bruit may be audible in or near the mass. It may arise from the mass or from an adjacent vessel. This gives valuable information about local blood flow.

Position of the mass

For the purposes of organisation, the abdomen is divided into nine regions as shown in Figure 17.1. The position of the mass needs to be specified in relation to one or more of these regions.

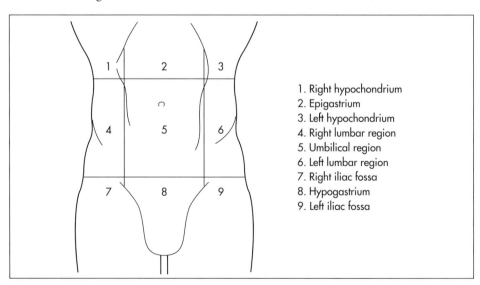

FIGURE 17.1: Schematic illustration of the nine abdominal regions.
(Based on Talley NJ and O'Connor S, Clinical Examination, 5th edn, Elsevier Australia.)

ABDOMINAL WALL MASSES

The position of the abdominal mass needs to be defined in relation to the abdominal wall. Masses of the abdominal wall are listed in Table 17.1.

To separate these from intra-abdominal masses, ask the patient to contract the abdominal musculature. Patients can be asked to lift their head from the examining couch with their hands behind their head, or to straight leg raise both their legs simultaneously. These manoeuvres always make definition by palpation of a mass in the intra-abdominal cavity less distinct. A mass in the abdominal wall that is superficial to the abdominal wall musculature will be thrown into relief by this manoeuvre.

Abdominal wall hernias are usually easily identifiable. A cough impulse is a requirement for diagnosis. The different types and their features are listed in Table 17. 1.

TABLE 17.1: Causes of abdominal wall masses

Lumps arising in the skin and subcutaneous fat (that could occur anywhere on the body)

- Lipoma
- Sebaceous cyst

Lumps arising in the skin and subcutaneous fat (specific to the anterior abdominal wall)

- Tumour nodule of the umbilicus (secondary to intraperitoneal malignancy, also called Sister Mary Joseph nodule)

Lumps arising in the fascia and muscle

- Rectus sheath haematoma (usually painful)
- Desmoid tumour (associated with Gardiner's syndrome; Chapter 20)

Hernia

Incisional	It has an overlying scar. The sac may be very much larger than the neck of the hernia
Umbilical	The hernia is through the umbilical scar. Those presenting at birth commonly resolve in the first years of life
Paraumbilical	The neck is just lateral to the umbilical scar. Patients usually present later in life
Epigastric	It occurs in the midline between the xiphoid process and the umbilicus. They are usually small (< 2 cm). They result when a knuckle of extraperitoneal fat extrudes through a small defect in the linea alba. Commonly irreducible and without an expansile cough impulse
Spigelian	A rare hernia found along the linea semilunaris at the lateral edge of the rectus sheath, most commonly a third of the way between the umbilicus and the pubis

Divarication of the recti

- Supraumbilical elliptical swelling of attenuated linea alba (no cough impulse)

RETROPERITONEAL MASSES

The retroperitoneal region is subdivided into five regions:

- a central column containing the great vessels and surrounding lymph nodes posteriorly and the pancreas and duodenum anteriorly;
- two lateral upper regions containing the kidneys and adrenals, and the ascending and descending colon; and
- two lateral lower regions which lie below the posterior brim of the pelvis and containing the ureters, the caecum and the lower descending colon.

Retroperitoneal masses do not move with respiration. Some of those in the upper lateral regions are *ballotable* to bimanual palpation. This sign is elicited by dipping the fingers of one hand into the renal angle while palpating the corresponding point on the anterior abdominal wall with the other. This manoeuvre may accentuate the mass felt with the hand on the anterior abdominal wall; the mass will be felt to move anteriorly. The classic ballotable mass is an enlarged kidney. (A mobile normal right kidney is sometimes ballotable in thin patients.) Other laterally placed masses, such as cancers of the ascending and descending colon, are rarely ballotable. Adrenal masses are not ballotable because they are situated above the inferior margin of the chest wall posteriorly. (An enlarged spleen is not ballotable. With enlargement the lower pole expands anteroinferiorly while the upper pole remains covered by the posterior rib cage posteriorly.)

Masses in the central column are covered by the spine and the erector spinae muscles posteriorly. Masses in the lower lateral regions are protected by the pelvis posteriorly.

INTRA-ABDOMINAL MASSES

Site

On the basis of position (Figure 17.1), one can start to define the organ of origin of an intra-abdominal mass as shown in Table 17.2.

The clinician should not expect to identify the origin of a palpable mass on the basis of its position alone. When the organs expand, they do not necessarily do so concentrically from a fixed point as described above for the spleen. Rather, their expansion is determined by the presence of surrounding structures, by special features of their retroperitoneal attachments and by the pathological process responsible for the organomegaly. The liver, for example, being limited by the diaphragm superiorly and laterally, tends to enlarge downwards and inwards. The uterus and bladder being limited by, as well as attached to, the pelvis inferiorly, tend to enlarge upwards in the midline. The kidneys, aorta and pancreas, being retroperitoneal, tend to expand from their original site in all directions. An enlarged segment of small bowel is usually not found in the upper three segments of the abdomen because the transverse mesocolon, the transverse colon and the greater omentum are attached to retroperitoneal tissues along a horizontal line at the level of the inferior border of the pancreas. These three organs tend to form a barrier restricting upward migration of small bowel masses.

The same pathological process can have differing effects on different organs and even on the same organ. Thus, a locally aggressive cancer of the sigmoid colon may become fixed to the posterior abdominal wall. Omental secondary deposits from a sigmoid primary tumour may be relatively mobile. Finally, the enlarged organ may come to fill several adjacent segments if the degree of enlargement is great. Thus, in the third trimester of pregnancy, an enlarged pregnant uterus can be expected to fill the hypogastrium, the periumbilical region and part of the epigastrium.

The following features are used to try and define the likely organ of origin (see Tables 17.3 and 17.4).

TABLE 17.2: Organ of origin of intra-abdominal masses by region

Right hypochondrium	Epigastrium	Left hypochondrium
Right lobe of liver	Stomach	Spleen
Gall bladder	Left lobe of liver	Pancreas*
	Pancreas*	Stomach
	Lymph nodes*	
	Aorta*	
Right lumbar region	**Periumbilical**	**Left lumbar**
Ascending colon*	Omentum	Descending colon*
Right kidney*	Transverse colon	Left kidney*
	Aorta*	
	Retroperitoneal nodes*	
Right iliac fossa	**Hypogastrium**	**Left iliac fossa**
Appendix	Bladder	Sigmoid colon
Caecum*	Uterus	Iliac aneurysm*
Iliac aneurysm*	Right and left ovary*	Left ovary*
Right ovary		Iliac nodes*
Iliac nodes*		
* Strictly retroperitoneal in position		

TABLE 17.3: Features of an abdominal mass that need to be defined

- Is it superficial or deep to the anterior abdominal wall?
- Does it have an expansive cough impulse?
- Is it single or multiple?
- What is the position of the mass?
- What are the shape and dimensions?
- Can all of the margins be palpated?
- What is the surface texture (smooth or irregular)? Are the margins sharp or blunt/indistinct?
- What is the consistency (hard, firm or soft)?
- Does the mass move spontaneously with respiration or does it move on palpation?
- Is it indentable?
- Is there tenderness?
- Is it resonant or dull?
- Is there pulsatility, or a bruit?
- Does it appear to go into the pelvis?
- Is the inferior margin palpable per rectum or per vagina?

TABLE 17.4: Clinical clues in the patient with an apparently asymptomatic abdominal mass

Mass position	Features on examination	Symptoms that may have been overlooked	Clinical examples
Right hypochondrium	Hard irregular, moves with respiration, can't get above it	Vaguely unwell, symptoms referable to primary tumour	Metastatic liver disease (e.g., pancreas, stomach, colon, lung, breast)
	Firm smooth, moves with respiration, can't get above it	—	Hydatid disease, fatty liver
	Globular, moves with respiration	Previous attack of cholecystitis	Mucocoele of the gall bladder
Epigastric	Hard, no movement with respiration, mobile or fixed	Anorexia, nausea, weight loss, symptoms of anaemia, mild symptoms of dyspepsia	Carcinoma of the stomach
	Hard, fixed (no movement with respiration), can't get above it	Anorexia, nausea, weight loss, vague epigastric or back pain	Carcinoma of the pancreas
	Hard fixed (no movement with respiration)	Vaguely unwell	Metastatic para-aortic lymphadenopathy
Left hypochondrium	Moves with respiration, can't get above it	—	Splenomegaly
Right lumbar	Ballotable	Symptoms of renal failure, vague ache in loin	Massive hydronephrosis, polycystic kidney
	Mobile/fixed, no movement with respiration	Symptoms of anaemia	Carcinoma of ascending colon
Periumbilical	Single/multiple, mobile ± ascites	Lassitude, weight loss, symptoms attributable to primary tumour	Metastatic omental tumour
	Mobile/fixed, no movement with respiration	Symptoms of anaemia	Carcinoma of transverse colon
	Pulsatile, immobile	Vague back ache	Aortic aneurysm
	Hard, fixed (no movement with respiration)	Vaguely unwell	Metastatic lymph nodes

TABLE 17.4: Clinical clues in the patient with an apparently asymptomatic abdominal mass *(continued)*

Mass position	Features on examination	Symptoms that may have been overlooked	Clinical examples
Left lumbar	Ballotable	Symptoms of renal failure, vague ache in loin	Massive hydronephrosis, polycystic kidney
	Mobile/fixed, no movement with respiration	Per rectum bleeding, change in bowel habit, symptoms of anaemia	Carcinoma of descending colon
Right iliac fossa	Mobile/fixed	Symptoms of anaemia, dull ache in right iliac fossa	Carcinoma of caecum
	Mobile, indentable	Constipation	Constipation
Hypogastrium	Globular, smooth, immobile, not palpable bimanually, pressure over it may induce desire to micturate	Difficulty with micturition	Chronically obstructed bladder
	Palpable bimanually, ± lobulated	Irregular and heavy menstruation, vague hypogastric pains, backache	Fibroids
	Palpable bimanually, perhaps slightly off midline	Vague lower abdominal ache	Benign or malignant ovarian cyst
	Globular, smooth, immobile, palpable bimanually	Missed menstrual period	Pregnancy
Left iliac fossa	Mobile, fixed	Per rectum bleeding, change of bowel habit	Carcinoma of sigmoid colon
	Mobile, indentable	Constipation	Constipation

Movement with respiration

Abdominal organs move with respiration because the diaphragm moves inferiorly with inspiration and back to its neutral position with expiration. Immediately below the diaphragm are the liver and the spleen. An enlarged liver or spleen can be expected to move inferiorly with each inspiratory effort. As well as moving inferiorly, the liver edge and the inferior pole of the spleen move medially in relation to the costal margin. Other organs in the upper abdomen do not move with respiration. As mentioned above, the retroperitoneal organs (pancreas, aorta, kidneys and lymph nodes) are relatively fixed posteriorly so that they are not displaced inferiorly with each movement of the liver and spleen, which slide over them. The hollow viscera inferior to the liver and spleen (the stomach, transverse colon and small bowel) also tend not to move much with respiration as the surrounding stomach and bowel is compressed by the rise in intra-abdominal pressure with inspiration. An enlarged gall bladder moves inferiorly with respiration as it is firmly attached to the liver. Similarly an inflamed or neoplastic mass just inferior to the liver, which is pathologically attached to the inferior surface of the liver but not to retroperitoneal structures, will also move inferiorly with respiration.

Relation to the costal margin and the brim of the pelvis

Palpation of the upper reaches of the abdominal cavity is prevented by the costal margins. Palpation of the pelvic cavity is restricted by the pubis. Thus, the full extent of hepatomegaly and splenomegaly is not appreciated by abdominal palpation. Unlike a mass in the transverse colon or omentum, the examiner will not be able to define a superior edge of an enlarged liver or spleen by palpation. Similarly, the examiner will not be able to define by abdominal examination an inferior margin of enlarged organs that lie in the pelvis (bladder and uterus).

Mobility

Most abdominal masses are relatively immobile if one tries to move them within the abdominal cavity with the fingers of one or two hands. On some occasions, this manoeuvre will result in movement of neoplastic masses involving the omentum, the transverse colon, the sigmoid colon and the small bowel. All of these organs are both anteriorly placed as well as loosely attached to the posterior abdominal wall by a mesentery. Inflammatory masses of the bowel (which are usually painful) tend to be less mobile because of local adhesions caused by the inflammatory process.

Shape, edge and consistency

The most common asymptomatic intra-abdominal mass is a segment of colon (Figure 17.2), usually caecum or sigmoid, loaded with faeces. A loaded colon tends to be tubular or sausage shaped. The surface may also be lobulated. The orientation of a caecum loaded with faeces is vertical, while that of sigmoid colon is oblique, parallel to the inguinal ligament. The diagnostic feature of colon loaded with faeces is that it can be indented or moulded; pressing a finger or thumb into the mass may leave an impression, which is subsequently discernible by the examining fingers.

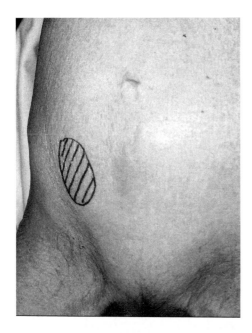

FIGURE 17.2: Hard non-indentable abdominal mass. This was caused by a caecal carcinoma.

The contour of malignant tumours may be vaguely nodular to palpation; benign tumours always have a smooth contour.

Malignant tumours tend to be hard in consistency, while benign tumours may be soft. One might think that necrosis of, or haemorrhage into, a malignant tumour should render the tumour soft. In fact, as the haemorrhage is usually contained within the tumour and the necrosis in the centre of the tumour is associated with oedema, the net result is that the tumour remains hard. The perceived consistency of a tumour is also dependent on the amount of soft tissue, such as a fatty abdominal wall, overlying the tumour. Thus, hard tumours may still be perceived as soft to abdominal palpation.

Single or multiple

If more than one mass is found, then the differential diagnosis is narrowed. The commonest cause is constipation. The next commonest cause is multiple peritoneal secondaries.

Tender or non-tender

An asymptomatic abdominal mass is unlikely to be tender. Tenderness implies inflammation, which may be due to infection, infarction or haemorrhage into the mass (Table 17.5).

Pulsatile or non-pulsatile

The commonest abdominal aneurysm is an abdominal aortic aneurysm. This is found in the midline just above the umbilicus. This mass expands laterally in both directions (*expansile pulsation*). It needs to be distinguished from a mass situated between the aorta and the anterior abdominal wall, which transmits the aortic pulsation anteriorly, but is not expansile laterally. If there is any doubt, then the patient can be asked to rest on his or her hands and knees while the mass is repalpated. If an overlying mass is mobile with respect to the posterior abdominal wall, then the mass may fall away from the previously underlying artery and will no longer transmit the pulsation.

Percussion note

Solid abdominal tumours are dull to percussion. If apparently enlarged, the upper level of liver in the mid-clavicular line should be determined by percussion and the liver span determined (normal < 12.5 cm).

Bruit or silent

Auscultation of the mass may reveal a bruit. Bruits are most commonly limited to systole and are caused by turbulence in a narrowed artery. A continuous or machinery bruit may be heard overlying an extremely vascular tumour. It signifies the presence of major arteriovenous shunting within the tumour. A bruit over the liver may also occur in acute alcoholic hepatitis or with an arteriovenous malformation.

Bimanually palpable on rectal or vaginal examination

Some masses within the lower half of the abdomen, particularly those in the hypogastrium, arise from the pelvic organs, in particular the bladder, uterus and ovaries. Such an origin may be suspected if the lower margin of the mass cannot be palpated because of the bony pubis. The mass should be further characterised by bimanual palpation. This is achieved by palpating the superior edge of the mass with one hand on the abdomen, while attempting to palpate the inferior edge with either the index finger of the other hand in the rectum (or the index and middle fingers in the vagina). For a bimanual rectal examination, the patient is positioned in the left lateral decubitus position with the hips and knees flexed. For a bimanual vaginal examination, the patient is positioned supine with the hips and knees flexed and the hips externally rotated

If the mass is palpable bimanually, then its size can be estimated, its surface characteristics more easily determined with the internally placed finger and its relationship to the uterus ascertained. The lower edge of the bladder cannot be appreciated per rectum or per vagina. An ovarian mass should be distinguishable from the uterus bimanually; the circular indentation of the cervix is used to identify the uterus.

Several other important observations may be made during the rectal examination. Firstly, the rectum may be loaded with faeces. This is consistent with the presence of one or more abdominal masses caused by constipation. Secondly, there may be evidence of peritoneal spread of a malignant tumour of the stomach, colon or ovary. The sign to seek is the presence of a hard, irregular and relatively fixed tumour mass anterior to the rectum at the tip of the examining finger on rectal examination (Blumer's shelf), but this is rare. Finally, one might note blood on the glove from a previously unsuspected colon cancer or the hard irregular mass of a rectal tumour (Chapter 20).

Having defined the features of the mass, the clinician should review the clinical history with a focus on symptoms that might be associated with possible clinical diagnoses. On specific questioning, symptoms that were previously overlooked by the patient might be recalled (see Table 17.6).

TABLE 17.5: Tender abdominal masses[1]

Position of mass	Features on examination	Diagnosis
Right hypochondrium	Localised, moves with respiration, can't get above it	Acute cholecystitis, empyema of the gall bladder Haemorrhage or infarction in a liver tumour (or cyst)
Right hypochondrium	Enlarged liver	Cholangitis Portal pyaemia Hepatic metastases Acute severe right heart failure
Epigastric	Immobile	Pancreatic pseudocyst, Pancreatic phlegmon Dissection in abdominal aortic aneurysm
Left hypochondrium	Enlarged spleen	Splenic infarct
Right loin	Enlarged kidney	Pyonephrosis Renal cell carcinoma
Periumbilical	Pulsatile	Dissection in abdominal aortic aneurysm
Right iliac fossa	Immobile	Appendix phlegmon/abscess Crohn's disease
Hypogastrium	Enlarged bladder Enlarged uterus Enlarged ovary	Acute urinary retention Haemorrhage or infarction in a fibroid Haemorrhage or infarction in an ovarian tumour/cyst Acute pyosalpinx
Left iliac fossa	Immobile, sometimes palpable bimanually	Acute diverticular phlegmon Diverticular abscess

1. Usually symptomatic

TABLE 17.6: Examples of vague symptoms that may only be revealed after the mass is uncovered

Non-specific symptoms
- Mild abdominal discomfort
- Lethargy, easy fatigueability
- Weight loss, anorexia
- Nausea, vomiting
- Bloating

Symptoms indicating an extra-abdominal consequence of the disease process
- Worsening angina due to cardiac decompensation caused by occult blood loss and iron deficiency anaemia
- Dyspnoea from a pleural effusion due to pulmonary spread of an abdominal malignancy
- Superficial thrombophlebitis due to paraneoplastic phenomena

Symptoms suggesting the disease process or organ
- Upper gut—heartburn, dyspepsia, dysphagia, early satiety
- Lower gut—altered bowel habit, blood, mucus or pus in stools, colicky abdominal pain
- Pancreas/biliary tree—pruritus, jaundice, steatorrhoea

Other signs on general physical examination

The physical examination is completed mindful of the working diagnosis, based on the finding of an abdominal mass. Specific examples of relevant positive findings are listed in Table 17.7.

TABLE 17.7: Examples of extra-abdominal signs that may be associated with an asymptomatic abdominal mass

Sign	Associated abdominal mass
Pallor	Gastrointestinal malignancy with occult bleeding
Wasting	Advanced malignancy
Signs of chronic liver disease (palmar erythema, spider naevi, gynaecomastia, testicular atrophy)	Splenomegaly associated with portal hypertension, hepatocellular carcinoma associated with cirrhosis
Hard, fixed irregular breast lump Hard supraclavicular lymph node Signs of pleural effusion	Hepatomegaly due to metastatic breast cancer Epigastric mass due to stomach cancer Mass of malignant origin or benign ovarian tumour (Meigs' syndrome)

OFFICE TESTS

Although the finding of occult blood on testing of the faeces provides supportive evidence that an abdominal mass might be due to a gastrointestinal malignancy, the result is neither sensitive nor specific (Chapter 9), and so it is of limited clinical usefulness in clarifying the cause of the mass. More definitive examinations are required. Similarly, the finding of blood or protein in the urine may focus attention on the urinary tract.

IMAGING

Plain radiology

A plain abdominal X-ray examination is of limited value in the assessment of abdominal masses. Consequently, this step is often omitted in favour of the more powerful imaging tools, ultrasound and CT scanning. Useful diagnostic information that might be gleaned from a plain abdominal X-ray film includes:

- Calcification in the wall of an arterial aneurysm;
- Plate-like or curvilinear calcification in the wall of a liver hydatid cyst (Figure 17.3A; Chapter 23);
- Calcification due to chronic pancreatitis associated with a pancreatic pseudocyst (Figure 17.3B); and
- Calcification in an ovarian mass.

  A plain chest X-ray examination must be performed. It may reveal:

- Rounded shadows due to pulmonary metastases; or
- A pleural effusion due to pulmonary metastases.

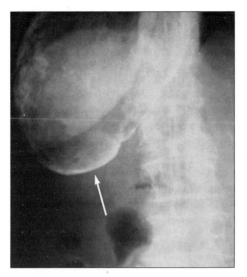

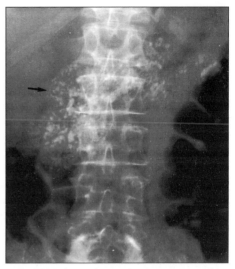

FIGURE 17.3A: Plain X-ray film showing calcium in the wall of a hydatid cyst.

FIGURE 17.3B: Plain X-ray film showing calcium in chronic pancreatitis.
(From Talley NJ and O'Connor S, Clinical Examination, *5th edn, Elsevier Australia.)*

Ultrasound and computerised tomography

These modalities should allow definition of which abdominal organ is enlarged; not uncommonly, the pathology responsible for the palpable mass will also be apparent. Each technique has particular advantages. Ultrasound discriminates well between cystic and solid lesions. CT scanning is better in obese people as adjacent structures can be separated visually by intervening lucent fat planes. Ultrasound images are often suboptimal in obese patients. Further, if the space between the anterior abdominal wall and the palpable mass contains gas-filled loops of bowel, these will cast posterior shadows and distortions on the ultrasound but not the CT image, making CT scanning the preferred technique in this situation (Chapter 21).

In practical terms, if the abdominal organ which holds the palpable mass cannot be determined on the basis of the performance of the first examination, whether ultrasound or CT, then the other examination is usually performed.

Finding of an enlarged organ on imaging

The next investigations depend on the results from ultrasound/CT scan(s).

Liver

Is the enlargement uniform or irregular? The possible causes of a diffuse and uniform enlargement are listed in Table 17.8. If the enlargement is irregular or patchy, then the clinician should determine whether the lump(s) is solid or cystic on ultrasound. The evaluation of lumps in the liver is discussed in detail in Chapter 23.

If the lesion(s) that has caused hepatomegaly is cystic, it is likely to be a simple cyst or a hydatid cyst.

If the lesion that has caused hepatomegaly is single and solid, it is likely to be a solitary secondary deposit or a hepatoma. The other single solid lesions discussed in Chapter 23 tend to be less massive and so do not cause hepatomegaly.

If the lesions that have caused hepatomegaly are multiple and solid, metastatic liver disease is the likely explanation. The next step is to establish the primary source. The common sources are colon, pancreas, stomach, breast and lung. A histological confirmation of the diagnosis should usually be sought. A biopsy of the primary tumour is preferred as the histology from the liver is often non-discriminatory. Further, the biopsy of primary tumour, whether by gastroscopy, colonoscopy, bronchoscopy or biopsy of a breast lump, is safer than liver biopsy. If the primary tumour cannot be found, then ultrasound- or CT-guided biopsy may be indicated.

Gall bladder

Gall bladder enlargement due to obstruction of the common bile duct (e.g., carcinoma of the head of the pancreas or ampulla of Vater) will usually be associated with jaundice (Chapter 21). A gall bladder may be palpably enlarged with a mucocele of the gall bladder, which may be relatively painless and non-tender. Enlargement due to carcinoma of the gall bladder is unusual.

TABLE 17.8: Causes of hepatomegaly

Diffusely enlarged and smooth

Massive
- Metastatic disease
- Alcoholic liver disease with fatty infiltration
- Myeloproliferative diseases (e.g., polycythaemia rubra vera, myelofibrosis)

Moderate
- The above causes
- Haemochromatosis
- Haematological disease (e.g., chronic myeloid leukaemia, lymphoma)
- Fatty liver (e.g., diabetes mellitus, obseity)
- Infiltrative disorders (e.g., amyloid)

Mild
- The above causes
- Hepatitis (viral, drugs)
- Cirrhosis
- Biliary obstruction
- Granulomatous disorders (e.g., sarcoid)
- HIV infection

Diffusely enlarged and irregular
- Metastatic disease
- Cirrhosis
- Hydatid disease
- Polycystic liver disease

Localised swellings
- Riedel's lobe (a normal variant—the lobe may be palpable in the right lumbar region)
- Metastasis
- Large simple hepatic cyst
- Hydatid cyst
- Hepatoma
- Liver abscess (e.g., amoebic abscess)

(Based on Talley NJ and O'Connor S, Clinical Examination, 5th edn, Elsevier Australia.)

Stomach

If the mass is thought to be gastric on CT, then gastric carcinoma or lymphoma is the likely diagnosis. Gastroscopy and biopsy should confirm the diagnosis. Visualisation of the stomach by ultrasound is poor. Further management of this asymptomatic tumour of the stomach will depend on the stage of the disease (Chapter 15).

Pancreas

On the basis of the ultrasound or CT, the clinician should know whether the lesion is cystic or solid. If it is cystic, then it is likely to be either a pseudocyst of the pancreas or a cystadenoma (rarely cystadenocarcinoma). For the diagnosis of pseudocyst, there should have been a definite prior episode of pancreatitis. The management of pancreatic pseudocyst is discussed in Chapter 4. The treatment of cystadenoma is surgical resection (Chapter 23).

If the lesion is solid, then pancreatic cancer is likely. On ultrasound, a pancreatic cancer has a characteristic hypo-echoic appearance. The CT scan should be examined for evidence of spread to the liver, to peripancreatic and portal lymph nodes, encasement of the portal vein and dilatation of the pancreatic duct. Most malignant tumours that have grown to the point where they are palpable on physical examination will be surgically incurable. Many of these tumours will also have resulted in obstructive jaundice (see Chapter 21). Tumours of the pancreatic head cause jaundice by obstructing the common bile duct in the pancreas. Primary tumours of the body and tail of the pancreas cause jaundice by obstruction of the bile ducts at the porta hepatis by metastatic portal lymph nodes. The management of pancreatic cancer is considered in Chapter 15.

Lymph nodes

Enlarged para-aortic lymph nodes producing an epigastric mass are likely to have arisen from a primary tumour elsewhere. The common sites of origin are stomach, colon, pancreas and testis. The origin of the lymphadenopathy should be established by investigation of the likely primary site (see above). If no primary site is found, then a guided percutaneous biopsy is reasonable. The biopsy may be non-diagnostic if the lymphadenopathy is due to malignant lymphoma (Chapter 23).

Spleen

The causes of splenomegaly are listed in Table 17.9. The most important gastroenterological cause of splenomegaly is portal hypertension. This is considered in detail in Chapter 22.

Kidneys

The common causes of an enlarged kidney are shown in Table 17.10.

Colon

Asymptomatic masses are likely to be secondary to constipation or tumours, mostly malignant. Smaller benign tumours may be apparent if they have caused intussusception; they also usually cause abdominal pain.

Faecal masses should disappear with purgation. Masses in the colon, as in the stomach, are poorly imaged by ultrasound. By the time they are palpable, the organ of origin can usually be determined by CT scan. However, the diagnosis is best determined by either barium enema or colonoscopy. Colonoscopy has an advantage over barium enema in that the diagnosis can be confirmed on biopsy. A malignant tumour is staged as described in Chapter 20.

Small bowel

A palpable small bowel mass will be apparent on CT. The causes of asymptomatic small bowel masses are shown in Table 17.11. Unlike the stomach and the colon, endoscopy of the small bowel is difficult. If further imaging of a small bowel mass is required then it is achieved by small bowel series or enema (see Figure 17.4) or capsule endoscopy. Biopsy, often involving small bowel resection, is the next step if there is no evidence of disease other than in the small bowel.

TABLE 17.9: Causes of splenomegaly and hepatosplenomegaly

Massive splenomegaly
- Haematological disease (e.g., chronic myeloid leukaemia, myelofibrosis)

Moderate splenomegaly
- The above causes
- Portal hypertension
- Haematological disease (e.g., lymphoma, leukaemia, thalassaemia)
- Storage disease (e.g., Gaucher's disease)

Small splenomegaly
- The above causes
- Infective (hepatitis, leptospirosis, malaria, bacterial endocarditis)
- Haematological disease (e.g., haemolytic anaemias, essential thrombocythaemia, polycythaemia rubra vera)
- Connective tissue diseases or vasculitis (e.g., rheumatoid arthritis, systemic lupus erythematosus, polyarteritis nodosa)
- Solitary cyst, polycystic syndrome, hydatid cyst
- Infiltration (amyloid, sarcoid)

Hepatosplenomegaly
- Chronic liver disease with portal hypertension
- Haematological disease (e.g., myeloproliferative disease, lymphoma)
- Infection (e.g., acute viral hepatitis, infectious mononucleosis)
- Infiltration (e.g., amyloid, sarcoid)
- Connective tissue disease (e.g., systemic lupus erythematosus)

(Based on Talley NJ and O'Connor S, Clinical Examination, 5th edn, Elsevier Australia.)

TABLE 17.10: Causes of unilateral kidney enlargement

- Hydronephrosis (may be bilateral)
- Polycystic kidney (may be bilateral)
- Simple cyst of kidney
- Renal cell carcinoma
- Pyonephrosis (may be bilateral)
- Acute renal vein thrombosis

(Based on Talley NJ and O'Connor S, Clinical Examination, 5th edn, Elsevier Australia.)

Omentum

The omentum only becomes palpable when it is infiltrated by tumour, usually by transperitoneal spread. The common sites of origin are colon, ovary, stomach and pancreas. Omental secondaries are usually associated with some degree of ascites. Tapping the ascites, with ultrasound guidance if the amount is subclinical, provides a specimen for cytological analysis (Chapter 18). Further treatment, except in the case of an ovarian tumour, will be palliative, as the demonstration of omental secondaries establishes that the disease is advanced. Gynaecological opinion should be sought if an ovarian source seems likely.

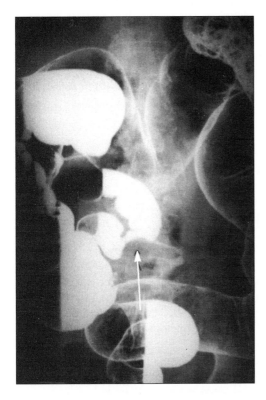

FIGURE 17.4: Small bowel tumour in the terminal ileum (due to a carcinoid).

TABLE 17.11: Causes of small bowel masses		
Cause	**Pathology**	**Comment**
Cyst	Mesenteric cyst	(fluid collection in the mesentery derived from remnants of reduplicated bowel)
Tumour	Benign Malignant	Lipoma Hamartoma (e.g., Peutz-Jegher syndrome) Adenocarcinoma Carcinoid tumour Lymphoma
Intussusception		(may have a polyp or tumour at its leading edge)
Inflammation	Crohn's disease	

Aorta

After an aneurysm has been detected, it is important to measure its width (side to side), because the risk of sudden rupture of the aneurysm is related to its width. While a reasonable estimate of the width can be made on clinical examination, ultrasound (or CT) is more accurate. It is also important to define whether the proximal extent of the aneurysm can be palpated; if the proximal end cannot be defined, then the aneurysm may involve the renal arteries, making subsequent repair more difficult. Again, the clinical impression can be substantiated on ultrasound. The management decision should be made by a vascular surgeon, but operative graft replacement or endoluminal grafting is usually indicated if the aneurysm is greater than 5–6 cm in diameter or if the patient has local tenderness over the aneurysm, suggesting than there is localised dissection in the wall.

Bladder

An enlarged bladder is nearly always an obstructed bladder and should be drained initially by urinary catheterisation.

Ovaries

Treatment of ovarian enlargement remains in the province of the gynaecologist. Specialist opinion should be sought when an enlarged ovary is discovered incidentally.

OTHER INVESTIGATIONS

Blood tests

The finding of an asymptomatic abdominal mass usually heralds the uncovering of a major clinical problem. A faecally-loaded colon is an obvious exception. Simple haematological and biochemical screening with a full blood count and urea, electrolytes and liver function tests often provides useful information about systemic consequences of the mass. Consequently, these screens are usually performed at the same time as the ultrasound or CT scans.

Further blood tests may be useful once the organ of origin and the likely pathological process are defined from the ultrasound or CT scan, as shown in Table 17.12.

Nuclear medicine

The use of radionuclide scanning in the anatomical assessment of abdominal masses and deduction of the likely pathological processes has declined with the advent of cross-sectional imaging, which can also be used to take targeted biopsies. In gastroenterological practice, radionuclide scans are only used when cross-sectional imaging has not allowed identification of the underlying pathological process and laparotomy may not be required for definitive therapy. They still have a place in the assessment of incidentalomas of the liver (see Chapter 23). A gallium scan can also be useful in the characterisation of an abdominal mass of inflammatory or lymphatic origin. A labelled white cell scan is occasionally useful in the assessment of inflammatory bowel disease and intraperitoneal collections of pus. In neither of these cases is the mass likely to be asymptomatic.

Tissue diagnosis

Whenever a mass is thought to be neoplastic, a definitive tissue diagnosis should be sought. This information is useful in assisting patients understand their prognosis and in selecting treatments, such as surgery, radiotherapy or chemotherapy.

As indicated above, the biopsy should be taken from the primary tumour if possible. This is pertinent for tumours of the stomach, colon, lung, breast and pancreas. For stomach, colon and lung, the biopsy is taken using an endoscopic technique. For breast and pancreas, it is by direct puncture, guided radiologically if the primary is impalpable.

Most liver masses can now be safely accessed by the percutaneous route. Bleeding and tumour rupture and dissemination can occur as a result of the procedure. Tumour cells can be seeded along the needle track. Hepatocellular carcinomas extending to the liver surface are at particular risk for these consequences of needle biopsy. Thus, specialist opinion should be sought before the radiologist is asked to perform a liver biopsy.

Tumour biopsy by laparoscopic or open operation may still occasionally be required to finalise a diagnosis if fine needle biopsy is unsafe (e.g., some hepatocellular carcinomas), or unlikely to yield diagnostic material (e.g., liposarcoma of the retroperitoneum).

TABLE 17.12: Further evaluation of abdominal masses by blood tests

Clinical diagnosis	Further blood test and rationale
Possible gastrointestinal malignancy	Carcinoembryonic antigen (CEA) (Chapter 15)
Possible hepatoma	Alpha-fetoprotein (AFP) (Chapter 15) Hepatitis B and C serology—seeking a cause of hepatoma
Significant liver replacement	Coagulation studies—prior to any intervention (e.g., biopsy) which might be complicated by excessive bleeding
Possible hydatid disease of the liver	Hydatid serology—to confirm the diagnosis, and to ensure that biopsy is not attempted as it might spread the disease (Chapter 23)
Pancreatic mass	CA-19-9 (Chapter 15) Endocrine screen depending on symptoms (insulin, gastrin, vasoactive intestinal peptide, glucagon)—endocrine tumours have a better prognosis than adenocarcinoma of the pancreas and management is different (Chapter 23)

Further reading

Grover SA, Barkuyn AN, Sackett DL. The rational clinical examination. Does this patient have splenomegaly? *J Am Med Assoc* 1993; 270: 2218–21.

McGee S. *Evidence-based physical diagnosis.* Philadelphia: Saunders, 2001.

Naylor CD. The rational clinical examination. Physical examination of the liver. *J Am Med Assoc* 1994; 271: 1859–65.

Talley NJ, O'Connor S. *Clinical Examination. A Systematic Guide to Physical Diagnosis,* 5th edn. Sydney: MacLennan & Petty, 2005.

chapter 18

ABDOMINAL DISTENSION

PRELIMINARY EXAMINATION OF THE ABDOMEN

The traditionally taught five causes of generalised abdominal distension, the 'five Fs', are: flatus, fluid, faeces, fetus and fat. To this list should be added a sixth, massive organomegaly or 'filthy big tumour'.

For the patient presenting with generalised abdominal distension, a preliminary abdominal examination is worthwhile before taking a detailed history to determine which of the 'six Fs' is the most likely cause. The reason for this departure from the usual sequence of history followed by examination is that history taking can be greatly simplified if the clinician has some prior idea of the underlying problem.

1. Flatus

The cause is gaseous distension of the bowel often secondary to a bowel obstruction or paralytic ileus. There is generalised hyper-resonance to percussion. Any fluid contained within the distended bowel associated with a bowel obstruction or ileus is clinically undetectable. It lies posteriorly with the patient lying supine and is not percussable. It is contained within bowel loops and cannot shift. Auscultation of the abdomen reveals hyperactive bowel sounds with mechanical obstruction and absent or just a few tinkly bowel sounds with paralytic ileus.

2. Fluid or ascites

Intraperitoneal fluid collection is associated with dullness to percussion in the flanks with the patient lying supine. The dullness is described as shifting dullness because the upper limit of the dullness moves in relation to the abdominal wall as the patient is rolled onto the side. Massive ascites is also associated with a fluid thrill felt in one flank after tapping in the other. The distension is less globally distributed with ascites than with gaseous distension of the abdomen, with the effect that the flanks tend to sag.

3. Faeces

Stool can accumulate in the colon to produce abdominal distension. This can cause gaseous distension of more proximal bowel. The degree of distension tends to be less than can occur with ascites or bowel obstruction. The faeces can be recognised as firm to hard lumps that are indentable when prodded with the tip of the examining finger (Chapter 17). The segments of colon overlying the brim of the pelvis on the left and right sides may be more prominent to the examining hand.

4. Fetus

Pregnancy and the associated enlarged uterus produce a globular firm mass, which arises out of the pelvis so that the examining hand cannot palpate an inferior border. In early pregnancy, the swelling is confined to the lower abdomen. The mass may reach as high as the epigastrium in late pregnancy. Further, bony fetal parts, such as the head and back, may be identifiable to palpation and fetal heart sounds may be heard on auscultation.

5. Fat

Within the abdomen, fat commonly produces abdominal distension. It is known colloquially as 'pot belly' or 'beer gut'. It does not have characteristic features on clinical examination except that other parts of the body are usually also obviously fat. Obesity is so prevalent that a previously obese patient may present with further distension due to one of the other 'five Fs'. Evaluation by physical examination is always more difficult under these circumstances.

6. Massive organomegaly

Features of massive organomegaly are covered in Chapter 17.

HISTORY AND FURTHER EXAMINATION

A classification of the causes of abdominal distension is presented in Table 18.1 and relevant symptoms are listed in Table 18.2. The duration of abdominal distension and its association with abdominal pain are key questions. Thus, one should not usually expect abdominal pain to be a feature, except with abdominal distension due to gas in bowel obstruction; with the other causes, there may be milder discomfort due to stretching of the parietal peritoneum or the capsule of an organ. Localised pain can occur with organ swelling. Similarly, the speed of development for most causes is slow, except with abdominal distension from gas, in which case it can be fast. Tense swelling of the abdomen due to fluid or a large tumour can cause increased intra-abdominal pressure leading to heartburn, nausea or vomiting, or dyspnoea (from elevation of the diaphragm). The specific clinical features for each cause are described below.

CLINICAL FEATURES

Gaseous distension of the bowel (flatus)

Mechanical obstruction of the bowel (small or large)

The distension is usually acute in onset and develops over hours to days. The obstruction may be open or closed. Examples of open obstructions are a band adhesion occluding the lumen of the small bowel and a cicatrising carcinoma of the sigmoid colon. With these, the distension is generalised. Examples of closed obstructions are sigmoid and caecal volvulus. The time frame of development is similar. The abdominal distension with a sigmoid volvulus is directed from the pelvis towards the right hypochondrium, because the sigmoid mesocolon is attached to the left false pelvis. The abdominal distension with a caecal volvulus is directed from the pelvis towards the left hypochondrium, because of the attachment of the caecum to the right false pelvis.

The distension is associated with other features of bowel obstruction, namely colicky abdominal pain, vomiting and constipation. The diagnosis and management of bowel obstruction is discussed in Chapter 4.

TABLE 18.1: Classification of causes of abdominal distension: the 'six Fs'		
Cause	**Example**	**Distension**
1. Flatus (gaseous distension)		
• *Bowel obstructed:*		
Open		Generalised
Closed	Sigmoid volvulus	Localised
	Caecal volvulus	Localised
• *Bowel not obstructed:*		
	Paralytic ileus	Generalised
	Pseudo-obstruction	Generalised
	Irritable bowel syndrome	Generalised
	Acute gastric dilatation	Localised
	Gas bloat	Generalised
2. Fluid (ascites)	(see Table 18.3 for detail)	Generalised
3. Faeces		Localised
4. Fat		Generalised
5. Fetus		Localised
6. Filthy big tumour (organomegaly)		
• Liver	(see Chapter 17)	Localised
• Spleen	(see Chapter 17)	Localised
• Ovary	Ovarian cyst	Localised
• Uterus	Fibroids	Localised
• Kidney	Polycystic kidney	Localised
• Hydronephrosis		Localised
• Bladder	Obstructed bladder	Localised
• Mesentery	Tumour	Localised
• Retroperitoneum	Tumour	Localised or generalised

Paralytic ileus

This is usually preceded by an abdominal operation. Operations involving retroperitoneal structures (e.g., repair of an aortic aneurysm), operations during which there is considerable handling of the bowel and prolonged operations are more prone to paralytic ileus. Irritation of the retroperitoneum as occurs with severe pancreatitis or a spontaneous retroperitoneal haemorrhage can precipitate an ileus. An intra-abdominal inflammatory process such as acute diverticulitis and biochemical disturbances such as hypokalaemia, hypomagnesaemia and uraemia can also precipitate an ileus. In contradistinction to a mechanical bowel obstruction, there is no colicky pain with paralytic ileus, just the discomfort associated with distending the parietal peritoneum. The condition settles spontaneously with correction or resolution of precipitating factors. Gastric decompression and fluid replacement (and sometimes intravenous hyperalimentation) are required while resolution occurs.

TABLE 18.2: Possible symptoms with abdominal distension	
Symptom	**Relevance/significance**

• Abdominal pain:
  - Abdominal tightness/ vague generalised ache
  - Colicky (periumbilical or lower abdominal)
	Non-specific
	
	Bowel obstruction

• Nausea/vomiting	Bowel obstruction
• Anorexia	Non-specific, malignancy, cirrhosis
• Loss of weight	Non-specific, malignancy, cirrhosis
• Bowel habit (recent and usual)	Bowel obstruction, constipation
• Respiratory symptoms	Secondary to elevation of the diaphragm
• Previous history of malignant disease	As a possible cause of ascites
• Alcohol or drug abuse	As a cause of liver disease and ascites
• Jaundice	Associated with liver disease
• Easy bruising/spontaneous bleeding	Associated with liver disease
• Missed menstrual cycle(s)	Pregnancy

Pseudo-obstruction

The time course of pseudo-obstruction is more protracted than with mechanical obstruction; the degree of distension may fluctuate considerably. Pseudo-obstruction is discussed in Chapter 6.

Irritable bowel syndrome

This may be associated with chronic fluctuating abdominal distension of moderate degree. This condition is considered in detail in Chapter 6.

Acute gastric dilatation

This is most commonly seen soon after major trauma (not necessarily abdominal trauma). Diabetes mellitus is another cause. The major manifestation is copious vomiting of coffee grounds, a mixture of gastric secretions and old blood. The condition is managed by decompression with a nasogastric tube and fluid replacement.

Gas bloat

This particular chronic problem can occur as a complication of anti-reflux surgery for gastro-oesophageal reflux. It results from air swallowing in a patient who has a diminished ability to belch because of their surgery. The degree of distension of stomach and bowel can vary considerably. It is generally worse postprandially. There is usually some degree of discomfort. This may vary from a vague feeling of fullness to a more localised epigastric discomfort to central abdominal colicky pain. It may be relieved to a degree by passage of flatus.

Ascites (fluid)

This usually develops gradually and continuously, with the onset over weeks to months, and is relatively painless. When the ascites is gross, there may be a vague discomfort caused by stretching of the abdominal wall and the parietal peritoneum. When ascites is painful, infected ascites, hepatoma or pancreatitis should be considered. There may be respiratory symptoms due to respiratory embarrassment with gross ascites or development of a pleural effusion (usually on the right due to a leak of fluid through the diaphragmatic lymphatics).

The main causes of ascites and their prevalence are listed in Table 18.3.

Cirrhosis. Eighty percent of patients with ascites have cirrhosis. The causes of cirrhosis are discussed in Chapter 22. Risk factors to enquire about include alcohol abuse, intravenous drug use, tattoos, blood transfusion and living in developing countries where the prevalence of hepatitis B is high. These patients may have splenomegaly due to portal hypertension as well as other stigmata of chronic liver disease including spider naevi, palmar erythema, testicular atrophy and gynaecomastia.

TABLE 18.3: Causes of ascites	
Cause	**Prevalence**
Cirrhosis	80%
Malignancy	10%
Heart failure	5%
Tuberculosis	1%
Other: hypoproteinaemia caused by starvation (kwashiorkor and malignancy) or excessive loss (protein-losing enteropathy, nephrotic syndrome); pancreatic ascites; chylous ascites	4%

Malignancy. Ten percent of patients have ascites secondary to malignancy. Most of these patients have a past history of malignancy. In some, abdominal distension is the presenting feature. There may be lymphadenopathy or other evidence of tumour spread.

Cardiac ascites. Cardiac ascites is secondary to severe right-sided heart failure, most commonly due to constrictive pericarditis. Other signs include an elevated jugular venous pressure, pulsatile tender hepatomegaly and peripheral oedema.

Hypoproteinaemia. Ascites due to hypoproteinaemia (e.g., from starvation, or excessive loss from protein-losing enteropathy or nephrotic syndrome) is minor in degree and associated with peripheral oedema.

Pancreatic ascites. This is only seen after severe acute pancreatitis or a blunt transacting injury to the pancreas.

Chylous ascites. Chylous ascites results from surgical trauma to cisterna chyli or rarely due to obstruction by lymphatic spread of tumour.

Faecal impaction of the colon (faeces)

This is a chronic problem caused by chronic constipation, and is most commonly seen in elderly persons. The various causes of constipation are considered in detail in Chapter 10. Abdominal distension is an uncommon feature of the most severe end of the spectrum. A history of infrequent, usually hard bowel actions is expected. A history of laxative abuse is also very common. Lower abdominal colicky pain may be associated. When such pain occurs it should be relieved by the passage of flatus or a large evacuation of the bowel.

Pregnancy (fetus)

This is associated with a menstrual-free period in women.

Abdominal distension due to obesity (fat)

This is painless and long-standing. The deposition of fat is in the mesentery of the bowel and the omentum to a greater degree, and in the anterior abdominal wall to a lesser degree.

Organomegaly

The presenting history of patients with organomegaly resulting in abdominal distension is covered in Chapter 17.

INVESTIGATIONS

The appropriate investigations to evaluate abdominal distension are detailed below.

Plain radiology of the abdomen

This will demonstrate bowel obstruction and paralytic ileus (Figures 18.1 and 18.2) as well as faecal loading. The fluid of ascites may give a 'ground glass' appearance, a non-specific vague increased whiteness to the abdominal cavity.

Ultrasound or CT of the abdomen

This will confirm the presence of ascites (Figure 18.3) and define organomegaly.

Blood tests

Liver function tests may indicate underlying chronic liver disease (Chapter 22). A pregnancy test will confirm the presence of pregnancy.

There is no specific relevant test for obesity. Measure the weight and height to calculate the body mass index (BMI = weight [kg] divided by height squared [m^2]). BMI $\geq$ 30 indicates frank obesity (Chapter 15). The diagnosis can usually be made on clinical grounds.

Of the various causes of abdominal distension, only ascites will be discussed in further detail in this chapter. Bowel obstruction is discussed in Chapter 4. Constipation is discussed in Chapter 10. Obesity and pregnancy are beyond the scope of this text.

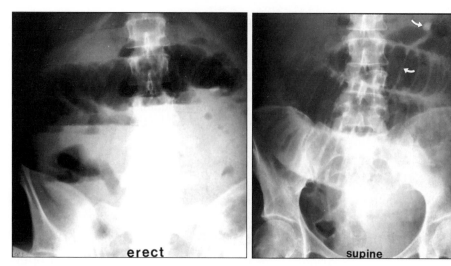

FIGURE 18.1: Plain abdominal X-ray film showing small bowel obstruction. There is dilatation of the small bowel. It is recognised as small bowel from its central position and its transverse mucosal bands—the valvulae conniventes (black arrow). Air-fluid levels are seen on the erect view. The supine view gives a better view of the distribution of the dilated loops. From the number and position of the displayed dilated loops, the obstruction would be at the level of the mid-small bowel. The round radio-opaque shadow in the left hypochondrium is a tablet (open arrow).

(From Talley NJ and O'Connor S, Clinical Examination, *5th edn, Elsevier Australia.)*

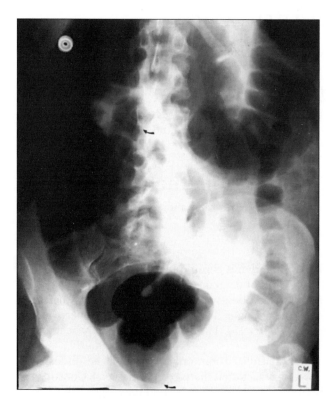

FIGURE 18.2: Plain abdominal X-ray film showing generalised ileus. The large bowel is filled with gas and is dilated except in the descending colon. Dilated small bowel is also seen in the right hypochondrium (arrow). As gas is seen around to the rectum (arrow), mechanical obstruction is excluded.

(From Talley NJ and O'Connor S, Clinical Examination, *5th edn, Elsevier Australia.)*

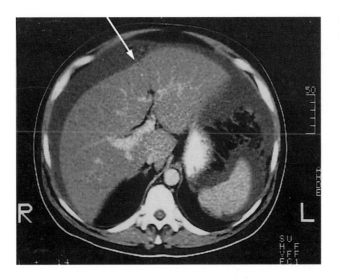

FIGURE 18.3: Abdominal CT showing ascites.

DIAGNOSIS OF ASCITES

There are two clinical steps to determining the cause of ascites. First, the clinical history and examination needs to be focused on elucidating which pathological process underlies the accumulation of ascites. Second, a sample of the ascites needs to be examined. The sample is aspirated and its appearance noted before it is sent to the laboratory for biochemical, cytological and microbiological analysis. Blood needs to be sent at the same time for estimation of the serum albumin level.

The features of ascitic fluid are summarised in Table 18.4.

TABLE 18.4: Characteristics of paracentesis fluid						
Aetiology	Colour	SAAG (g/L)	RBC (10^6/L)	WBC (10^6/L)	Cytology	Other
Cirrhosis	Straw	≥ 11	Few	< 250	–	–
Infected ascites	Straw	≥ 11	Few	≥ 250 polymorphs or ≥ 500 cells	–	+ve culture
Neoplastic	Straw/ haemorrhagic/ mucinous	< 11	Variable	Variable	Malignant cells	–
Tuberculosis	Clear/ turbid/ haemorrhagic	< 11	Many	> 1000 70% lympho-cytes	–	Acid-fast bacilli + culture
Cardiac failure	Straw	≥ 11	0	< 250	–	–
Pancreatic	Turbid/ haemorrhagic	< 11	Variable	Variable	–	Amylase increased
Lymphatic obstruction or disruption	White	< 11	0	0	–	Fat globules on staining
RBC = red blood cell count; SAAG = serum-ascites albumin gradient; WBC = white blood cell count.						

Appearance

Blood staining suggests malignancy or a traumatic ascitic tap, either current or past; turbidity or white fluid suggests infected or chylous ascites.

Serum-ascites albumin gradient

Calculate this by subtracting the ascitic fluid albumin from the serum albumin value; the serum-ascites albumin gradient (SAAG) correlates with portal pressure. If the SAAG is ≥ 11 g/L, then portal hypertension is the likely diagnosis (97% accurate). Peritoneal carcinomatosis, tuberculosis and pancreatic ascites have a gradient < 11 g/L (Table 18.5).

TABLE 18.5: Classification of ascites by serum-ascites albumin gradient (SAAG)	
SAAG: high (≥ 11 g/L)	**SAAG: low (< 11 g/L)**
Cirrhosis	Peritoneal carcinomatosis
Alcoholic hepatitis	Tuberculous peritonitis
Cardiac ascites	Pancreatic ascites
Massive liver metastases	Bile leak
Fulminant hepatic failure	
Cirrhosis plus another cause	

Other biochemistry

If pancreatic ascites is suspected, assess the ascitic amylase level, which is very high in pancreatic ascites. A low pH (< 7.35) suggests spontaneous bacterial peritonitis or systemic acidosis. The lactate level is elevated in spontaneous bacterial peritonitis. If chylous ascites is suspected, the diagnosis can be confirmed by staining the specimen for fat.

Cells

Examination of the ascites for polymorphonuclear cells is important to diagnose spontaneous bacterial peritonitis. A cell count ≥ 250×10^6 polymorphs/L (250 polymorphs/mm^3) or ≥ 500×10^6 white cells/L (500 cells/mm^3) is strongly suggestive of the diagnosis. The cause is usually a Gram-negative organism sensitive to treatment with a third-generation cephalosporin (e.g., cefotaxime).

Cytology

If the SAAG is less than 11 g/L or malignancy is otherwise suspected, a cytological examination looking for malignant cells should be performed after the sample has been centrifuged. Establishment of the primary site is usually not possible using this specimen.

Culture

As spontaneous bacterial peritonitis is insidious in onset and may have few associated symptoms and signs, a sample of ascites is always cultured. It is advisable to insert the specimen into blood culture bottles after collection to maximise the chance of a positive result. At the same time, the ascites should be cultured for acid-fast bacilli to diagnose the occasional case of tuberculous peritonitis.

MANAGEMENT OF ASCITES

This depends on the underlying diagnosis.

Liver disease

The management of ascites in liver disease is covered in Chapter 22.

Malignant ascites

It is important to try to establish the site of the primary tumour because systemic hormonal or chemotherapy can result in regression of the intraperitoneal tumour and the ascites, especially if the primary site is breast or ovary. Clinical re-examination of breasts and abdomen may be helpful. The investigations used to establish the common sites of the primary tumour, namely colon, stomach, pancreas, ovary and breast, are shown in Table 18.6.

In the event that the primary site is colon, stomach or pancreas, local therapy may be required to palliate the discomfort of distension. The therapeutic options are limited and none is really satisfactory. They include: a) repeated major paracentesis, which is time consuming and results in the development of hypoalbuminaemia and malnutrition; and b) peritoneovenous shunting, which can block and can be complicated by coagulopathy. However, not infrequently the best option is analgesia and general support.

TABLE 18.6: Investigations for primary tumour in patients with malignant ascites	
Site of primary	**Relevant investigations**
Colon	Colonoscopy and biopsy
Stomach	Gastroscopy and biopsy
Pancreas	Ultrasound ± CT scan ± fine needle aspiration EUS ± needle biopsy CA-19-9
Ovary	Pelvic ultrasound ± CT scan CEA, CA125
Breast	Mammography or fine needle aspiration cytology if palpable lump Breast biopsy and oestrogen receptors
CEA = carcinoembryonic antigen; CT = computerised tomography; EUS = endoscopic ultrasound.	

Cardiac ascites

The management is directed at treating the cardiac cause. This may involve pericardectomy if constrictive pericarditis is the underlying problem.

Pancreatic ascites

Pancreatic ascites usually settles with conservative management. This includes 'pancreatic rest' with total parenteral nutrition and suppression with the somatostatin analogue, octreotide. If the ascites fails to resolve over a number of weeks, endoscopic retrograde cholangiopancreatography should be performed to define the location of the disruption of the main pancreatic duct prior to a trial of pancreatic duct stenting or distal pancreatic resection.

Further reading

Runyon BA, Montano AA, Akriviadis EA *et al*. The serum-ascites albumin gradient is superior to the exudate/transudate concept in the differential diagnosis of ascites. *Ann Intern Med* 1992; 117: 215–20.

Runyon BA. Malignancy-related ascites and ascitic fluid "humoral tests of malignancy". *J Clin Gastroenterol* 1994; 18: 94–8.

Saadeh S, Davis GL. Management of ascites in patients with end-stage liver disease. *Rev Gastroenterol Disord* 2004; 4: 175–85.

Smith EM, Jayson GC. The current and future management of malignant ascites. *Clin Oncol* 2003; 15: 59–72.

Williams JW Jr, Simel DL. The rational clinical examination. Does this patient have ascites? How to divine fluid in the abdomen. *J Am Med Assoc* 1992; 267: 2645–8.

LUMP IN THE GROIN

The complaint of 'a lump in the groin' is commonly encountered in general clinical practice. The causes of this complaint are listed in Table 19.1. In the vast majority of cases, the cause is a hernia. The major clinical differentiation usually required is between a hernia and an enlarged inguinal lymph node. If a hernia is the problem, the clinician then has to decide whether it is inguinal or femoral.

One should be aware that patients do not always mean the inguinofemoral region when they refer to the groin. Thus, in the parlance of cricket, being 'hit in the groin' may mean the scrotum.

HISTORY

The painless lump

The lump in the groin may have been a chance finding by the patient and may not be associated with symptoms. Each of the conditions listed in Table 19.1 may present as a painless lump. Indeed, pain does not occur with a saphena varix, lipoma of the cord, encysted hydrocoele of the cord, hydrocoele of the canal of Nuck, or testicular maldescent. Hernias, inguinal lymphadenopathy and femoral aneurysms may or may not be associated with pain. Historically, the development of a hernia may have been preceded by groin pain after a heavy lift or 'strain'. However, many hernias appear without any such antecedent history.

The painful lump

Hernias can be associated with several types of pain.

Firstly, there may be a dull ache in the groin experienced when the hernia is filled with intra-abdominal contents, such as bowel or omentum. This ache is relieved by spontaneous reduction of the hernia, such as often occurs when the patient lies down. In these patients, the ache is typically worse at the end of a long, physically active day when the intra-abdominal contents have filled and distended the hernial sac.

Secondly, there is the pain secondary to venous congestion of the intra-abdominal contents of the hernial sac, caused by the constrictive effect of the neck of the hernia on venous outflow of the contents. This is a more severe, constant pain that may increase in intensity should venous congestion progress to arterial insufficiency (strangulation). In this circumstance, the hernia will not be reducible and will be locally tender to palpation. These symptoms and signs are related to inflammation in the tissues around the hernial sac.

Incarceration of the contents of a hernia within a hernial sac may be associated with intestinal obstruction, which is more commonly small bowel than large bowel. Small bowel obstruction is associated with central abdominal colicky pain (Chapter 4).

A painful enlarged lymph node is always inflamed. An inflamed lymph node is associated with a constant ache without abdominal symptoms. Not uncommonly, the cause of the inflamed lymph node, such as an infected ulcer or boil on the foot, will also be a source of pain.

A femoral artery aneurysm, or pseudoaneurysm, is rarely painful. This is because the rate of expansion of the aneurysm is usually slow. Rapid expansion is more common with a pseudoaneurysm than a true aneurysm, and can be associated with a dull ache. A false aneurysm is secondary to puncture or rupture of the artery, as can occur after angiography or penetrating trauma. If the puncture site does not close or seal, there is a communication between the lumen of the artery and the haematoma outside the artery. A true aneurysm is surrounded by attenuated arterial wall, while a false aneurysm is surrounded by a fibrous capsule.

Reducibility

There are three causes of a reducible lump: an inguinal hernia (most common); a femoral hernia; and a saphena varix (least common). A saphena varix is always reducible as it always disappears when the patient lies down. An inguinal hernia is commonly reducible, while a femoral hernia is less often reducible because the neck is usually narrow and rigid.

An incarcerated hernia is where the contents of a hernial sac are irreducible. This may lead to intestinal obstruction or even strangulation of the hernial contents (as above).

TABLE 19.1: Causes of a lump in the groin

Common causes

- Inguinal hernia
- Femoral hernia
- Lymph node

Other causes

- Saphena varix
- Femoral artery aneurysm/pseudoaneurysm
- Psoas abscess
- Lipoma of the cord
- Encysted hydrocoele of the cord (male)
- Testicular maldescent (male)
- Hydrocoele of canal of Nuck (female)

PHYSICAL EXAMINATION

Anatomical localisation of the lump

The initial step in the physical examination is to stand the patient to define whether the lump is in the inguinal or femoral region, whether or not there is a cough impulse and also observe if there is bilateral swelling. The two regions are separated by the inguinal ligament which stretches between the anterior superior iliac spine laterally and the pubic tubercle medially. Both of these bony prominences are readily palpable.

The other useful landmark to determine the precise position of lumps in the femoral region is the femoral artery, located just below the mid-inguinal point and identifiable by its pulsatile nature. The mid-inguinal point is situated midway between the anterior superior iliac spine and the pubic symphysis.

Figure 19.1 details the various groin lumps above and below the inguinal ligament.

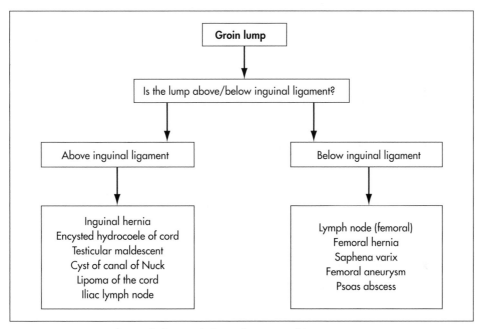

FIGURE 19.1: Groin lumps below and above the inguinal ligament

Lumps in the inguinal region (above inguinal ligament)

Inguinal hernias

Inguinal hernias exit from the abdominal cavity and then pass along the inguinal canal together with the spermatic cord in the male. The inguinal canal passes medially from the deep inguinal ring, the surface marking of which is the mid-inguinal point (see above) to the superficial inguinal ring, which is just above and medial to the pubic tubercle (Figure 19.2).

It is imperative to examine the patient complaining of a lump in the groin while the patient is standing because a hernia may only be apparent in this position. Having examined in the standing position, have the patient lie down and determine if the hernia is reducible—coughing should also cause it to return. By placing the fingers along the line of the inguinal canal and asking the patient to cough, a cough impulse may be elicited, which is a pathognomonic sign of an inguinal hernia. This sign refers to the sudden expansion of a bulge beneath the examining fingers, which occurs when the increase of intra-abdominal pressure blows some of the intra-abdominal contents out into the hernial sac. If the examiner believes that the sign has been elicited, then it is worth trying to elicit the sign on the contralateral side for two reasons. Firstly, inguinal hernias are not uncommonly bilateral. Secondly, the cough impulse of a hernia can be confused with a normal anterior movement of the whole of the lower anterior abdominal wall anteriorly with coughing. This anterior movement is not expansile.

Direct and indirect inguinal hernias

Inguinal hernias are defined as direct or indirect (Figure 19.2). With a direct hernia, the hernial sac enters the inguinal canal through a weakness in the tissues of the posterior wall of the inguinal canal. With an indirect hernia, the sac enters the inguinal canal through the deep inguinal ring. The distinction between the two types of inguinal hernias is of little practical importance. From the prognostic point of view, indirect hernias more commonly develop the complication of strangulation (a strangulated hernia is one in which the contents are ischaemic) as the neck is narrower. Indirect hernias more commonly pass down into the scrotum than do direct hernias. Direct inguinal hernias are more commonly bilateral and have a wider neck.

Some inguinal hernias, particularly the larger ones, may not reduce spontaneously but can be reduced with assistance. This manoeuvre is called taxis (pronounced *taksis*). It is achieved by making a funnel of one hand around the neck of the hernia, with the neck of the funnel being opposite to the neck of the hernia. Pressure is then applied by the other examining hand on the distal end of the hernia in the direction of the neck of the hernia. If the hernia is painful and tender, taxis should not be attempted and urgent surgical consultation arranged. Reduction of ischaemic bowel complicates the surgical management of the clinical problem.

Reducible or irreducible?

An irreducible inguinal lump may be: an irreducible inguinal hernia; a lipoma of the cord; an encysted hydrocoele of the cord (in males); a hydrocoele of the canal of Nuck (in females); a maldescended (ectopic) testis.

To sort out the diagnosis, it is imperative to first examine the scrotum to ensure that there are two testes present. If there is only one, then a maldescended testis is likely to be the diagnosis. The diagnosis can be confirmed with an ultrasound examination. The maldescended testis is most commonly located by palpation just superior to the pubic tubercle. An irreducible inguinal hernia is usually soft and may have a 'squelchy' feel to it.

An encysted hydrocoele of the cord within the inguinal canal should be suspected if traction on the ipsilateral testis causes the lump to move medially along the inguinal canal. An encysted hydrocoele of the cord distal to the superficial inguinal ring should be suspected on clinical examination by the presence of a transilluminable swelling in close proximity to the spermatic cord; this does not extend laterally into the superficial inguinal ring, making differentiation from an inguinal hernia relatively easy. If there is any doubt about the diagnosis of an encysted hydrocoele of the cord and a hydrocoele of the canal of Nuck, then the diagnosis can be confirmed by an ultrasound examination.

A lipoma of the cord cannot be distinguished from an inguinal hernia on clinical examination. It is a diagnosis made by the operating surgeon. Lipomas of the cord are also frequently associated with indirect inguinal hernias. The only possibility that needs to be considered is that the lump is not in the inguinal canal, but rather deep into it. Thus an enlarged external iliac lymph node might be palpable through the anterior abdominal wall, but only in a very thin patient.

Lumps in the femoral region (below inguinal ligament)

Figure 19.1 details the various groin lumps above and below the inguinal ligament.

Anatomy of the femoral region

The femoral region is inferior to the inguinal ligament. The reference point in the femoral region is the femoral artery, which is located inferior to the mid-inguinal point as a pulsatile longitudinal cord. Deep to the femoral artery is the psoas muscle, which passes posteriorly to attach to the lesser trochanter of the femur. Lateral to the femoral artery is the femoral nerve. Medial to it is the femoral vein into which drains the long saphenous vein. Medial to the femoral vein is the femoral canal through which a femoral hernia emerges from the abdominal cavity. The femoral canal usually contains just fatty tissue and a few tiny lymph nodes. Within the femoral region are the inguinal lymph nodes. They are divided into two groups, deep and superficial, depending on whether they are deep or superficial to the deep fascia. The deep group lie around the femoral vein. The superficial group are placed horizontally just below and parallel to the inguinal ligament or vertically along the line of the long saphenous vein.

Physical examination of the femoral region

Evaluate for the following:

1. **Single or multiple.** The only cause of multiple lumps in the femoral region are multiple enlarged lymph nodes. The presence of a single lump in the femoral region does not exclude an enlarged lymph node as the cause, as lymph nodes can enlarge individually or can expand as a matted mass.

2. **Reducible or irreducible.** If the femoral lump is reducible, then it is either a femoral hernia or a saphena varix. A saphena varix is always easily reducible. Pressure is not required if the patient goes from the standing to the supine position. Although a femoral hernia may be reducible, most are not reducible because the neck of this type of hernia tends to be small so that the contents easily become entrapped within the hernial sac.

3. **Mobile or immobile.** None of the common groin lumps is fixed to the underlying bony pelvis and hip joint, yet, as most are encased by the deep fascia of the thigh, they are relatively immobile. This is particularly so for a small irreducible femoral hernia, which is relatively fixed by bony and ligamentous structures around its neck. An enlarged inguinal lymph node is marginally more mobile than a femoral hernia in the transverse direction.

4. **The presence of a cough impulse.** The presence of this physical sign limits the diagnostic possibilities to a femoral hernia or a saphena varix. A saphena varix is a varicosity of the most proximal section of the long saphenous vein. It is associated with incompetence of the valve between the saphenous vein and the femoral vein. When the patient coughs, a palpable jet of blood spurts through the incompetent

saphenofemoral valve into the saphena varix. Tapping may be associated with the palpable transmission of the impulse to the saphena varix along the line of the long saphenous vein (a fluid thrill). A saphena varix is usually associated with incompetence of the long saphenous vein and, hence, the presence of varicose veins in the distribution of the long saphenous vein.

5. **Pulsatile or non-pulsatile.** If the femoral lump is pulsatile, then it is either an aneurysm or a pseudoaneurysm of the femoral artery.

6. **Tender or non-tender.** A femoral hernia may become tender if the vascularity of its contents is in any way impaired so that the contents and, subsequently, the neck and surroundings become inflamed. An inguinal lymph node will be tender if there is inflammation within the lymph node. A femoral artery aneurysm or pseudoaneurysm will be tender if there is inflammation in the surrounding tissues as a result of rapid expansion. A psoas abscess is not usually tender because the inflammation is typically chronic. This unusual lump more commonly lies lateral to the femoral artery and will often be associated with a flexion deformity of the hip because of chronic irritation and contracture of the major flexor of the hip, the psoas muscle. Further, there may be a pain in the flank as well as fever, and occasionally signs of femoral nerve irritation.

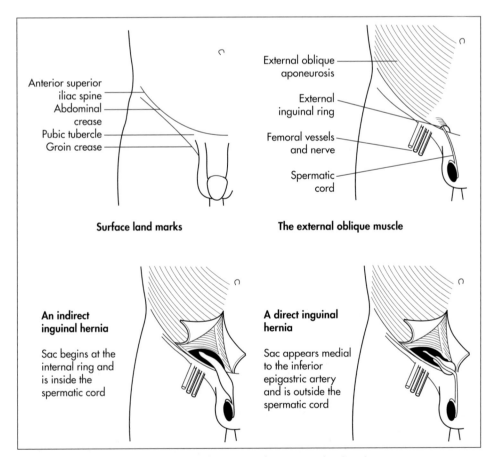

FIGURE 19.2: Anatomy of the inguinal region and important landmarks.
(Based on Browne NL, An Introduction to the Symptoms and Signs of Surgical Disease, 3rd edn. New York: Oxford University Press, 1977.)

Diagnosis remains uncertain

After the physical examination of the femoral region has been completed, the examiner may still not be sure whether the femoral lump is an enlarged lymph node or a femoral hernia.

The next step is to carefully examine the area drained by the inguinofemoral nodes as well as the reticuloendothelial system in general, as the enlarged lymph node may be part of a more generalised disease (e.g., lymphoma). As part of such a 'lymphatic look' it is vital to look carefully for a focus of infection or neoplasia as well as for any old scars that may represent a previously excised tumour. Tables 19.2 and 19.3 list all of the areas that should be included in your 'lymphatic look'.

An ultrasound may help to further define the nature of the lump.

TABLE 19.2: General lymphatic look

Reticuloendothelial system

- Cervical lymph nodes
- Supraclavicular lymph nodes
- Axillary lymph nodes
- Para-aortic nodes
- Liver
- Spleen

TABLE 19.3: Local lymphatic look

- Feet—including between the toes and on the sole of the foot
- Legs
- External genitalia
  - Male: penis and scrotum
  - Female: labia, vagina below level of hymen
- Perineal skin
- Anal canal—below level of mucocutaneous junction
- Buttocks
- Abdominal wall—to level of umbilicus
- Back—to level of umbilicus

MANAGEMENT OF GROIN LUMPS

Management of femoral and inguinal hernias

The preferred method of treatment is surgical repair (either open surgery or laparoscopic), the only method to cure an inguinal or a femoral hernia (see Figure 19.3). This has the benefit of relieving the inconvenience or discomfort of the hernia and, at the same time, preventing complications. Technically speaking, the hernia is always better to repair when it is small.

Questions that need to be addressed when an inguinal or femoral hernia is being considered for surgical repair are:

1. Is the hernia symptomatic?
2. What is the risk of strangulation?
3. What is the risk of a surgical repair in this patient?

The finding of a markedly tender lump in the groin is important. The differential diagnosis is usually between a strangulated hernia (inguinal or femoral) and an inflamed lymph node. For the clinician to decide that the cause is an inflamed lymph node, the primary focus of infection must be very apparent. Otherwise the diagnosis is an incarcerated hernia with contents of doubtful viability (strangulated) until proven otherwise. If there is any doubt about the viability of the contents of a hernia then surgical repair of the hernia must be performed urgently.

The situation is less pressing if the tenderness is only minor. A minor degree of tenderness in enlarged inguinal lymph nodes is relatively common. Frequently, the cause of a minor degree of lymphadenitis is not apparent and the symptoms and signs settle spontaneously with observation.

The repair of inguinal hernias in the very young (neonates and young children) should be performed electively, but as soon as possible because, at least in males, there is a risk that strangulation of the hernia may be associated with testicular infarction.

If the contents of a hernia are strangulated, then operative repair needs to be performed on an emergency basis. After initial fluid resuscitation, the hernia is opened and the viability of its contents are assessed. If the contents are viable, then the contents can be returned to the abdomen and the hernia repaired in a standard fashion. If the contents are non-viable, then they need to be resected and bowel continuity restored prior to the hernia repair.

The alternatives to surgical repair are observation alone and fitting a surgical truss. Observation alone might be considered if the patient is frail, particularly if the hernial sac is small and its neck wide. A surgical truss may relieve the dull ache of a hernia by maintaining the hernia reduced. The patient needs to be aware that, even if the truss is worn regularly, the hernia itself can cause significant discomfort and that permanent reduction is not guaranteed. Indeed, strangulation of a hernia can occur while the truss is fitted. In view of the limitations and problems with surgical trusses, most patients should have the hernia repaired surgically, especially as the procedure can be performed under local anaesthesia in most cases.

Management of an enlarged lymph node

An enlarged inguinal lymph node may be solitary, associated with other enlarged lymph nodes in the groin or associated with a more generalised process of the lymphatic system (see Figure 19.3).

Lymphadenitis

If the enlarged lymph node is secondary to a primary infection elsewhere, then it is appropriate to treat the primary infection.

If the enlarged lymph node is suspected to be part of a neoplastic process, then biopsy is indicated. Biopsy is performed to diagnose and stage the tumour. A biopsy is also required of the lesion thought to be the causative primary lesion. Fine needle aspiration cytology is reasonable in the first instance. Thereafter, a whole lymph node may need to be excised if the diagnosis is thought to be lymphoma.

If the diagnosis is metastatic tumour, then an 'en-bloc' dissection of lymph nodes in the groin may be performed as part of the treatment of the tumour. The most common example of this is radical clearance of groin nodes for metastatic melanoma in the inguinal lymph nodes after the primary has been adequately treated and when no distant metastases are apparent.

Generalised lymphadenopathy

If the inguinal lymphadenopathy is part of a more generalised lymphadenopathy, then an explanation for a generalised illness is required. Investigations under these circumstances may need to include:

- Full blood count;

- Erythrocyte sedimentation rate or C-reactive protein levels;

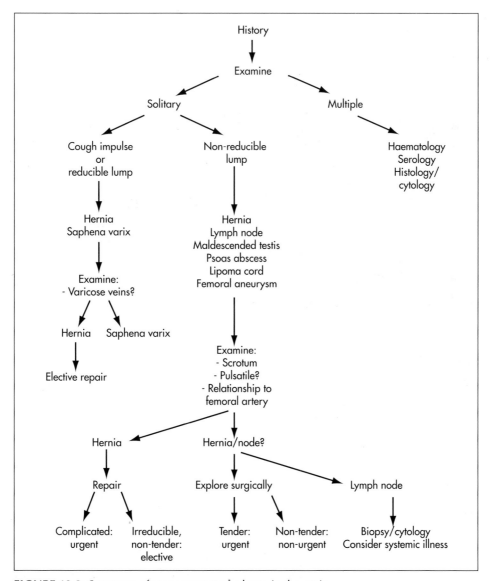

FIGURE 19.3: Summary of management of a lump in the groin.

- Chest X-ray examination;
- CT scan to look at those 'hidden' mediastinal and aortic lymph nodes;
- HIV status;
- Serological tests for infectious mononucleosis (e.g., mono spot test); and
- Other serological investigations for infection, such as toxoplasmosis and cytomegalovirus infections.

If the cause is not found by non-invasive investigations, then surgical biopsy may be required. Nodes other than inguinal lymph nodes are usually biopsied as non-specific inflammatory changes are commonly found in inguinal lymph nodes of normal patients.

Management of a saphena varix

The management of this lesion will be the management of incompetent veins in the leg. If the lesion is to be treated, then ligation of the saphenofemoral junction needs to be performed.

Management of a psoas abscess

A psoas abscess presenting as a groin lump is extremely uncommon. In the past, when tuberculosis of the spine was a condition commonly encountered in clinical practice, the 'cold abscess' (so described because of the lack of an associated acute inflammatory response and lack of pain and tenderness) could point in the groin usually lateral to the femoral artery. In current practice, the development of a psoas abscess is usually secondary to a posterior bowel perforation. The primary pathology may be rectrocaecal appendicitis, an inflammatory condition of the bowel such as Crohn's disease, diverticulitis or local invasion from an overlying colon cancer. The symptoms, loin pain and fever, generated by bowel organisms focally invading the psoas muscle are usually sufficient to demand clinical attention at an earlier stage. The diagnosis is usually confirmed by imaging the retroperitoneum by CT. Drainage of the abdominal abscess is performed either posteriorly or anteriorly, together with surgery for the primary problem.

Further reading

Avisse C, Delattre JF, Flament JB. The inguinal rings. *Surg Clin North Am* 2000; 80: 49–69.
Corder AP. The diagnosis of femoral hernia. *Postgrad Med J* 1992; 68: 26–8.
Kingsnorth A, LeBlanc K. Hernias: inguinal and incisional. *Lancet* 2003; 362: 1561–71.
McIntosh A, Hutchinson A, Roberts A, Withers H. Evidence-based management of groin hernia in primary care—a systematic review. *Fam Pract* 2000; 17: 442–7.
Nyhus LM, Condon RE. *Hernia*, 4th edn. Philadelphia: Lippincott, 1994.
Oishi SN, Page CP, Schwesinger WH. Complicated presentations of groin hernias. *Am J Surg* 1991; 162: 568–70.
Schumpelick V, Treutner KH, Arlt G. Inguinal hernia repair in adults. *Lancet* 1994; 344: 375–9.
Talley NJ, O'Connor S. Clinical Examination, 5th edn. Sydney: Churchill Livingstone, 2006.

chapter 20

RECTAL/PERIANAL MASS AND COLORECTAL CANCER

There are three ways a patient with a perianal or rectal mass may present:

1. The patient may have felt a lump;
2. The patient may present with some other anorectal symptom, such as pain, and a lump is found on physical examination; or
3. A mass may be found on routine physical examination.

The causes of a lump in the rectum or perianal region are listed in Table 20.1.

HISTORY

Establish when the lump was first recognised and whether it has changed over time. If the lump has been present constantly, this suggests a perianal lesion, while a lump that comes and goes suggests prolapse of a lesion from the rectum (e.g., haemorrhoids or rectal prolapse). One should also ask the patient whether he or she has tried to manually reduce the lump if it is external to the anus. Haemorrhoids are a classic example of a potentially reducible lump, but the differential diagnosis includes rectal prolapse and a hypertrophied anal papilla. An acute time course favours conditions such as thrombosed internal or external haemorrhoids. Tenderness suggests an infective process such as an ischiorectal abscess (Chapter 11).

If a rectal lump is found, ask about painful straining or feelings of incomplete rectal evacuation (when these two symptoms occur together causing a constant sense of the need to defecate they are called *tenesmus*); these complaints may occur with any irritating lesion of the rectum. Another key symptom is *rectal bleeding*. Never ignore rectal bleeding and assume it has a benign cause; bleeding should raise the suspicion of colorectal cancer. Less commonly, a solitary rectal ulcer secondary to prolapse of the rectum can cause bleeding and tenesmus. The passage of *mucus* may occur with benign or malignant tumours as well as ulceration. Systemic symptoms such as weight loss (e.g., with malignancy) or fever (e.g., with an abscess) may also help point towards the correct diagnosis. A history of menstrual bleeding associated with a tender lump suggests the rare perineal endometrial deposit. Ask about a family history of gastrointestinal disease and, in particular, colon cancer or polyps.

TABLE 20.1: Causes of a palpable mass in the rectum

- Rectal carcinoma
- Rectal polyp
- Hypertrophied anal papilla
- Diverticular phlegmon (prolapsing into the pouch of Douglas)
- Sigmoid colon carcinoma (prolapsing into the pouch of Douglas)
- Metastatic deposits at the pelvic reflection (Blumer's shelf)
- Primary pelvic malignancy (uterine, ovarian, prostatic or cervical)
- Mesorectal lymph nodes
- Endometriosis
- Solitary rectal ulcer syndrome
- Foreign body
- Faeces (indent)
- Presacral cyst
- Amoebic granuloma
- Vaginal tampon and even the pubic bone may be mistaken for a rectal mass

---

PHYSICAL EXAMINATION

Inspection

Careful inspection is crucial (see Chapter 11) but, importantly, one must expect to find an abnormality. Place the patient in the left lateral position with the buttocks well over the edge of the couch. Part the buttocks, looking for perianal skin tags which the patient may be aware of and may sometimes be associated with pruritus because of an inability to clean the area adequately. These are usually haemorrhoidal remnants, but they can occasionally be an indicator of systemic disease such as Crohn's disease (Chapter 13). A perianal haematoma may be visible, which is usually small (< 1 cm). Rectal prolapse can occur at any age; suspect this if the anus is patulous or gaping. Ask the patient to strain; perineal descent may be seen and sometimes prolapse may be demonstrated.

Palpation

To begin digital rectal examination, warn the patient, then apply gentle but firm pressure to the anal verge with the flat of the well lubricated right index fingertip. The initial contraction of the sphincter will relax after several moments and allow the finger in. The examination will be uncomfortable for the patient; if it is painful, desist. Note the resting muscle tone of the sphincter, and ask the patient to squeeze down on the examining finger to evaluate active tone. Note the anorectal ring where the external anal sphincter spreads out to become pelvic floor and the narrow anal canal (3 cm long) gives way to the spacious rectum. Palpate the coccyx between finger and thumb. This will lead you onto the pelvic floor; feel one side, then the other. Pronation and supination of the forearm may not give sufficient 'degrees of freedom' to the pulp of the index finger; change your angle of approach by squatting or sitting beside the examination couch to better feel the smooth mobility of normal mucosa over the midline groove of the prostate (in males).

Expect to feel a mass. If you feel a mass, determine its size, shape (e.g., polypoid, plaque, ulcer), consistency (soft, firm or hard; it may indent like faeces), surface texture (smooth or granular) and mobility. Tenderness of the lesion suggests an inflammatory process. Decide whether the lesion is mobile or fixed to surrounding structures, such as the prostate, pelvic floor or sacrum. Tethering implies that the pathological process has extended beyond the limits of the muscularis propria to involve the adjacent structure or organ. Fixation may occur as a result of fibrosis but usually indicates malignant infiltration.

Ask yourself: 'Will I be able to describe this mass in my notes or referral letter?' For example, 'on the left lateral wall of the rectum about 2 cm from the anorectal ring is a hard, fixed mass, 3 cm in diameter that does not indent'.

Occasionally you may feel a mass through the rectal wall; these arise most commonly in the sigmoid colon (e.g., a diverticular mass). Alternatively, there may be a hard, relatively immobile mass anterior to the rectum near the tip of the finger on deep palpation associated with a tumour which has spread from a primary elsewhere (such as in the stomach); this is termed a Blumer's shelf. Other masses that might be felt include a tampon or a pessary lying in the vagina, or lateral lumps from enlarged lymph nodes infiltrated with tumour from a primary rectal carcinoma.

Is it part of a benign or malignant process? As a general rule, benign processes are soft, while malignant processes are hard. Fixed, irregular lesions with friable mucosa are more often malignant. Blood on the examining finger is an important sign of friable mucosa.

SIGMOIDOSCOPY AND PROCTOSCOPY

These instruments may allow you to see the lesion that you have felt, exclude other impalpable lesions (e.g., multiple rectal polyps, or areas of ulceration that might be suggestive of inflammatory bowel disease) and take a biopsy of the lesion for histological examination.

The examination is most commonly performed with the patient in the left lateral decubitus position. In some centres, particularly those equipped with specialised tables, the examination is performed with the patient in the jack-knife position resting on the knees. Usually adequate clinical information can be achieved without rectal preparation. When the rectum is totally loaded it can be cleared by inserting an enema; full mechanical bowel preparation is not needed for this examination. Most patients will be anxious about proctoscopy or sigmoidoscopy. They need not see the instrument (Figure 20.1A and B). The examiner needs to reassure the patient, pointing out that the diameter of the instrument is less than the diameter of a large stool and that the examination will be discontinued if there is excessive discomfort.

With the patient in position, the uppermost buttock is lifted upwards and the lubricated instrument is gently inserted with the obturator in place in the line of the anal canal. Surprisingly, the line of the anal canal is toward the patient's umbilicus for the first 3–4 cm, then angles posteriorly. Once the instrument has been inserted into the lower rectum, the obturator is removed. The sigmoidoscope can usually be passed with deft insufflation (reassure the patient that you are putting the air in and not to be embarrassed) and minor deviations to the level of the rectosigmoid junction at about 15 cm from the anal verge. At the rectosigmoid junction there is usually acute angulation, which can make progression into the sigmoid colon more difficult. In older patients who are likely to have diverticular disease, it is always best to stop at this point

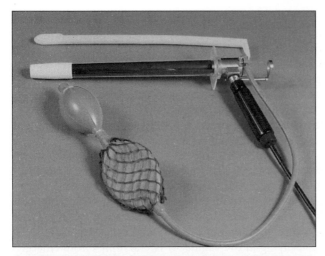

FIGURE 20.1A: Disposable rigid sigmoidoscope with bellows.

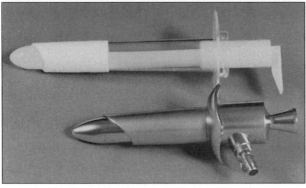

FIGURE 20.1B: Plastic disposable and metallic reusable proctoscopes. Note the oblique working end to visualise, inject or band haemorrhoids.

if there is any degree of difficulty. It is important to realise that the rectum is covered with peritoneum to a greater extent anteriorly than laterally or posteriorly. The limit of peritonealisation anteriorly is usually about 7–10 cm from the anal verge so one needs to be more careful with the depth of biopsy above the level of the peritoneal reflection to minimise the risk of rectal perforation. Biopsy may be best left to the specialist.

If further examination is required (e.g., colon cancer is confirmed), full colonoscopy should be performed at a later stage (see below).

TUMOURS OF THE COLON AND RECTUM

Colorectal cancer

Incidence

Colorectal cancer is common. The lifetime risk for colorectal cancer before age 75 is 1 in 18 for males and 1 in 26 for females. It is more common than breast cancer. Typically regarded as a disease of older patients, it does however occur in young and middle-aged persons. The risk of developing colorectal cancer under age 35 is 1% and under age 40 is 8%. If you as a clinician are suspicious that a patient may have colorectal cancer, you should have him or her investigated. Relatively young age should not be allowed to deprive a patient of the benefit of early detection and treatment. The incidence of colorectal cancer is slowly increasing and there is a slight trend towards more right-sided cancer.

Aetiology

Colorectal tumours can arise from any of the tissue elements found in the large bowel. The most common neoplasms develop from the mucosa (the columnar glandular lining of the large bowel) as premalignant adenomatous polyps, which can then develop into adenocarcinoma. Endocrine, lymphatic, smooth muscle and fatty neoplasms are rare.

Mutations in genes coding for proteins that regulate cell growth and behaviour are believed to lead to colon cancer. Western diets high in fat and low in fibre may play a role in increasing colonic cell proliferation through promoting increased bowel bile acid contact. The mutations may be inherited or acquired. Mutations were initially discovered in colonic polyps from patients with familial adenomatous polyposis and have since been found in sporadic colorectal cancer. Successive stages of the polyp-cancer sequence are marked by additional mutations.

The earliest mutations occur in a gene located on chromosome 5 called the APC (adenomatous polyposis coli) gene. Other mutations are found in one of the ras oncogenes (K-ras on chromosome 12) and in genes coding for proteins that inhibit growth (tumour suppressor genes), p53 on chromosome 17 and DCC (deleted in colorectal cancer) on chromosome 18. It is likely that further genes will be discovered that will serve as markers for tumour behaviour.

Hereditary non-polyposis colorectal cancer (HNPCC) is an autosomal dominant disease characterised by multiple cancers (colon as well as other sites, particularly endometrium and ovary) and early age of onset (the genetic mutation involves one of a family of DNA mismatch repair genes on chromosome 2 or 3—MSH2, MSH6, MLH1, PMS1, PMS2 and probably others). The most common mutations occur in MLH1 or MSH2. HNPCC can be identified historically (Amsterdam criteria):

- When three or more relatives have had colorectal cancer with one case being a first-degree relative to the other two;
- Colorectal cancer has involved at least two generations;
- With at least one case occurring before age 50 years; and
- Exclusion of familial adenomatous polyposis.

HNPCC contributes 1–4% of all colorectal cancer.

Genetic tests for mutations in the APC and other genes have been developed. Genetic understanding will have implications for screening, surveillance and probably therapy in the near future.

Sporadic colon cancer in a first-degree relative above age 55 is associated with twice the risk of developing colorectal cancer compared with the rest of the population. If one first-degree relative diagnosed before the age if 55 or two first/second degree relatives on the same side of the family diagnosed at any age are affected, the risk is increased up to six-fold.

Inflammatory bowel disease (particularly long-standing ulcerative colitis > 8 years) leads to an increased incidence of colon cancer (Chapter 13).

Polyps and the polyp-cancer sequence

Dysplastic proliferation of the mucosa leads to a heaping-up of the regular parallel 'tubular' glands and their cells, causing a polyp (adenoma). This is the stage that corresponds to a mutation in the APC gene. As long as the dysplastic cells are confined to their normal position above the muscularis mucosa, the adenomatous polyp is not malignant; this is because lymphatics rarely cross the muscularis mucosa. Adenomas grow in different microscopic patterns reflecting the extent of their de-differentiation from the parent glandular structure.

- Tubular adenomas—where the glandular structure is still discernible, although it may be branching and irregular (Figure 20.2).

- Villous adenomas—consist of fingers of lamina propria lined by dysplastic cells.

  The larger the polyp, the more likely it is to become cancerous (Table 20.2).

  Most colon cancers arise in a pre-existing adenoma. There are rare exceptions where colon cancers will arise in flat non-adenomatous epithelium. The pathologist recognises malignant change in a polyp when dysplastic cells infiltrate across the muscularis mucosa. Malignant spread then occurs both by direct extension along the bowel as well as through the muscle layers of the bowel wall to serosa and adjacent organs. Lymph nodes can be involved and distant spread may be lymph or blood borne.

TABLE 20.2: Proportion of patients with colonic polyps who develop carcinoma by size and type of polyp

Size of polyp	Tubular adenoma	Villous adenoma
< 1 cm	1%	10%
> 2 cm	25%	50%

Hyperplastic polyps have been typically considered an incidental finding with no potential for progression to colorectal cancer. However, there is a type of hyperplastic polyp known as hyperplastic polyposis, which has been shown to be associated with MS1-H cancer, possibly through a serrated adenoma pathway. Jass and Burt had proposed the following definition for hyperplastic polyposis:

- At least five histologically diagnosed hyperplastic polyps proximal to the sigmoid colon of which two are more than > 10 mm in diameter; or

- Any number of hyperplastic polyps occurring proximal to the sigmoid colon and in individuals who have a first degree relative with hyperplastic polyposis; or

- More than 30 hyperplastic polyps of any size distributed throughout the colon.

  There is no consensus on these criteria, but these patients are quite distinct because of the frequency, distribution and often large size of the hyperplastic polyps. These polyps may arise in patients with a family history of colorectal cancer, are often large and are found in the right colon. It is suggested that these patients are at risk of developing right-sided colorectal cancer and, therefore, should have a follow-up colonoscopy at a relatively short interval, i.e., 1–2 years.

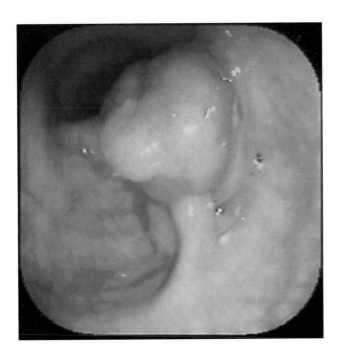

FIGURE 20.2: Tubular adenoma on a stalk.

Presentation

Various patterns of growth occurring at different sites within the large bowel ensure that a colorectal cancer can present with any symptom referable to the gastrointestinal tract; these include a recent change in bowel habit (constipation or diarrhoea), abdominal pain, bleeding (occult or major) or rarely an abdominal catastrophe (perforation or bowel obstruction). Other symptoms include weight loss, lethargy and those of disseminated metastatic disease (e.g., bone pain, jaundice, pathological fracture, and uncommonly thrombophlebitis migrans, skin nodules or acanthosis nigricans).

The classic *right-sided colorectal cancer* is soft and protuberant, and occurs in a part of the bowel where the lumen is large and the contents semisolid; anaemia is therefore more likely than obstruction. The classic *left-sided cancer* is annular, and stenoses a part of the bowel where the lumen is narrow and contents are firm; consequently, obstruction is more likely. Cancers may form a fistula into the bladder or elsewhere. Advanced cancers may be asymptomatic, while a very early caecal cancer may occasionally present with appendicitis having obstructed the appendiceal opening.

Diagnosis

Diagnosis is made on the basis of history, physical examination and special investigations (Table 20.3).

History-taking should include any family history of colon polyps, and colorectal or breast cancer. Has the patient had screening or surgery for bowel cancer in the past? Weight loss, recent change of bowel habit, rectal bleeding, abdominal pain and tenesmus are all indications for further investigation.

TABLE 20.3: Preoperative assessment of patients with colorectal carcinoma	
Investigation	**Comment**
Blood count, electrolytes, creatinine and liver function tests	Results probably will be normal; useful base-line assessment if major surgery planned
Carcinoembryonic antigen (CEA)	Useful—optional CEA is of no value in the preoperative diagnosis of colonic cancer or as a prognostic indicator CEA is of value in the follow-up of resected colonic cancer; a consistently rising titre suggests metastatic disease and further diagnostic evaluation is indicated
Chest X-ray	Useful—not necessary if patient is healthy or if CT chest is contemplated together with the CT abdomen/pelvis
Colonoscopy with biopsy of tumour	Essential unless patient presents acutely with bowel obstruction/perforation
Abdominopelvic CT	Essential especially if a laparoscopic colectomy is being considered
Transrectal ultrasonography (TRUS)	Essential for staging of rectal cancer which determines the course of management

Physical examination is directed towards making a diagnosis, assessing spread and detecting any other medical or surgical conditions likely to impact on treatment.

General examination should include evidence of muscle wasting, malnutrition or anaemia. Jaundice suggests hepatic metastases. Subcutaneous metastatic nodules may rarely be present. A left supraclavicular lymph node should be sought but is rare. Lung consolidation or pleural effusion will suggest lung metastases.

Abdominal examination may reveal distension due to ascites or bowel obstruction; there may be hepatomegaly due to secondary spread. A tumour mass may be palpable.

On digital rectal examination, a middle or lower-third rectal tumour or polyp will usually be palpable, but a higher cancer will not be unless it has prolapsed into the pouch of Douglas. The cervix, uterus, pubic bone and even a tampon may cause diagnostic confusion for the beginner.

The rectum is evaluated with a rigid 'sigmoidoscope'—a misnomer in that the sigmoid is not adequately seen with this 30 cm instrument. Full evaluation of the colon is necessary with either a barium enema or a colonoscopy to identify any tumours (Figures 20.3 and 20.4) and to rule out synchronous cancers. The bowel must be prepared (emptied of all stool) to see the wall clearly. Colonoscopy has the advantage of allowing tissue biopsies to be taken, and the disadvantage that it can cause rare bowel perforation.

Preoperative investigations should include a full blood count, electrolyte tests and liver function tests. Baseline carcinoembryonic antigen (CEA) can be sought to aid follow-up, although the benefit of this is controversial (Chapter 15). A chest X-ray examination may detect metastatic disease. If advanced disease is suspected, CT scanning of the abdomen may be useful; surgery may still be needed for palliation.

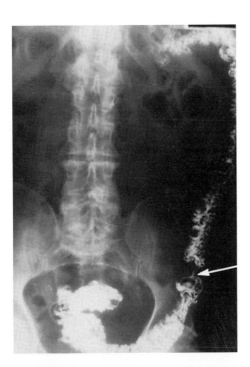

FIGURE 20.3: Apple-core lesion of the left colon due to colon cancer.

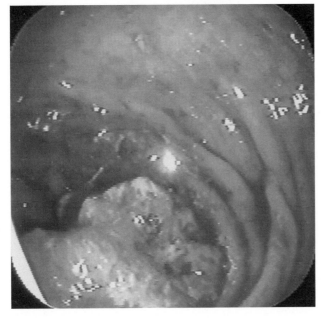

FIGURE 20.4: Colonic adenocarcinoma.

Staging

More advanced disease carries a worse prognosis. Our understanding of the natural history of tumour behaviour is reflected in staging systems, several of which have been developed. Staging systems are used for selecting appropriate treatment and estimating prognosis. Molecular genetic insights into tumour behaviour will probably allow more sophisticated staging systems. It is important to acknowledge that staging systems are descriptions only; the tumour does not know that it has been 'staged'.

Historically, the Dukes' classification is best known and is still widely used for colorectal cancer:

- Stage A: cancer limited to mucosa or submucosa (5-year survival: > 90%);
- Stage B: cancer extends into muscularis or serosa (5-year survival: 70–80%);
- Stage C: cancer involves regional lymph nodes (5-year survival: 30–60%);
- Stage D: distant metastases (5-year survival: 5%).

However, this classification is based solely on the pathologist's examination of the resected surgical specimen. The presence of residual tumour at the completion of operation after resection of the primary is a powerful prognostic factor that influences long-term survival, but is not recognised in the traditional Dukes' classification. Another approach to staging is the TNM classification (Table 20.4).

TABLE 20.4: TNM staging of colorectal cancer

Stage groupings	
Stage 0	Tis N0 M
Stage 1	Tis 1–2 N0 M0
Stage IIA Stage IIB	T3 N0 M0 T4 N0 M0
Stage IIIA Stage IIIB Stage IIIC	T1–2 N1 M0 T3–4 N1 M0 Any T N2 M0
Stage IV	Any T any N M1
T: primary tumour	
Tis	Carcinoma in situ; intraepithelial (within glandular basement membrane) or invasion of lamina propria (intramucosal)
T1	Tumour invades submucosa
T2	Tumour invades muscularis propria
T3	Tumour invades through the lamina propria into the subserosa or into non-peritonealised pericolic or perirectal tissues
T4	Tumour directly invades other organs or structures and/or perforates visceral peritoneum
N: regional lymph node	
NX	Regional lymph nodes cannot be assessed
N0	No regional nodal metastases
N1	Metastasis in 1–3 regional lymph nodes
N2	Metastasis in 4 or more regional lymph nodes
M: metastasis	
MX	Distant metastasis cannot be assessed
M0	No distant metastasis
M1	Distant metastasis

(Based on AJCC Cancer Staging Manual, 6th edn, New York: Springer Verlag, 2002, with permission.)

Treatment

Polyps are usually removed colonoscopically and examined histologically. If cancer is found in the polyp, further surgical resection of that segment of bowel may be indicated. However, a resection may not be indicated if there is:

- a clean margin of excision;
- well or moderately differentiated cancer; and
- absence of lymphatic or venous invasion.

Indeed, we need to take the health of the patient into account as well.

Most colorectal cancer will be amenable to surgical excision. Chemotherapy and radiotherapy have a role in advanced disease.

Surgical treatment aims to remove the tumour and a margin of normal bowel in continuity with draining lymph nodes and blood vessels. Restoration of intestinal continuity is usually possible. If the anus and sphincter complex need to be excised to ensure adequate cancer clearance, intestinal continuity will not be restored and the cut end of bowel will be brought out onto the abdomen as a colostomy. Patients who had laparoscopically assisted colectomy have a similar survival rate to those who had open colectomy at four years follow-up. Laparoscopically assisted colectomy also produced better clinical outcomes, such as early recovery, less pain and reduced length of stay. It is believed that there will be reduced incidence of small bowel obstruction and incisional hernia in the long term.

In the case of familial adenomatous polyposis (FAP) or dysplastic change in ulcerative colitis (Chapter 13), the entire colon is 'at risk' and should be removed; the rectum can be preserved in some circumstances, although this is a calculated risk and it must be watched closely.

Traditionally, surgery takes place electively with a fully prepared (clean) bowel. More recently, it was shown that fully prepared bowel is not needed. In fact, it is beneficial not to prepare the bowel in most colectomies as it avoids dehydration and improves patients' clinical outcomes. If the bowel is obstructed or the operation has to be done as an emergency (e.g., for bleeding or perforation), the surgeon may not be happy to join the bowel and will form a temporary colostomy.

Small cancers and polyps readily accessible through the anus can sometimes be removed locally. However, local excision of T_2 rectal tumour has been shown to have a poor outcome.

At surgery, the surgeon will make a thorough search for spread of the cancer (especially to the liver). In exceptional circumstances, it is possible to resect that part of the liver containing the metastatic disease, although this is best done at a second operation up to six months later. Resection of metastatic disease will only be undertaken if further investigations (angiographic, CT or PET scanning) directed at detecting small metastatic deposits confirm that all metastases can be safely removed.

Rarely a cancer will be too advanced to remove surgically and palliative bypass, colostomy or medical palliation alone will be the only options.

Follow-up

Colon cancer

Follow-up after the colon is cleared of polyps is directed at detection of post-surgical complications, new colon cancers (metachronous disease) or tumour recurrence. Three-monthly visits for the first year, six-monthly visits for the second year and annual visits thereafter is a typical regimen, although its benefit has not been proven. Colonoscopy should be done at one year and, if the colon is still free of polyps and cancer, colonoscopy should be repeated every 3–5 years.

Adenomatous polyps

If adenomatous polyps are found with no evidence of cancer and removed colonoscopically, the colonoscopy (and polypectomies) should be repeated at intervals depending on the number of polyps, size of polyps, any dysplastic change, completeness of the examination and completeness of the polypectomy. Therefore, the interval can vary from three-monthly to five-yearly. In general, the finding of multiple adenomas (≥ 3) should lead to a follow-up colonoscopy within three years; a five-year interval is reasonable if there were one or two small adenomas. Hyperplastic polyps do not require follow-up unless there is hyperplastic polyposis.

Family history of colon cancer

Members of the patient's family are at increased risk of developing a colon cancer and should be screened. Guidelines are constantly changing and it depends on the risk category.

Category 1—those at or slightly above average risk

- Faecal occult blood testing annually from the age of 50.
- Consider flexible sigmoidoscopy every 5 years from the age of 50.

Category 2—moderately increased risk

- Colonoscopy every 5 years starting at age 50, or at an age 10 years younger than the age of first diagnosis of colorectal cancer in the family, whichever comes first. Sigmoidoscopy plus double-contrast barium enema is an acceptable alternative for colonoscopy if the latter is unavailable.
- Consider faecal occult blood testing in intervening years.

Category 3—those at potentially high risk

- Members of a family with a known genetic predisposition (FAP or HNPCC).
- FAP family members should have a flexible sigmoidoscopy annually from the age of 10–15 years to 30–35 years and flexible sigmoidoscopy every three years after the age of 35 years.
- HNPCC family members should have a colonoscopy every 1–2 years beginning at the age of 25 years or 5 years earlier than the youngest affected member of the family (whichever is the earlier). Faecal occult blood test may be offered in the intervening years. Genetic testing is available for some of the genes responsible for the microsatellite instability. This will imply more frequent colonoscopy for the confirmed individuals.

Adjuvant treatment

The risks and potential benefits of adjuvant treatments such as chemotherapy and radiotherapy must be balanced against the probability that surgery alone has cured the patient. Putting it simplistically: if there is a chance that cancer cells remain in the patient after surgery, chemotherapy may help control the cells and decrease the chance of further disease. Resection of an advanced cancer, for example one that has spread to lymph nodes or through the bowel wall, may be an indication for chemotherapy; whereas resection of an early cancer, confined to the bowel wall and not involving lymph nodes, will not justify the expense, inconvenience and side effects of adjuvant therapy. The advantage of chemotherapy for the subgroup of patients with moderately advanced disease has been convincingly demonstrated. Fluorouracil and levamisole decrease cancer recurrence by more than 40% and mortality by one-third in patients with Dukes' C-stage cancer.

The use of combined chemoradiotherapy is applied to the cancer located at ≤ 10 cm from the anal verge and of an advanced stage T_3/T_4, N_1/N_2 determined from preoperative investigation. Resection of an advanced cancer of the rectum, where there is the theoretical risk that cancer cells remain, may be an indication for radiotherapy to the pelvis. Chemoradiotherapy may also be indicated preoperatively to 'shrink' the tumour when it is obvious from preoperative investigations that the tumour is locally advanced. Preoperative chemoradiotherapy is preferred over postoperative chemoradiotherapy and it has been shown to reduce local recurrence (by half) and improve survival.

FAMILIAL ADENOMATOUS POLYPOSIS

FAP is caused by an inherited autosomal dominant gene located on chromosome 5q. Polyps usually appear in the second decade of life. These patients usually have no symptoms until colon cancer develops. More than 95% of patients will have polyps on sigmoidoscopy by the age of 30 years, so the condition can usually be diagnosed by sigmoidoscopy in adults. The number of polyps in a colectomy specimen of a patient with FAP averages approximately 1000. Colorectal cancer inevitably occurs in patients with FAP, occurring approximately 10–15 years after the first onset of polyps. Members of families with FAP can be evaluated by examining the presence of genetic markers using DNA extracted from their white blood cells. The protein truncation assay is applied first. This allows greater than 90% probability estimates for first-degree relatives by the age of 10–15 years.

The presence of more than 100 polyps on sigmoidoscopy that are adenomas histologically establishes the diagnosis (Figure 20.5). Such patients should be referred to a centre of expertise because it can be difficult to detect cancer early in these cases.

Surgical management is the only acceptable approach unless there are other contraindications. The options are:

- total removal of the rectum and colon (proctocolectomy) with ileostomy (which requires an ileostomy bag) or creation of an ileal pouch connected to the anal canal (ileoanal pouch). This can now be performed laparoscopically; or

- colectomy only with rectal preservation and subsequent regular surveillance for removal of rectal polyps. This is performed in some leading colorectal centres because it avoids the problems of ileostomy and problems associated with an ileal pouch. However, a few cases of rectal cancer have been reported to develop in spite of close surveillance.

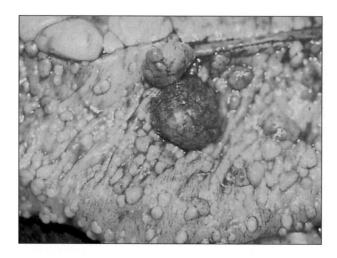

FIGURE 20.5: Familial adenomatous polyposis. Note the numerous polyps.

Medical management may be a useful adjunct in some cases. Non-steroidal anti-inflammatory drugs have been shown to lead to partial regression of polyps but complete regression does not occur.

There is a variant of FAP, previously known as Gardener's syndrome, that consists of all the features of FAP plus a number of extracolonic manifestations that may include desmoid tumours (non-metastasising fibrous tumours, commonly found in the abdominal wall in surgical wounds), osteomas (which can affect the long bones, skull and mandible), lipomas, fibromas, dental abnormalities (e.g., extra teeth) and, rarely, neoplasms of the biliary tree, liver, adrenal or thyroid.

Both the classical and variant types of FAP can cause proximal small bowel adenomas, classically involving the duodenal papillae, which have malignant potential. For this reason, some authorities also recommend annual screening with upper endoscopy after colonic adenomas appear in these patients. One study has shown a moderate gain in life expectancy from regular upper endoscopy.

ANAL CANAL CANCER

Anal canal cancer is more commonly seen in women, although carcinoma of the anal margin is more common in men (Figure 20.6). Together, these are rare tumours constituting only 3–4% of anorectal malignancies. There is a strong association between anal canal cancer and sexually transmitted diseases including HIV infection and condyloma acuminata caused by the human papilloma virus.

Anal canal cancer arises at or above the dentate line from transitional zone epithelium, the remnant of the cloacal membrane of early embryonic growth. However, this zone is not fixed in its relationship to other common landmarks. It may extend in the adult for a variable distance over the anal columns into the lower rectum, and it is composed of a variety of epithelia, including stratified squamous non-keratinised, stratified columnar or cuboidal and simple columnar epithelium. This partly explains the confusion that exists in the histological classification of this tumour.

Most tumours of the upper anal canal are poorly differentiated squamous cell carcinomas (SCC), usually showing little keratin production. Other tumours include basaloid carcinoma and malignant melanoma.

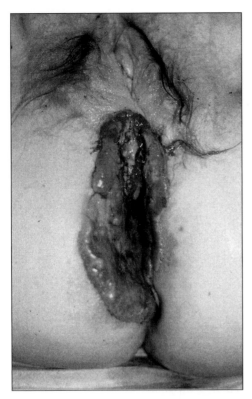

FIGURE 20.6: Cancer of the anus.

Carcinoma of the lower anal canal, below the dentate line is commonly a well differentiated squamous cell carcinoma situated at the anal margin where the modified skin of the pecten becomes continuous with normal hair-bearing skin.

The treatment of anal canal cancer is primarily chemoradiotherapy. Radical surgery is reserved for persistent or recurrent tumour.

Further reading

Calvert PM, Frucht H. The genetics of colorectal cancer. *Ann Intern Med* 2002; 137: 603–12.

Fuchs CS, Giovannucci EL, Colditz GA *et al*. A prospective study of family history and the risk of colorectal cancer. *N Engl J Med* 1994; 331: 1669–74.

Giardiello FM, Hamilton SR, Krush AJ *et al*. Treatment of colonic and rectal adenomas with sulindac in familial adenomatous polyposis. *N Engl J Med* 1993; 328: 1313–6.

Hyman NH, Anderson P and Blasyk H. Hyperplastic polyposis and the risk of colorectal cancer. *Dis Colon Rectum* 2004; 47: 2101–4.

Jass JR, Burt R. Hyperplastic polyposis. In: Hamilton, SR, Aaltonen LA (eds), *WHO International Classification of Tumors 3rd edn. Pathology and Genetics of Tumors of the Digestive System.* Berlin: Springer-Verlag: 135–6.

Kapiteijn E, Marijnen CAM, Nagtegaal ID *et al*. Preoperative radiotherapy combined with total mesorectal excision for resectable rectal cancer. *N Engl J Med* 2001; 345: 638–46.

Levin B. Inflammatory bowel disease and colon cancer. *Cancer* 1992; 70: 1313–6.

Lynch HT, de la Chapelle A. Hereditary colorectal cancer. *N Engl J Med* 2003; 348: 919–32.

Mandel JS, Bond JH, Church TR *et al*. Reducing mortality from colorectal cancer by screening for fecal occult blood. *N Engl J Med* 1993; 328: 1365–71.

Nelson H, Sargent DJ, Wieand HS *et al*. A comparison of laparoscopically assisted and open colectomy for colon cancer. *N Engl J Med* 2004; 350: 2050–9.

NHMRC. Guidelines for the prevention, early detection and management of colorectal cancer (CRC). Canberra: Commonwealth of Australia, 1999.

Sinicrope FA, Sugarman SM. Role of adjuvant therapy in surgically resected colorectal carcinoma. *Gastroenterology* 1995; 109: 984–93.

Stern HS. Contributions of molecular genetics to the clinical management of colorectal cancer. *Am J Surg* 1996; 171: 10–5.

Vasen HF, Bulow S, Myrhoj T *et al.* Decision analysis in the management of duodenal adenomatosis in familial adenomatous polyposis. *Gut* 1997; 40: 716–9.

Winawer S, Fletcher R, Rex D *et al.* Colorectal cancer screening and surveillance: clinical guidelines and rationale—Update based on new evidence. *Gastroenterology* 2003; 124: 544–60.

Winawer SJ, Zauber AG, Ho MN *et al.* Prevention of colorectal cancer by colonoscopic polypectomy. *N Engl J Med* 1993; 329: 1977–81.

Acknowledgement

Much of the material in this chapter was originally written by PH Chapuis and J Cartmill and has been adapted for the revised edition.

chapter 21

JAUNDICE AND PRURITUS

INTRODUCTION

Jaundice refers to the yellow discolouration of the body that occurs as a consequence of hyperbilirubinaemia. As bilirubin levels rise in the blood, jaundice first becomes noticeable in the sclera and with further rises, the skin, and mucous membranes. This becomes readily apparent when the serum bilirubin level rises above 50–75 µmol/L (normal: 3–15 µmol/L). It is most often associated with hepatobiliary disease and when cholestasis is present it may be associated with pruritus. The history and physical examination of the patient with suspected liver disease, and an approach to abnormal liver function tests is discussed in Chapter 22. This chapter focuses on bilirubin physiology and the clinical approach to patients with clinical jaundice. Biliary or pancreatic malignancy, gallstone disease and alcoholic liver disease are common causes of jaundice presenting to hospital.

Background physiology

Hyperbilirubinaemia can follow either increased production and/or decreased excretion of bilirubin. Bilirubin metabolism is summarised in Figure 21.1. Under normal conditions, 80% of serum bilirubin is generated by senescent red blood cells which are broken down by the reticuloendothelial system in the spleen, liver and bone marrow. The remaining 20% of serum bilirubin arises from the catabolism of other haem-containing proteins (e.g., cytochrome, myoglobin and haem-containing enzymes) and ineffective erythropoiesis. The haem (ferroprotoporphyrin IX) moiety is oxidatively cleaved to biliverdin and then bilirubin. As bilirubin is hydrophobic, its transport in the serum is dependent on it being tightly bound to albumin. This unconjugated bilirubin is delivered to the liver where it is conjugated to produce a water soluble product suitable for biliary excretion. This process is carried out by endoplasmic reticular enzymes, UDP-glucuronyl transferase.

Hepatocytes take up and conjugate 30% of available bilirubin on each pass of the blood. Conjugated bilirubin is then secreted into bile canaliculi by an active transport mechanism. It subsequently flows with the bile through the intrahepatic biliary system to the common bile duct and then into the small intestine. In the gastrointestinal tract it is either deconjugated or metabolised to urobilinogen by gut bacteria. Conjugated bilirubin is not reabsorbed by the bowel although some urobilinogen is absorbed and undergoes enterohepatic circulation. Faecal urobilinogen gives stools their colour.

Clinically, hyperbilirubinaemia and, therefore, jaundice may be considered as predominantly unconjugated following overproduction, inadequate hepatic uptake or defective conjugation or mixed unconjugated, and conjugated with hepatocellular disease, impaired canalicular excretion or biliary obstruction (Figure 21.1). The proportions of conjugated and unconjugated bilirubin detected in the serum depend on the point of the obstruction or overloading. Haemolysis or reabsorption of a haematoma leads to an unconjugated hyperbilirubinaemia as the pigment production exceeds the hepatocytes' capacity to take up and excrete bilirubin. Similarly, situations that impede that uptake and/or rates of conjugation will lead to increases in serum unconjugated bilirubin.

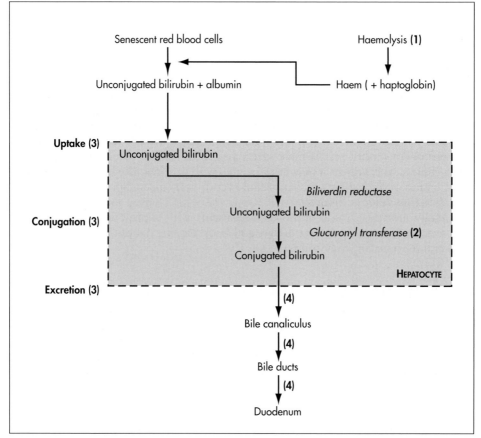

FIGURE 21.1: Schematic representation of the bilirubin pathway.
Increased haemolysis (1) overwhelms the hepatocytes' ability to conjugate bilirubin and excrete the conjugated form, leading to increased serum levels of unconjugated bilirubin. Low levels of glucuronyl transferase (2) (e.g., Gilbert's disease) cause decreased conjugation. Hepatocellular dysfunction (3) causes decreased uptake, conjugation, and excretion with increased unconjugated bilirubin and conjugated bilirubin. Post-hepatic obstruction (4) from stone or tumour prevents passage of bilirubin through the bile ducts into the bowel, leading to increased serum levels of conjugated bilirubin.

Primary hepatocellular diseases produce increases in both serum conjugated and unconjugated bilirubin as uptake, conjugation and excretion are affected. Transport across the canalicular membrane into the bile ductules, the rate-limiting step for excretion of bilirubin, tends to be particularly impaired leading to the accumulation of conjugated bilirubin and its diffusion back into the serum. There may be parallel increases in the levels of unconjugated bilirubin due to decreased rates of conjugation or portal-systemic shunting of blood around the liver.

On the other hand, obstruction of the bile ducts results in a predominantly conjugated hyperbilirubinaemia as uptake and conjugation continue, while secretion into the biliary system is compromised. As noted above, unconjugated bilirubin is tightly bound to albumin so it cannot be filtered by the kidneys, while the more water soluble conjugated bilirubin is only 60% bound and some is filtered. Thus, the urine becomes dark in those with obstructive jaundice. Finding bilirubin in the urine by dipstick indicates the presence of conjugated bilirubin.

Measurement of serum bilirubin

The normal range for serum bilirubin is 3–15 µmol/L in adults. Bilirubin is classified as *direct* (conjugated) and *indirect* (unconjugated). This terminology is derived from the commonly used assay, which makes use of a diazo reaction. Diazotised aromatic amines cleave the bilirubin molecule into two identical molecules, which are bound to the azo compound. The concentration of these can then be measured spectrophotometrically. In an acidic aqueous media, conjugated bilirubin reacts 'directly' with azo compound; whereas unconjugated bilirubin requires the addition of an accelerator molecule such as alcohol, thus reacting 'indirectly'.

In adults, the measurement of direct and indirect fractions of bilirubin is not routine but may sometimes be clinically useful when the total serum bilirubin concentration is less than 50–90 µmol/L. Levels greater than this will most often be due to conjugated hyperbilirubinaemia.

Chronic overproduction from haemolysis (intravascular and extravascular) and ineffective erythropoiesis can increase bilirubin loads by up to eight times the normal level, but the hepatocytes are capable of increased conjugation rates to meet the demand. However, in acute severe haemolysis, such as sickle cell crisis or paroxysmal nocturnal haemoglobinuria, bilirubin production can rarely overwhelm the hepatocytes and lead to unconjugated hyperbilirubinaemia greater then 90 µmol/L. Impaired hepatocellular function in the setting of chronic overproduction can also cause indirect serum bilirubin levels greater than 90 µmol/L (Chapter 22).

JAUNDICE—A CLINICAL CLASSIFICATION

The causes of jaundice are typically classified into three groups corresponding to the site of impaired bilirubin metabolism: prehepatic, hepatic and post-hepatic (cholestasis/obstruction). This classification is clinically useful when evaluating patients with jaundice or hyperbilirubinaemia. The liver function test profiles and clinical presentations can be helpful in differentiating between these groups (Table 21.1). Based on this information one can identify the likely level of impaired bilirubin metabolism, narrow the differential diagnosis and determine the most appropriate investigation to establish the diagnosis.

TABLE 21.1: Clinical features and liver function test profiles in hepatic (hepatocellular) and cholestatic (or obstructive) jaundice

	Suggests hepatocellular jaundice	Suggests obstructive jaundice
Clinical features	Nausea, anorexia, fatigue, myalgia, known infectious exposure, IV drug use, blood transfusions, alcohol, medication abuse, positive family history of liver disease or jaundice	Pain, pruritus, dark urine, pale stools, fever, past biliary surgery, weight loss, older age
Transaminases (AST, ALT)	++ (> 3 x normal)	+ (< 3 x normal)
Alkaline phosphatase	Normal to increased (< 3 x normal)	++ (> 3 x normal)
INR or prothrombin time after vitamin K	Does not correct	Corrects if extrahepatic obstruction

ALT = alanine aminotransferase; AST = aspartate aminotransferase; INR = international normalised ratio.

Prehepatic jaundice

Isolated unconjugated hyperbilirubinaemia (when other liver function tests are normal) is a common clinical problem. Patients typically present with mildly elevated serum bilirubin but normal levels of serum transaminases and alkaline phosphatase (refer to Chapter 22 for a detailed discussion of liver function tests). The serum bilirubin is almost entirely unconjugated. Hepatocellular function and biliary excretion are normal.

Intermittent jaundice may occur but the patient has no hepatobiliary symptoms and physical examination is normal. The two most likely causes are: 1) Gilbert's disease (often detected on routine blood screens performed on fasting individuals who show no other signs of liver disease); and 2) haemolysis.

Hepatic jaundice

Hepatic jaundice may be acute or chronic in origin. These patients have different clinical presentations and liver function test profiles, but there may be considerable overlap. The level of hyperbilirubinaemia can vary greatly and it is seldom a clue to the diagnosis (Chapter 22).

Obstruction or cholestasis

Obstructive jaundice occurs when the flow of bile through the extrahepatic biliary tree is impaired, usually by mechanical obstruction caused by a gallstone or tumour. Intrahepatic cholestasis reflects the failure of hepatocytes to effectively excrete conjugated bilirubin. This may be caused by an adverse drug reaction, viral hepatitis (particularly hepatitis A) and certain chronic liver diseases (e.g., primary sclerosing cholangitis and primary biliary cirrhosis).

The clinical features and liver function test abnormalities produced by cholestasis and obstruction are similar. Both may present with prominent jaundice, dark urine and pale stools. Pruritus may also be present if the cholestasis or obstruction is long-standing. In general, the serum alkaline phosphatase level is usually greater than three times the normal level, transaminases are usually less than three times normal, and serum bilirubin concentration is elevated. The INR may be raised (prothrombin time or photopaenic areas in the liver scan picture, e.g., colon carcinoma metastases. Liver cell adenomas also tend to be photopaenic.

Labelled red cell scan. This is particularly useful in the diagnosis of hepatic haemangiomas. A sample of a patient's own blood is withdrawn and mixed with a radioactive marker that attaches to the red cells. The blood is then injected back into the patient and the patient is scanned. Haemangiomas typically show progressive accumulation of radiolabelled red blood cells (focal 'hot' spot(s)).

Biliary scan. Here the injected contrast agent is taken up by liver cells (hepatocytes) and rapidly excreted into the bile. This is most commonly used in the diagnosis of acute cholecystitis by identifying cystic duct obstruction (absent visualisation of the gall bladder). This test is occasionally useful in the characterisation of liver masses containing hepatocytes if the diagnosis remains unclear after cross-sectional imaging, liver-spleen scanning and labelled red cell scanning. Masses that do not contain hepatocytes will not take up the radiolabelled tracer, e.g., colon carcinoma metastases. A mass which contains hepatocytes, but which has an inadequate biliary drainage apparatus, may take up and hold the radiolabelled tracer and appear as isodense at first, but later it may appear as a delayed hot spot after the normal liver has cleared the radiolabelled tracer into the biliary tree, e.g., focal nodular hyperplasia.

Other radionuclide scans for liver masses. A gallium scan can highlight certain lesions, including lymphoma, metastatic melanoma, hepatoma and inflammatory collections. Unfortunately, this scan has limited usefulness for liver lesions because the gallium is also taken up by normal liver parenchyma. Neuroendocrine tumours (e.g., carcinoid) including their liver metastases concentrate 111-indium pentetreotide (octreotide scan).

Other radionuclide scans for other abdominal masses. Other tracers are available for specific circumstances, but are uncommonly used as initial investigations. These include radioiodine-labelled MIBG for phaeochromocytoma and paraganglioma, labelled white cell scans for inflammatory bowel disease and inflammatory collections and positron emission tomography (PET) for some carcinomas.

Invasive diagnostic procedures in the diagnosis of hepatic masses

The need for invasive investigations depends on the certainty of the initial scan diagnosis, the risk that the diagnostic possibilities pose to the patient, the likelihood that treatment may be needed or be possible, acceptance of an investigation and treatment plan and its risks to the patient, and the capacity of the patient to tolerate any treatment necessary. The highest order diagnosis possible should be sought for potentially treatable lesions in patients likely to be able to tolerate and benefit from treatment, but invasive investigations should only be undertaken with appropriate specialist advice and as part of an overall management plan.

Angiography. Selective cannulation of either the coeliac or superior mesenteric arteries is now rarely required to obtain high quality images of liver lesions. Most commonly, all the information that is required for clinical decision-making is available from the arterial and portal venous phase of the triple-phase CT scan.

Endoscopy. This is of particular value when the hepatic lesion is thought to be a metastasis and a gastrointestinal tract primary is being sought. Endoscopic ultrasound of the pancreas with biopsy may be appropriate if the liver lesion is thought to be a pancreatic metastasis.

Biopsy. Biopsy is occasionally required to finalise the diagnosis and the treatment plan. Remember that even though the risks are usually low, biopsy of a liver mass by any method will entail some risk. The risks include bleeding from lesions, which can be very vascular, and tumour spread by seeding along a biopsy track or by tumour rupture. Thus, needle biopsy of liver masses is usually avoided if there is any likelihood that the tumour might be vascular or if the tumour might be malignant and amenable to subsequent surgical excision with a view to cure. It is not performed by and large for cystic lesions as it is unlikely to alter management, and may even lead to peritoneal spread of hydatid disease. The possibility of surgical excision biopsy should be considered for liver adenomas, some hepatomas and some liver metastases.

RETROPERITONEAL MASSES

The retroperitoneum is a common source of incidental scan-detected masses. Tissues of origin may include lymph nodes, mesenchyme and nerves of the sympathetic chain or of the somatic neural network.

Lymph node masses. These may be reactive or inflammatory in nature. These changes in lymph nodes are most commonly caused by localised inflammation somewhere in the draining field but can be part of a diffuse inflammatory response. The nodal enlargement is usually modest, non-progressive and temporary. Malignant retroperitoneal lymphadenopathy may be quite bulky, particularly when due to malignant lymphoma (Figure 23.6). It is usually progressive, though it may fluctuate, particularly early in the course of the disease. In patients with lymphoma, close questioning may uncover suggestive symptoms (e.g., fever, rash, pruritus) and careful

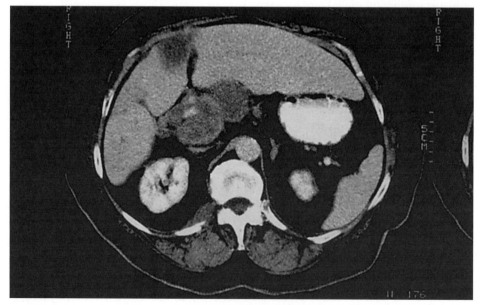

FIGURE 23.6: Para-aortic lymphadenopathy and liver metastases on CT scan. The nodes were due to colon cancer deposits. The patient presented with an epigastric mass and change in bowel habit.

examination may detect enlarged lymph nodes in the groin, axillae or neck. In patients with metastatic disease, there may be a history of a mole or lump, which may have been ignored or previously removed. Some of the more common primary sites include the colon, the stomach, the pancreas and the testes. There may be symptoms arising from, or signs in, an organ draining to the site. There may be non-specific symptoms, such as lethargy or weight loss as seen with many malignancies.

Benign mesenchymal tumours. Benign mesenchymal tumours, such as lipomas, are often asymptomatic, sometimes in spite of considerable bulk. However, all must be suspected of being malignant (sarcomas). Most retroperitoneal mesenchymal tumours are silent until they metastasise or become large enough to be palpable or produce local symptoms by their bulk. The development of symptoms or of a mass is usually slow.

Initial investigations of a retroperitoneal mass should include a full blood count, erythrocyte sedimentation rate and a chest X-ray examination. If the mass is in lymph nodes, the diagnosis may be suggested by blood count changes consistent with infection or a lymphoproliferative disease. Remember that retroperitoneal masses may also be extra-adrenal endocrine tumours, particularly those close to the kidney, and can be functional. An endocrine tumour should be screened for if the patient has a personal or family history of an endocrine neoplasm or has been hypertensive and experiencing episodes of palpitations (e.g., phaeochromocytoma), or episodes of flushing and diarrhoea (e.g., carcinoid). If an endocrine tumour is a possibility, a search for other endocrine tumours should also be undertaken, particularly in the thyroid, parathyroid and adrenal glands (multiple endocrine neoplasia; Table 23.5). Invasive investigations must be avoided until the secretory status of the tumour has been ascertained.

Metastatic carcinoma in the retroperitoneal nodes denotes disseminated disease that cannot be cured by surgery. Other simple investigations such as a tumour marker screen and a chest X-ray examination may help characterise and stage the disease, but will not be specifically diagnostic (Chapter 15). Diagnosis is generally established by biopsy of the metastases or the primary tumour and treatment is generally non-surgical. However, biopsy should be approached with caution. If the lesion is a lymphoma or a mesenchymal tumour, needle biopsy may well be non-diagnostic and, if it is a sarcoma, it may compromise subsequent treatment by seeding along the needle track. Detailed scanning should be undertaken for all suspected mesenchymal tumours, but biopsy of potentially sarcomatous lesions is best deferred until the advice of a surgical oncologist has been sought.

Biopsy of the retroperitoneal mass may be indicated if the history, examination and index scan do not suggest an endocrine tumour or a sarcoma, the mass does not involve the vascular tree, there is no diagnostic evidence of a lymphoproliferative disease on the haematological screen, the chest X-ray examination is clear and there is no more easily accessible mass to biopsy such as a groin or axillary node. If the lesion is a carcinoma, a needle biopsy will usually be diagnostic. If it is due to a lymphoma, the pathologist may still not be able to differentiate benign reactive changes from a lymphoma unless an incisional or excisional node biopsy is done. If lymphoma in retroperitoneal nodes is suspected but not definitely diagnosed on needle biopsy, it may be advisable to proceed to a gallium scan and referral to a haematological oncologist before committing the patient to an open biopsy. Although lymphomas are commonly gallium avid, gallium scans are not specific for lymphoma. Several other conditions including inflammation and malignant melanoma may also cause a positive gallium scan. Other manoeuvres such as bone marrow biopsy or lymph node biopsy in the neck, axilla or groin may remove the need for an abdominal operation to make the diagnosis of lymphoma after discovery of a retroperitoneal mass.

TABLE 23.5: Multiple endocrine neoplasia (MEN)

All these syndromes are autosomal dominant

MEN I

Hyperplasia, adenoma or carcinoma of:
- Parathyroid
- Pituitary
- Pancreatic islets (adrenal cortex and thyroid may also be involved)

MEN II
- Parathyroid
- Medullary carcinoma of thyroid
- Phaeochromocytoma (frequently bilateral)

MEN III

Features of MEN 11 and dysmorphic features:
- Neuromas on conjunctiva, tongue, buccal mucosa
- Marfanoid habitus
- Pigmentation

(Based on Talley NJ, Internal Medicine, MacLennan & Petty, with permission.)

Mesenteric masses

Mesenteric cysts are benign and generally of no clinical consequence. They are uncommon but, of those that are diagnosed, an increasing number are discovered incidentally during abdominal scanning. They must be differentiated from solid mesenteric masses and from aneurysms of the mesenteric vessels. Mesenteric cysts can usually be diagnosed as such on ultrasound. Solid mesenteric masses are generally due to lymph nodes or mesenchymal neoplasms and their investigation may be approached in the same way as for retroperitoneal masses. Duplex ultrasound will identify most aneurysms by demonstrating the blood flow within them. If doubt persists after duplex ultrasound has been performed, triple-phase CT scanning may be performed.

Primary cancer of the peritoneum

This occurs as a mesothelioma or as a primary peritoneal carcinoma, a condition very similar to ovarian carcinoma. They are uncommon conditions that usually present with abdominal symptoms and signs. They are rarely incidental scan findings. A background history of asbestos exposure should be sought. The diagnosis may be made on cytology from samples of peritoneal fluid or needle biopsy, but open biopsy is frequently required.

Further reading

Ahmed A, Cheung RC, Keeffe EB. Management of gallstones and their complications. *Am Fam Physician* 2000; 61: 1687–8.

Carling T. Multiple endocrine neoplasia syndrome: genetic basis for clinical management. *Curr Opin Oncol* 2005; 17: 7–12.

Levy MJ, Clain JE. Evaluation and management of cystic pancreatic tumors: emphasis on the role of EUS FNA. *Clin Gastroenterol Hepatol* 2004; 2: 639–53.

Metcalfe MS, Wemyss-Holden SA, Maddern GJ. Management dilemmas with choledochal cysts. *Arch Surg* 2003; 138: 333–9.

Rubens DJ. Hepatobiliary imaging and its pitfalls. *Radiol Clin North Am* 2004; 42: 257–78.

Schipper HG, Kager PA. Diagnosis and treatment of hepatic echinococcosis: an overview. *Scand J Gastroenterol* Suppl 2004; (241): 50–5.

index

Acute fatty liver of pregnancy

This condition occurs in approximately 1 in 13,000 pregnancies. It carries with it a high fetal and maternal mortality. A brief non-specific prodrome may rapidly progress to fulminant hepatic failure. The onset is in the third trimester, generally after 32 weeks of gestation. Twin, male and primipara pregnancies are at greater risk of acute fatty liver.

Nausea and vomiting are features of the clinical illness. Polydipsia may occur in association with diabetes insipidus. There may be abdominal pain. This can be epigastric or centred in the right upper quadrant. Malaise and fatigue is followed by pruritus and jaundice that rapidly progresses to liver failure. Ascites occurs in 50% of cases. Encephalopathy, hypoglycaemia, coagulopathy and renal failure follow. The mortality, without hepatic transplantation, is greater than 80% in advanced cases.

Commonly there is mild hypertension, oedema and proteinuria, suggesting a possible relationship to pre-eclampsia. Haematology reveals leucocytosis, thrombocytopaenia and evidence of microangiopathic haemolysis. Creatinine is elevated with a greater elevation in uric acid levels. Bilirubin and ALP levels are raised, while serum transaminase levels are 300–500 U/L. Hypoglycaemia and coagulopathy may be severe and represent major management problems.

Abdominal ultrasound scans have poor sensitivity in identifying acute fatty liver but are of use in excluding Budd-Chiari syndrome and gallstones. If necessary, a fine-needle aspiration biopsy will confirm the diagnosis. However, once the clinical diagnosis is made, performing a biopsy could waste valuable time and in so doing adversely affect the outcome.

The treatment of acute fatty liver of pregnancy is emergency delivery of the fetus. This reduces the mortality to approximately 20%. It is of note that the mother's condition may worsen after delivery. Liver transplantation may be required. There is no chronic disease following recovery. Recurrent acute fatty liver with subsequent pregnancies is not expected, but has rarely been reported.

Benign intrahepatic cholestasis of pregnancy

This condition presents with pruritus and jaundice, often in the third trimester of pregnancy. Liver function tests are 'cholestatic' but the mother is otherwise well. Occasionally there may also be a significant rise in serum transaminase levels. The condition resolves with delivery. There is a strong genetic predisposition. Recurrence with subsequent pregnancy and during oestrogen therapy is likely. Cholestasis of pregnancy is associated with increased fetal loss. Severe symptomatic cases with progressively rising levels of serum bile acids or abnormal liver function results should be considered for early delivery. Symptomatic treatment of the pruritus has limited success.

Ursodeoxycholic acid has been shown to be effective in relieving the maternal symptoms and appears to reduce fetal mortality. Numerous other measures have been tried in the control of the pruritus. These include cholestyramine, evening primrose oil, antihistamines, rifampicin, opiate antagonists, phenobarbitone and S-adenosylmethionine. The effectiveness and safety in pregnancy of all these agents has not been objectively established.

Pre-eclampsia and the HELLP syndrome

Liver disease occurs in approximately 10% of cases of pre-eclampsia. In general, hepatic injury is secondary to the underlying condition, and reflects advanced disease. Pre-eclamptic signs may be mild. Symptoms include right upper quadrant and epigastric pain, nausea and vomiting. Jaundice, often mild, occurs in 40% of those affected. ALT levels are, in general, greater than 500 U/L.

Most maternal deaths are from cerebral pathology, but hepatic involvement may contribute to death when infarction, haemorrhage or haematoma formation (with or without rupture) occurs.

A special case of pre-eclampsia is the HELLP syndrome. This syndrome consists of **H**aemolysis, **E**levated **L**iver function tests and **L**ow **P**latelets. There is a microangiopathic haemolytic anaemia. Early aggressive management with delivery is appropriate.

Further reading

Aithal PG, Day CP. The natural history of histologically proved drug-induced liver disease. *Gut* 1999; 44: 731–5.

Cabre E, Rodriguez Iglesias P, Caballeria J *et al.* Short and long term outcome of severe alcohol-induced hepatitis treated with steroids or enteral nutrition: a multicenter randomized trial. *Hepatology* 2000; 32: 36–42.

Chitturi S, Abeygunasekera S, Farrell GC *et al.* NASH and insulin resistance: insulin hypersecretion and specific association with the insulin resistance syndrome. *Hepatology* 2002; 35: 373–9.

Czaja AJ. Current concepts in autoimmune hepatitis. *Ann Hepatol* 2005; 4: 6–24.

Fried MW, Shiffman ML, Reddy KR *et al.* Peginterferon alfa-2a plus ribavirin for chronic hepatitis C virus infection. *N Engl J Med* 2002; 347: 975–82.

Giannini EG, Testa R, Savarino V. Liver enzyme alteration: a guide for clinicians. *CMAJ* 2005; 172: 367–79.

Gines P, Uriz J, Calahorra B *et al.* Transjugular intrahepatic portosystemic shunting versus repeated paracentesis plus intravenous albumin for refractory ascites in cirrhosis: A multicenter randomized comparative study. *Gastroenterology* 2002; 123: 1839–47.

Harrison SA, Bacon BR. Hereditary hemochromatosis: update for 2003. *J Hepatol* 2003; 38: S14–23.

Heathcote J, Main J. Treatment of hepatitis C. *J Viral Hepat* 2005; 12: 223–35.

Kamal SM, Fouly AE, Kamel RR *et al.* Peginterferon alpha-26 therapy in acute hepatitis C: impact of onset of therapy on sustained virological response. *Gastroenterology* 2006; 130: 632–8.

Kamath PS, Wiesner RH, Malinchoc M *et al.* A model to predict survival in patients with end-stage liver disease. *Hepatology* 2001; 33: 464–70.

Lau GK, Piratvisuth T, Luo KX *et al.* Peginterferon alfa-2a, lamivudine and the combination for HBeAg-positive chronic hepatitis B. *N Eng J Med* 2005; 352: 2682–95.

Marcellin P, Chang TT, Lim SG *et al.* Adefovir dipivoxil for the treatment of hepatitis B e-antigen-positive chronic hepatitis B. *N Engl J Med* 2003; 348: 808–16.

Menon KV, Kamath PS. Managing the complications of cirrhosis. *Mayo Clin Proc* 2000; 75: 501–9.

Neuschwander-Tetri BA, Caldwell SH. Nonalcoholic steatohepatitis: summary of an AASLD single topic conference. *Hepatology* 2003; 37: 1202–19.

Okano N, Yamamoto K, Sakaguchi K *et al.* Clinicopathological features of acute-onset autoimmune hepatitis. *Hepatol Res* 2003; 25: 263–70.

Ratziu V, Giral P, Charlotte F *et al.* Liver fibrosis in overweight patients. *Gastroenterology* 2000; 118: 1117–23.

Roberts EA, Schilsky ML. Practice guidline on Wilson disease. *Hepatology* 2003; 37: 1475–92.

Rosado B, Kamath PS. Transjugular intrahepatic portosystemic shunts: an update. *Liver Transpl* 2003; 9: 207–17.

Sanyal AJ, Genning C, Reddy KR *et al*. The North American Study for the treatment of refractory ascites. *Gastroenterology* 2003; 124: 634–41.

Sherman M. Screening for hepatocellular carcinoma. *Best Pract Res Clin Gastroenterol* 2005; 19: 101–8.

Siegel CA, Silas AM, Suriawinata AA, van Leeuwen DJ. Liver biopsy 2005: when and how? *Cleve Clin J Med* 2005; 72: 199–201, 206, 208.

Talwalkar JA, Kamath PS. An evidence-based medicine approach to beta-blocker therapy in patients with cirrhosis. *Am J Med* 2004; 116: 759–66.

Valla D-C. The diagnosis and management of Budd-Chiari syndrome: consensus and controversies. *Hepatology* 2003, 38: 793–803.

Velazquez RF, Rodriguez M, Navascues CA *et al*. Prospective analysis of risk factors for hepatocellular carcinoma in patients with liver cirrhosis. *Hepatology* 2003; 37: 520–7.

Yamamoto K, Terada R, Okamoto R *et al*. A scoring system for primary biliary cirrhosis and its application for variant forms of autoimmune liver disease. *J Gastroenterol* 2003; 38: 52–9.

chapter 23

INCIDENTALOMA:
AN UNEXPECTED ABNORMALITY DETECTED ON ABDOMINAL IMAGING

In this chapter the approach to unexpected abdominal masses detected on scanning is examined. These are defined as masses detected in a patient in whom no symptoms or signs indicating the likelihood of such a mass are known at the time the scan is performed.

This situation arises intermittently during investigation for a separate complaint, or haematological or biochemical abnormality. The unexpected finding on abdominal imaging should stimulate a review of the previous history and physical examination, usually with greater focus triggered by the new-found knowledge.

At present, unexpected findings usually result from ultrasound scanning and computerised axial tomography (CT) as these are the most commonly used scans. Magnetic resonance imaging (MRI) is less widely available. As techniques become more sensitive and readily available, the problems reviewed in this chapter will become more common.

Masses commonly presenting as incidental scan findings discussed in this chapter include gall bladder stones and polyps, stones in the bile ducts, dilated bile ducts (including choledochal cysts), pancreatic masses, solid and cystic liver masses, retroperitoneal lymph node masses and mesenteric masses.

Most patients and their relatives associate the discovery of an incidentaloma with the presence of cancer. In fact, the majority of lesions encountered this way are benign, unrelated to the symptom or sign that triggered the scan in the first place and are of little or no risk to health. In most, the diagnosis is immediately apparent. Some require further investigations, and only a minority require treatment.

PRINCIPLES OF ORGANISING THE INVESTIGATIONS

Abdominal masses discovered on scanning can be cystic or solid. The differentiation of cystic from solid masses may not be clear on the initial scan. Differentiation is best done with ultrasound if there is any doubt. Simple cysts are quite common in the liver and kidney and are also seen in the pancreas and mesentery of the bowel. Simple cysts rarely require further investigation or treatment. Parasitic cysts, post-traumatic cysts and pseudocysts need careful assessment; not all require treatment. All solid or mixed solid and cystic lesions require investigation to clarify the diagnosis. While the majority are benign, some are malignant.

The investigation of incidentalomas is a two-stage process entailing non-invasive and invasive investigations (Table 23.1). Initially, a thorough review of the clinical history and examination with particular focus on the types of pathology that might have caused the incidentaloma is indicated. Enquire particularly about disease risk factors and symptoms suggesting a process that may have involved the organ secondarily. Then, an equally thorough physical examination including a careful and complete examination outside the involved system is needed. Next, obtain a few simple, non-invasive investigational tests.

TABLE 23.1: Approach to investigation of incidental, scan-detected abdominal masses

Stage 1. Non-invasive investigations

- Review history
- Repeat physical examination
- Non-specific blood tests (full blood count, biochemistry)
- Specific blood tests (tumour markers, immunological, hormone assays)
- Ultrasound to differentiate cystic from solid (if not already certain)
- Other non-invasive scans to clarify anatomical and functional details relevant to involved organ

Stage 2. Invasive investigations

- Invasive imaging
- Endoscopy ± biopsy
- Laparoscopy ± biopsy
- Ultrasound- or CT-guided biopsy

The initial investigations usually include non-specific investigations such as a full blood count and biochemical screening. More specific investigations may be needed such as tumour markers, immunological testing for specific disease processes that might be the cause as well as assays for specific hormones that might be being produced by the mass.

Another cross-sectional scan of the type that revealed the mass may be necessary, particularly if the original scan did not give optimal imaging detail of the lesion and its anatomic relationships, or if the lesion is small and the differentiation of a cystic from a solid mass has not been clearly made. CT and ultrasound are often complementary to one another in this phase. If the original scan was of poor quality, it might need to be repeated.

Non-invasive contrast radiology relevant to the organ or site implicated on the scan such as barium meal, small bowel series or barium enema, magnetic resonance cholangiopancreatography (MRCP), CT cholangiography and nuclear scans need to be considered. These may be helpful in diagnosing the nature of the mass, as well as indicating the degree of functional compromise caused to the organ involved.

It will not always be necessary to proceed to the second stage of invasive investigations, which include imaging procedures such as arteriography, endoscopic procedures and biopsies. All of these incur some risk, discomfort and expense. The need to do this and the pattern of investigations chosen depend on the findings at stage 1.

GALL BLADDER AND BILIARY TREE

Asymptomatic gallstones

Most gallstones that are asymptomatic and are discovered as an incidental finding on abdominal scanning remain asymptomatic. Approximately 10% of patients with asymptomatic stones develop symptoms within five years of diagnosis, and approximately 20% by 20 years. The rate of symptom development is maximal in the early years after diagnosis. This then tapers off to an annual rate of 1–2% of asymptomatic patients becoming symptomatic.

Only about 10% of gallstones are calcified, leading to a low detection rate on abdominal X-ray examinations. However, the sensitivity and specificity of ultrasound for the detection of stones in the gall bladder (cholelithiasis) is high (> 90%) so that most asymptomatic incidental gallstones are found in this way.

In general, the risks of cholecystectomy for asymptomatic gallstones outweigh the benefits, so observation alone is usually recommended. If the stones become symptomatic, cholecystectomy is indicated. Usually the index presentation is with biliary colic; only 10% present with acute cholecystitis, which most often resolves with non-operative treatment, so that elective cholecystectomy can be performed subsequently in most cases. It is argued by some that the chances of presentation with acute cholecystitis are higher if the gallstone(s) is larger than 2.5 cm so that such patients might be offered prophylactic cholecystectomy. An argument in favour of prophylactic cholecystectomy is also made for diabetic patients with asymptomatic gallstones because the risks of acute cholecystitis are higher in these patients. Special consideration may also be indicated for certain high-risk patients, such as those with haemolytic diseases, those undergoing non-hepatic transplantation, and very young patients.

The risk of gall bladder cancer is increased by stones, but remains very low. This risk was once used as a justification for prophylactic cholecystectomy in asymptomatic patients. However, that argument is difficult to sustain because the risk of operation is greater than the risks of gall bladder cancer for most patients. A special case has been made for patients with porcelain gall bladder (see Figure 23.1), where chronic infection resulting in calcification of the gall bladder wall is associated with a higher than average risk of developing gall bladder cancer.

Polyp(s) in the gall bladder

Polyps in the gall bladder are usually asymptomatic. They may be detected during upper abdominal ultrasound. They are differentiated on ultrasound from stones by their lack of mobility when the patient is moved as they are attached to the gall bladder wall and by the lack of acoustic shadowing behind them. The risk that a polyp is a small, unsuspected carcinoma increases as the size of the polyp increases. For this reason, polyps greater than 1 cm are generally removed by cholecystectomy. The chance that a small carcinoma has been unearthed is addressed by repeating the ultrasound in 3–6 months in which time a carcinoma, but not a polyp, would be expected to have increased in size.

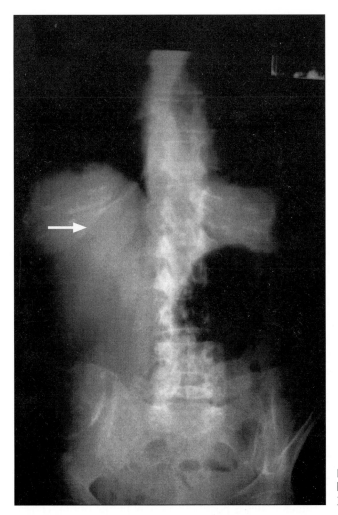

FIGURE 23.1: Porcelain gall bladder on plain abdominal X-ray examination.

Asymptomatic dilatation of the common bile duct and asymptomatic stones in the common bile duct

The upper limit of common bile duct size as seen on ultrasound scan in normal patients less than 60 years is 6 mm. The limit increases by 1 mm per decade thereafter. A previous uncomplicated cholecystectomy can also be associated with dilatation of the common bile duct by several millimetres. Other causes are listed in Table 23.2. These possibilities need to be elucidated, if present. The likelihood of one of the significant causes being present is increased if the dilatation is associated with abnormal liver function tests, so these are performed first. The likelihood of a malignant cause is increased if the tumour marker CA-19-9 is elevated, so this too should be checked. Thereafter consideration needs to be given to better imaging of the bile duct. The choice lies between the two non-invasive techniques, MRCP and CT cholangiography, and endoscopic retrograde cholangiopancreatography (ERCP). The last option is invasive but carries with it the advantages of endoscopic sphincterotomy and thereafter clearance of bile duct stones, dilatation of a stricture and biopsy of a carcinoma of the ampulla or brush cytology of a carcinoma of the bile duct. On many occasions one of the non-invasive modalities will be chosen first just to make sure that a subsequent ERCP with its attendant risks is really necessary.

TABLE 23.2: Causes of a dilated bile duct

- Normal variant
- Post cholecystectomy
- Unsuspected bile duct stone
- Sphincter of Oddi stenosis
- Occult bile duct stricture
- Previous bile duct injury
- Early carcinoma of the pancreas, carcinoma of the bile duct or carcinoma of the ampulla
- Extrinsic compression of the bile duct by a primary or secondary neoplasm

---

Stones in the common bile duct, particularly if they are at its lower end, can be difficult to detect on ultrasound because the stones may be behind the duodenum and be obscured by overlying duodenal or small bowel or colonic gas. Choledocholithiasis can also be asymptomatic. Small stones may pass spontaneously. However, the incidence of serious complications, such as obstructive jaundice and pancreatitis, is around 20% over five years. Consequently, removal of stones in the common bile duct is generally recommended even if they are asymptomatic.

The standard treatment for choledocholithiasis before the development of ERCP was open surgical exploration of the common bile duct, usually during cholecystectomy. At present, the most common treatment for common bile duct stones that do not pass spontaneously is ERCP, endoscopic sphincterotomy and endoscopic stone extraction. Laparoscopic clearance of bile duct stones is possible and may be the option chosen rather than endoscopic clearance particularly if there is bile duct dilatation and the gall bladder is still in situ. Thus a two-stage treatment (ERCP and subsequent surgical removal of the gall bladder) can on occasions be condensed into a single procedure to remove the gall bladder and clear the bile duct laparoscopically.

Choledochal cysts

Choledochal cysts represent a range of pathological bile duct dilatation patterns including single or multiple dilatations of the extrahepatic or intrahepatic biliary tree, or of both, in the absence of a pre-existing outflow obstruction (Table 23.3). Though the cysts are not primarily caused by bile duct obstruction, strictures, tumours or stones, these problems may develop in association with them over time. This, in turn, may lead to complications such as obstructive jaundice, infection in the biliary tree (cholangitis), impaired hepatic function and bile duct cancer.

Choledochal cysts are most common in infancy. However, 20% present in adulthood. They are much more common in women (80%) than men. A popular hypothesis to explain their occurrence is that they are associated with an anomalous junction of the common bile duct and pancreatic duct. This anatomical arrangement allows mixing of pancreatic juice and bile within the bile ducts. Exposure of the pancreatic exocrine secretions to the bile leads to activation of the pancreatic digestive enzymes, perhaps eventually leading to weakening and dilation of the duct. This may also induce the epithelial changes which predispose these patients to bile duct cancer.

In adults, a few choledochal cysts are discovered while still asymptomatic. The discovery of intrahepatic or extrahepatic bile duct dilation consistent with a choledochal cyst necessitates further investigation, initially by assessment of liver function and then by MRCP or CT cholangiography. Masses associated with choledochal cysts may be biliary cancers. These may develop outside the liver in the extrahepatic bile ducts or gall bladder or they may arise in the liver from the small, intrahepatic bile ducts.

TABLE 23.3: Todani classification of choledochal cysts		
Site of cyst(s)	**Classification**	**ERCP findings**
Extrahepatic	I	Solitary fusiform cyst
	II	Supraduodenal diverticulum
	III	Intraduodenal diverticulum (choledochocoele)
	IVB	Multiple extrahepatic cysts
Extrahepatic and intrahepatic	IVA	Extra and intrahepatic cysts
Intrahepatic	V	Multiple intrahepatic cysts (Caroli's disease)
ERCP = endoscopic retrograde cholangiopancreatography.		

Surgical excision is usually undertaken for extrahepatic choledochal cysts. Multiple intrahepatic cysts may not be amenable to surgical excision and drainage. These are usually treated with endoscopic or percutaneous tubes (stents) in the bile ducts if biliary drainage is impaired. The cycle of chronic obstruction and recurrent biliary sepsis can lead to liver failure and necessitate hepatic transplantation.

PANCREATIC MASSES

Unexpected masses in the pancreas may be cystic or solid and may be derived from stromal, exocrine or endocrine elements of the pancreas or from lymph glands lying in, or adjacent to, the pancreas. Historically a past history of epigastric pain is sought, which might correspond to a previous episode of pancreatitis. Other epigastric pains or back pain would be relevant, as would a history of nausea or weight loss. Physical examination may reveal an epigastric mass, although this is unlikely unless the lesion is very large. Thereafter, cystic masses are differentiated from solid masses by ultrasound scanning.

Most asymptomatic cystic lesions of the pancreas are simple cysts. These are usually unilocular, lined by simple one-layered epithelium and contain serous fluid. They do not grow or develop other complications and require no treatment. The difficulty is to be confident that a cyst is a simple cyst and not a cystic neoplasm or a pseudocyst. If doubt exists then endoscopic ultrasound provides a more detailed image as well as the potential for cyst aspiration for biochemical analysis of the cyst fluid for amylase and tumour markers. The specimen can also be examined cytologically.

The other common cystic mass in, or more commonly adjacent to, the pancreas is a *pseudocyst* (Chapter 4). This occurs as an accumulation of amylase rich fluid most commonly in the lesser sac in the weeks to months following an attack of acute pancreatitis. The nature of the cyst may be suggested by the presence of calcium deposits elsewhere in the pancreas. Uncomplicated pseudocysts smaller than 5 cm are usually suitable for observation alone as they commonly resolve spontaneously; they should be followed up with repeat scanning. Larger pseudocysts usually do not resolve spontaneously and usually require drainage. This can often be achieved by endoscopic drainage through the posterior wall of the stomach. Alternatively, a drain can be inserted into the pseudocyst through the anterior and then the posterior wall of the stomach under CT control. Subsequently, some weeks later, the radiologist will separate the drainage system into two parts: a drain from the pseudocyst into the stomach, and an external gastrostomy. Some pseudocysts are not suitable for either technique and require surgical drainage into the stomach (cystogastrostomy) or into a loop of small bowel (cystojejunostomy).

The common cystic neoplasms are *mucinous cystadenoma* (cystadenocarcinoma) and *serous cystadenoma*. These are multilocular and commonly have solid elements or irregularities or thickening of their walls. Clinical distinction between these lesions is important but difficult. The presence of tiny flecks of calcium within the wall increases the chance that the lesion is a serous cystadenoma. If the lesion can be demonstrated to be a serous cystadenoma then no treatment is required, as the lesion is benign with no malignant potential. If the lesion is a mucinous cystadenoma, then if the patient is fit and well, resection should be considered as some of these lesions are malignant even though they may look histologically benign.

Another common cause of a mixed cystic and solid mass is a *pancreatic adenocarcinoma* (Figures 23.2A and B), which is predominantly solid with cystic elements arising from necrosis or haemorrhage. Biopsy by endoscopic ultrasound should be considered to establish the diagnosis. Other rarer mixed solid and cystic lesions are microcystic adenomas and papillary and cystic tumours.

Non-cystic (solid) pancreatic masses may be due to pancreatic tumours or local nodal enlargement. Very small pancreatic head and body masses can be difficult to diagnose. Lymph nodes are usually of low density on CT and MRI, do not increase over time, and do not show malignant or neuroendocrine features if subjected to needle biopsy and cytological assessment.

Endocrine neoplasms of the pancreas may be secretory or non-secretory (Table 23.4). They also may appear as small, low density lesions on CT scanning. The secretory types usually present with symptoms caused by an excess of the secreted compound. They are rarely true incidental findings. Small non-secretory endocrine tumours of the pancreas may be detected as incidental scan findings. As with lymph nodes, investigation and management can be difficult, as the true nature of the lesion can be difficult to clarify. In general, they grow very slowly or not at all, are seen as low density masses within the substance of the pancreas on scanning and show cells consistent with a neuroendocrine origin on cytology.

By far the most common pancreatic neoplasms are *adenocarcinomas* derived from the exocrine pancreas (Chapter 15). Adenocarcinomas of the head of the pancreas are rarely detected at an asymptomatic stage. If resection is not an option, then biopsy, either at endoscopic ultrasound or by the percutaneous route, should be considered as occasionally such a lesion will happen to be a small lymphoma—a lesion with a much better prognosis and much more amenable to non-surgical therapies such as chemotherapy and radiotherapy. Rarely, *autoimmune pancreatitis* will present clinically as a pancreatic mass; serum IgG4 levels are often elevated.

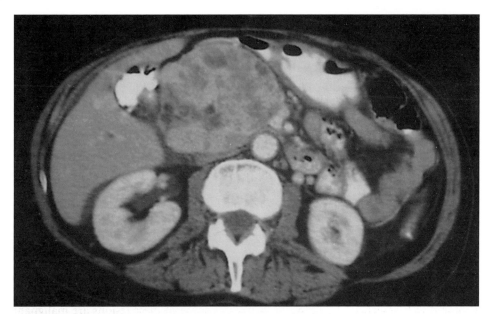

FIGURE 23.2A: Pancreatic carcinoma on CT.

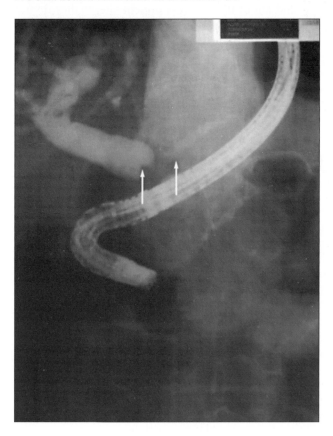

FIGURE 23.2B: Pancreatic carcinoma of the head of the pancreas causing the double duct sign on ERCP due to obstruction of the pancreatic and common bile duct.

TABLE 23.4: Endocrine tumours of the pancreas

Type	Clinical features	Hormone secreted	Malignancy rate
Gastrinoma	Dyspepsia (Chapter 5) Diarrhoea	Gastrin	60–90%
VIPoma	Diarrhoea Flushing Weight loss	VIP	> 60%
Glucagonoma	Diarrhoea Dermatitis (necrolytic migratory erythema) Diabetes mellitus Weight loss	Glucagon	50–80%
Somatostatinoma	Diarrhoea	Somatostatin	> 70%
Insulinoma	Symptoms of hypoglycaemia: fasting confusion, irritability, weakness, palpitations, sweating	Insulin	< 10%

VIP = vasoactive intestinal polypeptide.

Adenocarcinomas of the body and tail of the pancreas present late, as they do not involve the bile duct or coeliac plexus until the disease is quite advanced. Even when discovered while asymptomatic, pancreatic body and tail carcinomas are usually not resectable and generally are incurable.

Hydatid disease can involve the pancreas and cause cysts just as it does in the liver. The radiological features are curved plates of calcification in cyst walls and grape-like daughter cysts within large cysts. Hydatid disease in the pancreas is a marker of disease dissemination.

LIVER MASSES

Cystic

The great majority of cystic hepatic lesions are non-neoplastic. Most are simple cysts, which require no further investigation or treatment, unless they cause worrying symptoms or there is doubt about the diagnosis. Simple cysts have thin, smooth, epithelium-lined walls and contain serous fluid. They do not connect with the biliary tree. They vary in size, ranging from only just detectable on scan (5 mm) to greater than 20 cm and palpable. They may be single or multiple. The multiple form is known as *polycystic liver disease* and may be associated with polycystic renal disease. Liver cysts are more common in women than men. Abdominal ultrasound scanning is the most useful diagnostic tool. Needle biopsy is rarely indicated and hydatid disease must be absolutely excluded first, as cyst needling may result in leakage and dissemination causing acute hypersensitivity reactions and disease spread. Solitary simple cysts rarely require treatment. Very large cysts may sometimes cause abdominal discomfort or pain. Very occasionally they may cause abnormal liver function test profiles or even jaundice by compression of the bile duct. Polycystic liver disease may cause enormous enlargement of the liver and may be a cause of pain, hepatomegaly, jaundice and impaired liver function.

Other hepatic cysts may be due to *hydatid disease* or, very uncommonly, *hepatic cystadenoma* or *cystadenocarcinoma*. Viable hydatid cysts may be encountered as incidental scan findings, particularly in people from areas where the disease is endemic. A farming background and a history of contact with sheep and dogs is common. Such contact may have occurred during childhood and may not always be clearly remembered. Hepatic hydatid cysts often have plate-like or curvilinear calcification in their walls. This may be clearly visible on plain abdominal X-ray examination or on CT scans. Non-viable hydatids may show up on scans or on plain X-ray examinations as heavily calcified lesions with little or no cystic component remaining. Provided other potentially viable hydatid cysts are excluded on the abdominal scan and chest X-ray examination, further investigations or treatment are not usually required to diagnose 'dead' hydatid cysts, as long as the cyst has been obliterated. Scans of viable hydatid cysts show no calcification or incomplete calcification and non-uniform density due to daughter cysts or hydatid debris within the main cyst. Hydatid serology may be positive in the presence of a non-viable cyst and is occasionally negative in the presence of a viable cyst. A positive test is a useful way of confirming that a patient has had hydatid disease at some time, but is not diagnostic of active hydatidosis. Potentially viable hydatid cysts require careful investigation, even if they are truly asymptomatic, because of the risk of rupture into the peritoneal cavity. Cysts that are completely intrahepatic may simply be kept under observation after treatment with an anthelmintic agent (albendazole). Cysts that are large, involve the surface of the liver, become infected, are associated with compromise of liver function or are symptomatic usually need treatment. Cysts that discharge into the biliary tree may present with jaundice and are usually treated by endoscopic drainage of the bile duct. Otherwise, the treatment of hydatids in the liver is usually surgical and usually performed after a course of an anthelmintic agent to reduce the risk of postsurgical recurrence.

Solid

The finding of a solid hepatic lesion does increase the likelihood of malignancy. However, approximately 75% of solid liver lesions presenting as incidentaloma(s) are benign and non-neoplastic. The majority are hepatic *haemangiomas* (Figure 23.3). Hepatic haemangiomas are not neoplasms and, unless large and involving the surface of the liver, are an uncommon source of symptoms. Haemangiomas, particularly the larger ones, can thrombose leading to episodes of upper abdominal discomfort. Most instances of rupture and bleeding of hepatic haemangiomas have resulted from ill-advised attempts at needle biopsy. Spontaneous rupture or rupture due to external violence is rare. On ultrasound, haemangiomas are usually very echogenic. This may not show clearly in small lesions (< 2 cm). Giant haemangiomas (> 4 cm) often show quite variable, non-diagnostic echo patterns on ultrasound. The radiolabelled red cell scan is diagnostic in most cases, though lesions less than 2 cm may be too small to resolve, and those that are partly calcified or in which thrombosis has occurred may give equivocal results. Triple phase, dynamic CT or contrast enhanced MRI may then be diagnostic, showing slow filling of the lesion from its periphery followed by retention of contrast within it. Angiography is not indicated for diagnostic purposes.

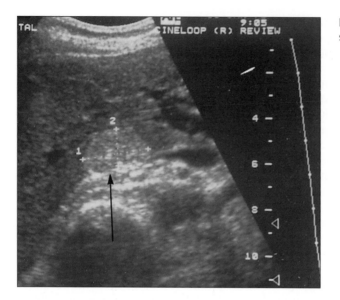

FIGURE 23.3: Ultrasound scan of a haemangioma.

Another innocent solid lesion of the liver is a *fibronodular hyperplasia* (FNH). This has no 'malignant potential' and can be observed once the diagnosis is made with confidence. Unfortunately, there are no tumour markers to identify the lesion. However, it can often be identified by its characteristic appearance on dynamic or triple phase CT scan. It can exhibit a central scar with radiating prongs. When followed sequentially after intravenous injection of contrast agent it can be shown to have a central feeding vessel which fills first. Thereafter there is a blush within the rest of the lesion as perfusion occurs from the feeding vessel. This appearance needs to be distinguished from that of the fibrolamellar variant of hepatocellular carcinoma. Distinguishing features in favour of FNH are elevation of alpha-fetoprotein and the presence of a central feeding vessel. A liver biopsy may be required to confirm that the lesion is an FNH.

Liver cell adenoma, formerly called 'pill' adenoma because of its association with the taking of oral contraceptive pills, also has a solid often homogeneous appearance on cross-sectional imaging. The risk that such lesions can bleed and rupture into the peritoneal cavity usually results in consideration of surgical excision. In an asymptomatic patient this difficult surgical decision is compounded by the risk, even though small, that this lesion may turn malignant. A percutaneous biopsy is usually avoided partly because the specimen can be very hard for the pathologist to interpret, and bleeding may result. Another reason is that puncture of the lesion can result in spillage of tumour if the lesion happened to be a malignant hepatoma, and not suspected because the patient had not been infected with hepatitis B or C and because there was no underlying cirrhosis. Again the measurement of alpha-fetoprotein can be useful in this context, as a high reading can alert the clinician to the possibility that the lesion is a hepatoma. A hepatoma might also be suspected by the presence of a satellite lesion protruding from the main lesion.

In summary, the majority of solid lesions remaining after a haemangioma has been excluded are benign neoplasms. The lack of specific imaging characteristics often makes separation of benign from malignant lesions difficult. All must be regarded as possibly malignant at the outset, particularly in older persons, when the liver or a liver mass is palpable, when liver function is disturbed or when there is a history of hepatitis B or C. A careful physical examination should include the skin (for melanoma), breast, lungs, lymph nodes, as well as the anus, and abdomen for other abdominal masses. If a lesion can be found outside the liver, the diagnostic problem may be more simply and safely solved by biopsy of that lesion, than by invasive investigation of the liver. A chest X-ray examination should be carried out looking for a lung primary or metastases, and upper and lower gastrointestinal tract endoscopy should be considered, particularly if the serum carcinoembryonic antigen (CEA) level is elevated, looking for stomach or colon cancer (Figure 23.4).

In review, clinical, biochemical and imaging characteristics are useful in assessing the risk of malignancy but none of these can reliably distinguish benign from malignant neoplasms. The index of suspicion rises for the presence of a malignant mass according to the number of risk factors present (Figure 23.5).

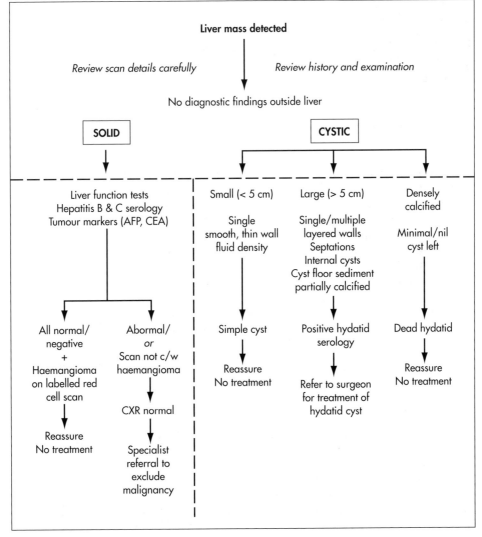

AFP = alpha-fetoprotein; CEA = carcinoembryonic antigen; CXR = chest X-ray

FIGURE 23.4: Investigation of the incidental, scan-detected space-occupying lesion in the liver.

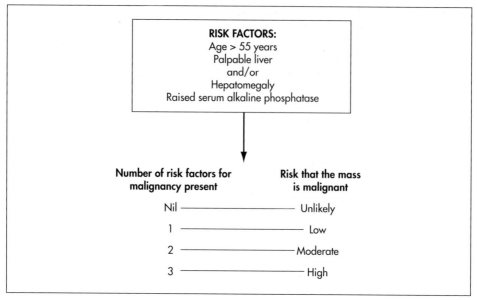

FIGURE 23.5: Solid hepatic mass: indicators of malignancy. Used as a simple screen, these factors allow a reasonable assessment of the likelihood that an incidentally discovered, solid hepatic mass is malignant. The more positive risk factors for malignancy in an incidentally found liver mass, the higher the likelihood of malignancy.

The focal presence or absence of an accumulation of fat within the liver can give the appearance of an incidentaloma of the liver on CT scanning. Such occurrences, commonly in segment four of the liver adjacent to the ligamentum teres, are usually recognised by the radiologist by their radiological characteristics.

Rare liver lesions include teratomas, large biliary adenomas and myxomas. Small biliary adenomas are commonly seen during abdominal operations, but are usually too small to be seen on scanning.

Radioactive pharmaceutical imaging in the investigation of hepatic masses

Radionuclide scans exploit the capacity of certain tissues to selectively concentrate radioactive labelled tracer. Different tracers are utilised to highlight different lesions as a result of selective uptake. The use of radioisotope scanning in the detection and anatomical assessment of abdominal masses has declined with the advent of cross-sectional imaging. However, some radionuclide scans can give additional useful information on the constituent tissues and the functional characteristics of an abdominal mass.

Liver/spleen scan. Here the radiopharmaceutical is bound to a colloid, which is taken up by the reticuloendothelial cells (Kupffer cells) of the liver to give an outline of the whole organ. This whole-organ affinity for the colloid carrying the radioactive marker can then be used to delineate masses that do not contain Kupffer cells as 'cold'

History

A presentation of ascites in a patient known to have chronic liver disease often heralds end-stage disease. Similarly, people with unrecognised cirrhosis can come to medical attention with the development of ascites. The history is of progressive abdominal distension, often with peripheral oedema. This can progress rapidly and be associated with significant abdominal discomfort. History should note details of known liver disease or, in de-novo cases, historical evidence of the cause of liver disease. Acute hepatic disease is possible when the history is short, so note risk factors for viral hepatitis and vascular disease. History should also seek evidence of cardiac, renal or malignant disease (Chapter 18).

Examination

Ascites is usually readily identified on physical examination. The demonstration of shifting dullness is not possible with volumes < 2 L. Smaller amounts of fluid can be found by the finding of periumbilical percussion dullness with the patient on hands and knees. In obese patients, physical examination for ascites can be difficult and inconclusive. In such cases abdominal ultrasound examination is indicated.

Signs of chronic liver disease (Table 22.1) are expected in patients presenting with ascites and cirrhosis. Peripheral oedema is often present. Other complications of chronic liver disease or of the underlying condition may be present. Their absence should raise the possibility of acute hepatic disease or non-cirrhotic portal hypertension. Alternatively, there may be a non-hepatic cause for the ascites. Physical examination may identify other causes of ascites, including cardiac failure and malignant disease. A pleural effusion, particularly on the right, may be present. Umbilical hernias commonly occur in patients with ascites and surgical repair in this circumstance carries a high mortality.

Investigation

The diagnosis of the cause of ascites and exclusion of spontaneous bacterial peritonitis by paracentesis (tapping the peritoneal fluid) is mandatory. The gradient of albumin concentration between the serum and the ascitic fluid is particularly useful. A gradient ≥ 11 g/L strongly suggests portal hypertension (as with cirrhosis). On the other hand, a gradient < 11 g/L suggests malignancy or infection. If the patient is known to have cirrhosis, a low serum–ascites albumin gradient raises the possibility of spontaneous bacterial peritonitis or the development of hepatocellular carcinoma (Chapter 18).

Abdominal ultrasound scans with Doppler studies will document the ascitic fluid and the state of the portal and hepatic vessels.

Mechanisms

Ascites forms in the patient with portal hypertension and marked splanchnic vasodilatation that occurs consequent to cirrhosis. This, in turn, reduces effective arterial blood volume, activating endocrine systems responsible for volume retention; sodium is retained by the kidneys increasing the blood volume and producing ascites. There is an increase in aldosterone production, and a reduction in its removal, often accompanied by inappropriate levels of antidiuretic hormone. There is no convincing evidence to support a role for reduced vascular oncotic pressure due to hypoalbuminaemia in the pathogenesis of ascites.

Management

Symptomatic ascites is initially managed with fluid and sodium restriction (no added salt). If this fails to control the ascites, spironolactone, up to 400 mg/day, can be used. It must be noted that spironolactone will take several days to have an effect. A loop diuretic, such as frusemide, may then be added in resistant cases, initially at 20–40 mg/day. Careful monitoring of renal function and serum electrolytes is needed as renal impairment and electrolyte disturbances followed by hepatic decompensation with encephalopathy can be precipitated by this therapy.

In profound ascites, paracentesis can also be used. Large volumes of ascitic fluid can be safely removed, especially if peripheral oedema is present; albumin should be infused during large-volume paracentesis (> 3 L).

There is evidence that intravenous albumin may be of value in the therapy of ascitic patients when used in combination with diuretics or paracentesis and during treatment for spontaneous bacterial peritonitis or the hepatorenal syndrome.

Refractory ascites is an indicator of a poor prognosis. TIPS may be of value in the control of refractory ascites. The success of TIPS is tempered by portosystemic encephalopathy and shunt occlusion. The patient's suitability for liver transplantation should be considered.

Peritoneovenous shunts can be used but are fraught with problems including infection, blockage and stimulation of the coagulation cascade (causing disseminated intravascular coagulation).

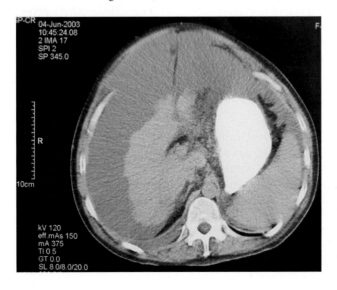

FIGURE 22.3: CT scan showing marked ascites in a patient with cirrhosis secondary to excessive alcohol consumption. Note the small liver, large spleen and ascites.

ASCITES, FEVER AND PAIN: SPONTANEOUS BACTERIAL PERITONITIS

Spontaneous bacterial peritonitis is nearly always an indicator of severe liver disease. It carries a poor short- and long-term prognosis. There is a greater risk of this complication when the ascitic protein level is low. *It may be asymptomatic initially.*

History and examination

The presenting features of spontaneous bacterial peritonitis are ascites with fever, abdominal pain, jaundice, confusion and abdominal tenderness, but there may be no symptoms. There may be a history of severe acute or chronic liver disease. Ascitic fluid is a prerequisite for this condition. There is likely to be large-volume ascites, but it is possible even when peritoneal fluid is not clinically detectable. Signs of peritonitis may be absent, and death rapid. As few as 10% of patients will have rebound tenderness or shock at presentation.

Management

Ascitic fluid must be sampled and examined in all patients with ascites and a recent decompensation (Chapter 18); this should be done on admission regardless of clinical signs. Of all cirrhotic patients with ascites admitted to hospital, 12–15% will have spontaneous bacterial peritonitis. An ascitic polymorphonuclear leucocyte count ≥ 250 cells/L is indicative of the condition. Ascitic fluid cultures should be collected and the samples inoculated into blood culture bottles, at the bedside. Cefotaxime is adequate antibiotic therapy in most cases.

Common organisms include *Escherichia coli*, *Streptococcus pneumoniae* and *Klebsiella*. Spread to the peritoneum appears to be via the blood. Bacteria may also breach a mucosal barrier, as occurs during gastrointestinal haemorrhage or instrumentation.

The lower the ascitic fluid protein concentration, the more likely spontaneous bacterial peritonitis becomes. Peritoneal macrophage dysfunction and reduced opsonic capacity of ascitic fluid may allow progression of colonisation of infection.

Secondary peritonitis following perforation of a viscus needs to be excluded, as this would also require surgical intervention. Such surgery would carry a very high mortality. Cirrhotic patients with ascites and secondary peritonitis can also display a paucity of clinical signs.

HEPATIC ENCEPHALOPATHY IN THE CIRRHOTIC PATIENT

The precise mechanisms responsible for this process are unclear. Under normal circumstances, the liver detoxifies neuroactive nitrogenous metabolites that pass into the portal system from the gastrointestinal tract. With the loss of functional hepatocytes and/or portosystemic shunting of blood, these 'toxins' reach the systemic circulation where they may alter central nervous system function.

History and examination

The clinical features and grades of hepatic encephalopathy are shown in Table 22.8.

Encephalopathy in cirrhotic patients may occur in a subclinical form, demonstrable only by psychometric testing. Although not easily identified, this chronic, low-grade deficit can adversely affect the patient's functional capacity and quality of life.

Hepatic encephalopathy accompanying severe, acute liver disease carries a grave prognosis and is accompanied by the clinical features of acute disease. In chronic

liver disease with appropriate clinical features (above), milder, overt long-term encephalopathy may be found. Insomnia can be an early feature. A reversal of normal sleep patterns (sleeping during daylight hours and waking at night) is suggestive of early encephalopathy. More profound encephalopathy accompanies acute episodes of decompensation (e.g., infection, gastrointestinal bleeding) or progression to end-stage liver failure. Drug effects (especially sedatives), electrolyte abnormalities (diuretics), constipation, dietary protein load and renal failure should also be considered as precipitants (Table 22.9).

TABLE 22.8: Grades of severity of hepatic encephalopathy

Grade	Clinical features
I	Personality and mood changes, disturbed sleep pattern, poor hand writing, fetor, asterixis
II	Mild disorientation, inappropriate behaviour, slurred speech, ataxia, hyporeflexia
III	Disoriented, amnesia, somnolent but rousable, incoherent speech, marked asterixis, hyper-reflexia, clonus, rigidity
IV	A. Responsive to painful stimuli, hypotonia, hyporeflexia, hyperventilation B. Unresponsive, decorticate/decerebrate posture

---

TABLE 22.9: Factors (and possible mechanisms) that may precipitate hepatic encephalopathy in chronic liver disease

- Gastrointestinal bleeding (increasing ammonia and other toxin load)
- High dietary protein intake or constipation (increases ammonia and other toxins)
- Electrolyte disturbances, e.g., after diuretics (hypokalaemia increases the renal production of ammonia, while alkalosis increases the amount of ammonia and other toxins that cross the blood–brain barrier)
- Infection
- Deteriorating liver function, e.g., alcoholic binge, development of hepatoma
- Drugs, e.g., sedatives
- Metabolic, e.g., hypoglycaemia, hypoxia, hypercapnia, anaemia, myxoedema

---

Infection may be present without fever, leucocytosis or localising signs. A systematic search for evidence of sepsis is required, with a chest X-ray examination and cultures of blood, urine, ascites and sputum.

Portosystemic shunting, surgical or spontaneous, also often results in hepatic encephalopathy. Serum ammonia levels are useful in detecting unsuspected significant portosystemic shunts, as are Doppler ultrasound studies.

Management

Management of hepatic encephalopathy attempts to improve the underlying condition, together with supportive measures and the reduction of the amount of 'toxins' entering the circulation from the intestine. A low protein diet is appropriate. Treatment is directed at any precipitating event, such as sepsis or gastrointestinal bleeding. The addition of lactulose, to acidify the colonic contents and act as a cathartic, is helpful. Alterations in nitrogen, fatty acid and glutamine metabolism of colonic bacteria may also contribute to the activity of this agent. Lactulose decreases the psychometric abnormalities associated with subclinical encephalopathy as well as improving clinically overt encephalopathy. Neomycin suppresses the production of 'toxins' by bowel bacteria and is as effective as lactulose. The combination of these two agents is unlikely to provide added benefit. Patients should not be permitted to become constipated and great care must be taken with the use of medications. Zinc, which may increase the capacity to metabolise ammonia, can be useful in malnourished patients. Hepatic transplantation will reverse the condition.

LIVER DISEASE IN PREGNANCY

In normal pregnancy, serum levels of AST and ALT are not altered, but the GGT level is reduced. ALP levels, on the other hand, may double after three months. Serum albumin concentration is reduced slightly by haemodilution.

Hepatic diseases during pregnancy are generally managed as if the patient were not pregnant. Liver disease in pregnancy can conveniently be divided into disease which is incidental to the pregnancy, disease which is exacerbated by the pregnancy, and pregnancy-specific disorders (see Table 22.10). Severe chronic liver disease reduces fertility such that decompensated chronic liver disease is not common in pregnant women. Pregnancy does not preclude hepatic transplantation for acute hepatic failure. Furthermore, past hepatic transplantation does not prevent subsequent successful pregnancy.

History

Patients presenting with liver disease in pregnancy require prompt assessment and close follow-up because severe life-threatening illness may rapidly follow a seemingly mild prodrome.

Timing of the onset of illness should be noted. Hyperemesis gravidarum evolves early in the pregnancy. Cholestasis of pregnancy, acute fatty liver and pre-eclampsia usually occur in the third trimester.

In cholestasis of pregnancy, itch is a predominant feature. There may be a history of a similar problem in previous pregnancies or after taking oral contraceptives.

Nausea and vomiting with abdominal pain, especially in late pregnancy, indicate a need for complete and careful assessment for pre-eclampsia and acute fatty liver, especially if there is right upper quadrant pain. However, right upper quadrant pain at any stage in pregnancy could reflect a hepatitic process, biliary disease, a change in a hepatic mass lesion or vascular disease (Table 22.10).

Drug and alcohol consumption must be considered, and history of potential exposure to infectious agents sought.

TABLE 22.10: Liver disease in pregnancy

Disease	Cause	Comment
Incidental to pregnancy	Viral hepatitis	Most common cause of liver disease in pregnancy
	Alcohol related	—
	Autoimmune chronic active hepatitis	Most prevalent in females of reproductive age
Related to pregnancy (possibly influenced by hormones present in pregnancy)	Complicated gallstone disease	Bile ducts enlarge in pregnancy, tend to regress after delivery
	Hepatic adenoma	May enlarge and bleed, rare
	Focal nodular hyperplasia	May enlarge
	Budd-Chiari syndrome	Hepatic venous outflow obstruction
Specific to pregnancy	Severe hyperemesis gravidarum	Intractable vomiting causing ketosis; elevated aminotransferases
	Benign intrahepatic cholestasis	See text
	Acute fatty liver of pregnancy	See text
	Pre-eclampsia (HELLP)	See text

Examination

Scratch marks with or without jaundice are the physical findings in cholestasis of pregnancy. Hypertension and proteinuria (on urinalysis) and hyper-reflexia suggest pre-eclampsia. Jaundice, right upper quadrant tenderness and hepatomegaly are non-specific but warrant intensive investigation. Signs of hepatic decompensation with fulminant hepatic failure, progressive jaundice, encephalopathy, haemorrhage, or sepsis may mark preterminal disease. Conditions not specifically associated with pregnancy present with the same clinical features as are seen in the non-pregnant patient.

Investigation

Elevations in serum ALP levels may be predominant in cholestasis and biliary disease. Serum transaminase levels can also rise in these conditions. Evaluation of serum bile acid levels is helpful in the assessment of cholestasis of pregnancy.

Marked elevations (> 1000 U/L) of transaminase levels are likely to indicate viral hepatitis. Levels greater than 500 U/L may accompany pre-eclampsia; while in acute fatty liver, transaminase levels generally are between 300 and 500 U/L.

Assessment of the full blood count, blood film and coagulation profile is vital in liver disease in late pregnancy. Abnormalities in these mark severe life-threatening disease (e.g., acute fatty liver of pregnancy, or HELLP syndrome), requiring prompt intervention.

When acute fatty liver or severe pre-eclampsia is considered likely, the need for urgent intervention (delivery) is determined on the basis of the clinical assessment and basic blood test results. In less urgent circumstances, organ imaging with ultrasound may be used to exclude gallstones or hepatic mass lesions, or with Doppler studies, vascular disease (e.g., Budd-Chiari syndrome). Where the clinical setting is suggestive, viral and autoimmune serology should also be considered.

SPECIFIC HEPATIC DISEASES

Viral hepatitis

Hepatitis A (HAV). The hepatitis A virus is an RNA picornavirus transmitted by the faecal-oral route. It is not cytopathic to the hepatocyte; liver injury occurs as a consequence of T lymphocyte activity. The incubation period is 15–45 days (mean: 30 days). In the pre-icteric phase there is viraemia, and the virus is also present in saliva and urine. Faecal viral shedding occurs late in the incubation period and extends for approximately two weeks. Viral shedding ceases about the time the patient becomes icteric. Vertical transmission is not a feature.

Hepatitis A is a self-limiting acute illness. The diagnosis is established by finding IgM antibodies to the hepatitis A virus in the presence of an acute hepatitic illness. This virus does not cause chronic liver disease. There is a prodromal illness in 85% of icteric cases. Overall mortality is 0.1%, but this increases with age to approximately 1% in those over 40 years. Serum transaminase levels often reach several thousand units per litre and may remain elevated, at a much lesser extent, for months after the acute illness settles. Especially in adults, 10–20% of cases develop a relapsing course over several months. Occasionally, protracted cholestasis may develop which can benefit from cholestyramine or corticosteroid therapy.

The proportion of symptomatic cases increases with age. In toddlers, approximately 10% of cases are symptomatic. On the other hand, between 50 and 70% of adults develop the symptomatic illness. The incidence of severe hepatitis and fulminant hepatic failure increases with increasing age. However, more than 60% of cases with hepatitis A fulminant hepatic failure survive without liver transplantation. In Australia there is a reduction in childhood exposure to hepatitis A, and so a reduction in immunity in the young adult population. There is little immunity in adults younger than 30 years. Overseas travel to areas of high prevalence carries a risk of acquiring hepatitis A (even if travel is restricted to five-star hotels).

Vaccination is effective and should be considered for those at risk. Those at risk include travellers, plumbers and sewer workers, paediatric nurses and child care staff, and people exposed during local epidemics. Vaccination could also be offered to food handlers who, if infected, would represent a risk to others. People with compensated chronic liver disease should consider vaccination, as acute hepatitis A infection could precipitate a life-threatening decompensation. The use of passive immunity using pooled immunoglobulin is of limited temporary value.

Hepatitis B (HBV). Hepatitis B virus is a hardy, highly infectious DNA virus. There is an incubation period of 30–180 days (mean: 60–90 days) (Figure 22.4). Acute hepatitis occurs in approximately 25% of those who acquire the virus, with approximately 1% developing fulminant hepatic failure. Most cases are asymptomatic and recover completely, unaware of the infection. In hepatitis B infection, liver injury is mediated by T lymphocytes; the virus itself does not seem to cause hepatocyte death.

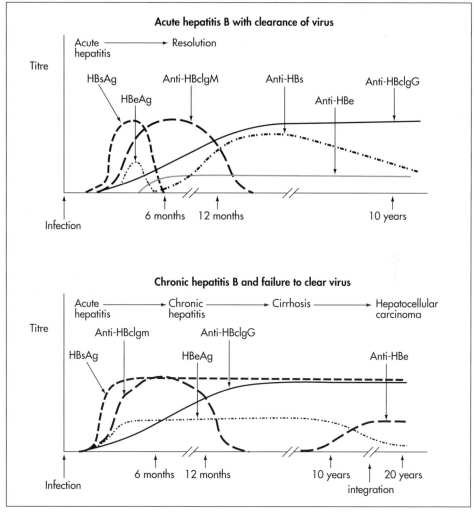

FIGURE 22.4: Hepatitis B serology in acute infection with viral clearance and chronic infection without viral clearance.
(Based on the Australian Gastroenterology Institute.)

Five to 10% of adults who acquire hepatitis B progress to chronic infection (Figure 22.5). In these, the prognosis is dependent on the degree of liver injury and the duration of infection. Between 70 and 90% evolve a 'carrier state' or immune tolerance, and the disease progresses slowly. The remainder develop more rapidly progressive disease. Eventually, chronic hepatitis B results in cirrhosis and/or hepatocellular carcinoma. Well-compensated, chronic hepatitis B liver disease has a five-year survival of 84%. Five-year survival in decompensated chronic hepatitis B is only 14%. Progression from milder forms of chronic hepatitis to more aggressive disease and to cirrhosis may occur. It is also possible for a patient with chronic hepatitis B to spontaneously clear the virus, mounting an immune response to the virus. This is usually associated with an episode of clinical hepatitis and is associated with loss of viral antigens and the development of antibodies. After a period of chronic infection, hepatitis B virus DNA may integrate into the hepatocyte genome, preventing its complete removal and predisposing to hepatocellular carcinoma. Worldwide, this virus is the major cause

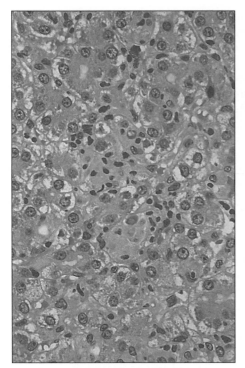

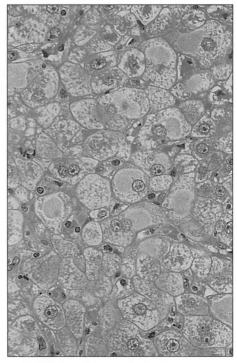

FIGURE 22.5A: Viral hepatitis, acute, classic type. The inflammatory infiltrate has a perivenular accentuation, which is typically seen in the early phase of acute viral hepatitis.

(From Kanel and Korula, Liver Biopsy Evaluation, *2000, Saunders, with permission.)*

FIGURE 22.5B: Viral hepatitis, chronic, type B. The haematoxylin-eosin (H & E) stain shows discrete intracytoplasmic inclusions having a finely granular 'ground-glass' appearance, with peripheral cytoplasmic clearing. This staining characteristic represents proliferation of the endoplasmic reticulum synthesising the hepatitis B antigen (HBsAg) particles.

(From Kanel and Korula, Liver Biopsy Evaluation, *2000, Saunders, with permission.)*

of hepatocellular carcinoma. Supercoiled hepatitis B DNA within hepatocytes is also resistant to removal by current therapies.

The tests used in the assessment of viral hepatitis B infection are outlined in Table 22.4.

The hepatitis B virus is physically resilient and extremely infectious. It is present in most body fluids of those infected and can readily be transmitted to close contacts. People living in the same house as the patient are at risk and should be vaccinated. Sharing needles among intravenous drug users, sexual exposure and inadequately sterilised skin piercing equipment (e.g., tattooing) carry a very high risk of transmitting the virus. Vertical transmission readily occurs. This is usually at the time of birth, and immunisation provides good protection for the infant. The presence of hepatitis B infection also needs to be considered in patients born in areas were there is a high prevalence, such as southern and eastern Europe and South East Asia.

Passive immunity against hepatitis B can be achieved with an injection of hyperimmune immunoglobulin directed against hepatitis B (HBIG) within 72 hours of exposure. Active immunity through a course of three injections of surface antigen

is safe and effective. However, a small proportion of individuals are not capable of mounting a response to this vaccine. This is especially a problem with increasing age, in immunocompromised persons, those on dialysis and obese individuals.

When there is chronic hepatitis B, therapy with lamivudine, adefovir and/or interferon alfa (5 million units daily for 16 weeks) should be considered, although cure (clearance of the virus) is not achieved. Those with chronic hepatitis, raised ALT and the presence of HBV DNA or hepatitis B e antigen (HBeAg) are suitable. Response to therapy may be marked by a 'flare up' of clinical symptoms.

Side effects of *interferon* include a flu-like syndrome early, and later headaches, weight loss, alopecia, and bone marrow suppression; depression may also occur. With interferon, higher ALT levels, recent acquisition of the virus and low HBV DNA titres are associated with good long-term responses. Thirty to 50% of selected cases lose circulating HBV DNA and HBeAg and become anti-HBeAg positive. Clearance of surface antigen is possible in a small proportion of patients. Improvement may continue for years after the completion of treatment. Five to ten per cent of patients relapse over five years after treatment. Interferon therapy is generally not useful if there is combined infection with hepatitis C or D. Response in the presence of HIV infection is poor.

Lamivudine is generally well tolerated over years of therapy, with response rates similar to those for interferon. Long-term lamivudine therapy is associated with the development of resistant mutants (YMDD variant). Long-term lamivudine or *adefovir* therapy is required to maintain hepatitis B virus suppression but is associated with concerns over adverse effects, resistance and costs. Relapse is common on drug withdrawal and it remains unclear as to how long such treatment should be continued. Although therapy combining pegylated interferon and lamivudine has been shown to be more effective in suppressing the virus than monotherapy, response rates (seroconversion) remain disappointing.

Liver transplantation is a therapeutic option in those with end-stage chronic hepatitis B. If the patient is HBV DNA negative, a good response to transplantation is possible. On the other hand, liver transplantation into a HBV DNA-positive patient is often followed by severe recurrent disease, often rapidly progressing to graft destruction (fibrosing cholestatic hepatitis). Antiviral therapy prior to transplantation may improve outcomes.

A number of *mutant varieties of hepatitis B* have been identified. A 'precore' mutant, which does not produce e antigen, may be associated with more severe acute hepatitis and fulminant hepatic failure. The serum of patients infected with this variant is negative for e antigen but positive for surface antigen and HBV DNA. Another form of hepatitis B has evolved an alteration in the surface antigen that allows it to escape the immunity afforded by antibodies to this antigen (and thus vaccination).

Hepatitis D virus (HDV). Hepatitis D virus infection can only occur in the presence of hepatitis B. This RNA virus uses the hepatitis B surface antigen as part of its own structure, making it totally dependent on hepatitis B. Hepatitis D occurs as either a co-infection, when acquired together with hepatitis B, or as a superinfection, when acquired by a chronic carrier of hepatitis B. Transmission of the virus is similar to that of hepatitis B. The combined infection produces more severe liver injury and a worse prognosis. *Therapy with interferon or liver transplantation is of limited value.*

Hepatitis C virus (HCV). Hepatitis C virus is an RNA virus, which is thought to be directly cytopathic to the hepatocyte (Figure 22.6). Prior to routine screening for this virus, it was responsible for at least 90% of cases of post-transfusion non-A non-B hepatitis. The carrier rate in the general population is unclear, but is probably between 0.2 and 1%. The incubation period for acute hepatitis C is 15–160 days (mean: 50 days). In the majority of cases, the acquisition of hepatitis C virus is not associated

with an acute symptomatic illness. However, chronic infection is common, occurring in up to 80% of infected cases. Of those who acquire hepatitis C, approximately 10-15% develop severe liver disease, which can take decades to develop. Hepatic failure and hepatocellular carcinoma may then follow. Significant hepatitis or liver injury (on liver biopsy) can be associated with normal serum ALT levels. Conversely, some people with mild histological liver damage have serum ALT levels greater than two or three times the upper limit of normal. From this it is apparent that ALT measurements are of limited value in the assessment of the severity of hepatitis C virus infection.

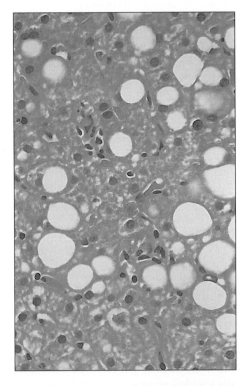

FIGURE 22.6A: Viral hepatitis, chronic, type C. Mild microvesicular fatty change is usually present.
(From Kanel and Korula, Liver Biopsy Evaluation, *2000, Saunders, with permission.)*

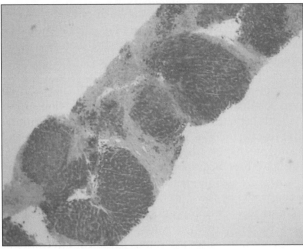

FIGURE 22.6B: Cirrhosis in a patient with chronic hepatitis C. Note regenerative nodules of hepatocytes separated by thick bands of fibrous tissue.

Hepatitis C virus appears to infect and replicate in both hepatocytes and mononuclear cells. Its antigenic structure is variable and appears able to escape immune surveillance. Furthermore, there are multiple genotypes (varieties) of the virus. Prior or current infection with hepatitis C virus does not protect an individual from acquiring further hepatitis C infections. One patient may harbour a number of varieties of hepatitis C virus. The genotype will influence the severity of the infection, response to therapy and its prognosis.

Transmission of hepatitis C in Western society is primarily by sharing needles. In the past, blood transfusion was a major mode. Other modes of parenteral transmission are possible, e.g., needlestick injuries. Sexual transmission is unlikely but seems more possible when another sexually transmitted disease or HIV/AIDS is present. Under normal circumstances, the risk of sexual transmission is very low, approximately 0.1% per year in a monogamous sexual partnership. Vertical transmission is also unusual, occurring in approximately 5% of cases, particularly when the maternal viral load is high. Alcoholics are also at higher risk of acquiring hepatitis C.

Risk factors for the progression of hepatitis C infection to more significant liver injury include excessive alcohol consumption, the presence of fatty liver, acquisition of the virus after the age of 40 years, male gender and co-infection with human immunodeficiency virus or hepatitis B.

Alpha-interferon (especially the pegylated preparations, given by once-weekly injection) in combination with *oral ribavirin* can be very effective in patients with chronic hepatitis C. Response to treatment is more likely with HCV genotypes 2 and 3, histologically less hepatic fibrosis, shorter duration of infection and lower viral titres. Moreover, the viral genotype may influence the severity of the disease and the viral titres. Patients with cirrhosis are less likely to respond to interferon and ribavirin therapy, but significant benefit can still be achieved.

In general, those without cirrhosis and genotypes 2 and 3, can expect a sustained virological response (the loss of HCV RNA from the blood and cure in most) in 80% or more who complete 24 weeks of treatment. Patients with genotype 1 will require treatment for 48 weeks and can reach response rates of over 30%.

Interferon alone appears effective against acute hepatitis C.

Liver transplantation is a therapeutic option in end-stage hepatitis C. Viraemia is common following transplantation. Among transplanted patients, 75–90% will develop chronic hepatitis C at 2–3 years (usually within one year).

Hepatitis C is responsibly for approximately 25% of hepatocellular carcinoma across the world. The incidence is increasing in Western countries and surveillance should be considered in cirrhotic patients. It is of note, however, that antiviral therapy reduces the risk of developing this malignancy.

Hepatitis E virus (HEV). Hepatitis E virus is an enterically transmitted RNA virus. This virus is endemic to India, South-East Asia and Africa. It may also be endemic in the tropical Northern Territory of Australia. Hepatitis E infections occur sporadically or as epidemics. As with hepatitis A infection, the illness is self-limiting and recovery full; no chronic liver disease follows. There is a risk of fulminant hepatic failure especially if acquired during pregnancy, where the mortality approaches 20%. In Australia, most recorded cases have been acquired in overseas endemic areas. The travel history should therefore be noted. Person to person transmission does not seem to occur. The diagnosis can be confirmed by the detection of IgM antibodies against the virus. The antigenic structure of this virus appears stable, and thus an effective vaccine is theoretically feasible.

Hepatitis G is transmitted by blood transfusion and causes persistent infection but does not appear to cause disease.

NON-ALCOHOLIC FATTY LIVER DISEASE AND STEATOHEPATITIS

Non-alcoholic fatty liver disease (NAFLD) is the most common cause for abnormal liver function tests in Australia, USA and UK. The prevalence of approximately 20% has been increasing dramatically over recent years as average body weights of these communities increase. It is often associated with mild (usually up to twice the upper limit of normal) rises in serum transaminase levels, often with elevated GGT levels. Typical patients are overweight with the features of the metabolic syndrome. Thus, strong associations exist with obesity, Type 2 diabetes, hypertension and dyslipidaemia. There is commonly a family history of Type 2 diabetes and evidence of insulin resistance.

When associated with hepatic inflammation (non-alcoholic steatohepatitis), NAFLD can unusually progress to produce significant hepatic fibrosis and eventual cirrhosis (Figure 22.7). Insulin resistance is likely to be the major pathogenic mechanism by which fatty liver occurs in these patients. A subsequent insult or 'second hit' (e.g., endotoxaemia) is thought to precipitate the more aggressive inflammatory steatohepatitis.

Usually there is fatty infiltration of the liver on ultrasonography, with no other apparent cause for abnormal liver function test results. In the typical case, liver biopsy is not necessary. However, if a biopsy is performed, this condition may have histological findings indistinguishable from alcoholic liver injury. Careful history-taking and viral serology are required to clarify the diagnosis in uncertain cases. A carbohydrate deficient transferrin test will be negative (Table 22.11), but no other biochemical features are diagnostically helpful. High BMI, age greater than 50 years, ALT greater

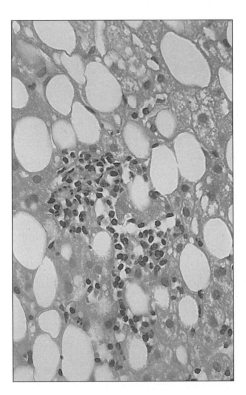

FIGURE 22.7: Non-alcoholic steatohepatitis. The majority of liver cells show a microvesicular fatty change associated with variable degrees of necroinflammatory change.
(From Kanel and Korula, Liver Biopsy Evaluation, *2000, Saunders, with permission.)*

TABLE 22.11: Tests useful in alcoholic liver disease	
Test	Comment
Erythrocyte mean cell volume (MCV)	Round macrocytes, low specificity
Gamma-glutamyl transpeptidase (GGT)	Enzyme-induced by ethanol, level related to long-term prognosis, sensitive but low specificity
Urate, high density lipoprotein and triglycerides	Elevated, low specificity
Carbohydrate deficient transferrin (CDT)	Sensitive and specific, reflects regular excessive ethanol consumption within previous two weeks

than twice the upper limit of normal and triglycerides greater than 1.7 mmol/L have been associated with a greater risk of hepatic fibrosis in NAFLD.

Management is directed towards weight loss and exercise, which can improve insulin sensitivity. When successful, this can result in biochemical and histological improvement. Sudden weight loss may be accompanied by further rises in serum transaminase levels. The rate of weight reduction should be less than 1 kg/week. When the patient's weight fluctuates, the transaminase levels may vary in parallel. Clearly, optimal diabetes control is essential. When hyperlipidaemia is present, it should be managed as usual with diet and medications (e.g., statins) as normally indicated. The use of metformin, ursodeoxycholic acid and thiazolidinediones requires further investigation.

Other causes of hepatic steatosis include excessive alcohol consumption, recent profound weight loss, hyperalimentation, intestinal bypass surgery and thyroid dysfunction. In these cases the condition is asymptomatic and may be discovered when an abnormal liver function profile or hepatomegaly is detected incidentally.

Certain drug toxicity reactions, fatty liver of pregnancy and Reye's syndrome are also associated with hepatic steatosis, but cause clinically apparent illnesses.

Alcoholic liver disease

Although alcohol is a direct hepatotoxin, a patient's nutritional state and genetic make-up will influence the degree of hepatic injury caused by excessive intake of this agent. Alcohol-induced liver injury is generally classified into fatty liver (Figure 22.8), alcoholic hepatitis and cirrhosis. The mainstay of therapy is abstinence from alcohol.

In general fatty liver is considered reversible if excessive alcohol consumption is ceased. Recovery and good hepatic function is expected. However, if drinking continues, the degree of fatty change is a prognostic indicator of significant long-term liver injury. Clinically there is hepatomegaly. There are no peripheral signs of chronic liver disease. Serum transaminases and especially GGT levels are moderately raised. When serum AST levels are two or more times greater than the ALT level, alcoholic liver disease is more likely the cause. (This does not apply in the presence of cirrhosis.) Fatty infiltration may be apparent on ultrasonography.

In alcoholic hepatitis there is active inflammatory injury to the liver. This may be mild, even subclinical, or severe and life-threatening. The severe form is typified by a mild fever, jaundice, neutrophil leucocytosis, moderate elevations of serum transaminase levels (usually < 300 U/L) and tender hepatomegaly. There may be a hepatic bruit. Liver failure with encephalopathy, ascites, gastrointestinal bleeding (often from oesophageal varices) and sepsis may occur.

Treatment is in general supportive. If the patient is malnourished, aggressive nutritional support may improve the short-term outcome; high-kilojoule, high-protein diets are appropriate.

Corticosteroids may improve short-term survival in those with severe acute alcoholic hepatitis and jaundice, a prolonged INR or encephalopathy but no gastrointestinal bleeding. In these patients enteral nutritional supplementation may also improve survival. Furthermore, pentoxifylline (400 mg tds) has been shown to improve survival in severe acute alcoholic hepatitis by reducing the risk of developing the hepatorenal syndrome. Antioxidants have been shown not to be of benefit.

Cirrhosis caused by alcohol consumption is similar clinically to that of other causes. Liver injury can progress to cirrhosis after overt alcoholic hepatitis or in the absence of clinically apparent hepatitis. If alcohol consumption continues, there may be superimposed alcoholic hepatitis and rapid progression to decompensated, end-stage liver disease and death.

It is important to note that severe alcohol-related liver disease can be associated with a substantial reversible component if alcohol is stopped. Hepatocyte function will improve and, with the resolution of hepatocyte swelling, portal hypertension can also ameliorate. With abstinence a remarkable degree of recovery may occur, even though it is possible for liver injury to progress once drinking has ceased.

Propylthiouracil may be of some value in alcoholic liver disease, increasing survival, but it is not widely used. Colchicine may be of benefit in cirrhosis, but data are limited and conflicting.

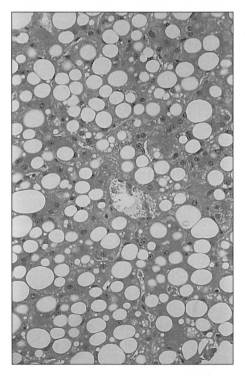

FIGURE 22.8: Alcoholic fatty liver. The majority of hepatocytes show a microvesicular fatty change in an active alcoholic.
(From Kanel and Korula, Liver Biopsy Evaluation, 2000, Saunders, with permission.)

Liver transplantation is a valid therapy, particularly in decompensated post-alcoholic cirrhosis where the long-term outcomes are similar to those of transplantation for other conditions. However, the patient's condition can improve to such a degree with abstinence that transplantation is not required. Care must be taken to exclude alcohol-related injury to other major organs, such as the brain and heart, prior to considering transplantation.

The prevalence of hepatitis C virus is greater in alcoholics than in the general population. The reason for this is not clear. However, the consumption of excessive amounts of alcohol accelerates hepatitis C-associated liver disease. Interface hepatitis (previously known as piecemeal necrosis, where the inflammatory process involving the portal tracts extends into the hepatic acinus/parenchyma) seen on liver biopsy in an alcoholic is likely to be due to hepatitis C infection.

In assessing a patient's alcohol consumption, an estimate of the number of grams of ethanol consumed per day is useful. The National Health and Medical Research Council of Australia recommends that consumption by a male should not exceed an average of 40 g per day, with two alcohol-free days per week. Females should not exceed an average of 20 g per day. Alcohol consumption above these levels is associated with increasing risk of injury. Aim to identify those individuals at risk. Once identified, brief counselling is often effective in reducing alcohol consumption towards safer levels. When applied by the general practitioner, this approach is effective in reducing a community's overall alcohol consumption and reducing alcohol-related social and physical trauma and pathology. 'Skid row'-type alcoholics will not respond to this approach. These severe cases may require more intensive management, but are much less likely to respond favourably.

Systematic questionnaires in relation to alcohol dependency are useful. A number of screening questions have been devised. One of the simplest is the CAGE screening test. In this, patients are asked if they ever felt:

- they needed to **C**ut down their drinking;
- **A**nnoyed by others criticising their drinking;
- **G**uilty about drinking; or
- the need for an **E**ye opener in the morning.

The greater the number of positive responses, the more likely the patient is to have an alcohol dependency problem.

The GGT level could be used to monitor abstinence, but it is non-specific (Table 22.11). GGT levels should normalise over 2–5 weeks of abstinence. Up to one-third of heavy drinkers do not have a raised GGT level. An isolated binge does not usually elevate the GGT level. The carbohydrate deficient transferrin (CDT) test is of more value but is not readily available. The CDT test detects a variant of transferrin in the serum that carries fewer sialic acid moieties than the usual form. The presence of CDT reflects the consumption of excessive amounts of alcohol. Levels rise after several weeks of excessive drinking and remain elevated for approximately two weeks after drinking has ceased.

Haemochromatosis

This is the most common genetic disorder in the Australian Anglo-Celtic population. Untreated, this condition produces iron overload, significantly reducing life expectancy. Moreover, haemochromatosis treated before there is end-organ damage is associated with a normal life expectancy. Patients often present because of the incidental finding of abnormal liver function test results or iron studies, or come to medical attention

after a relative has been diagnosed. Adequate screening and an accurate diagnosis are essential in first- and second-order relatives of confirmed cases.

One of the most common presenting symptoms is unexplained fatigue. Haemochromatosis may be present in 1% of patients in diabetic and rheumatological outpatient clinics, where they may go unrecognised. Cardiac failure in the presence of a cardiomyopathy is another presenting feature, albeit unusual.

Clinically apparent advanced haemochromatosis presents between 50 and 70 years of age (Figure 22.9). The male to female ratio is 4–5:1. Presenting features may include unexplained hepatomegaly, fatigue, loss of libido and hypogonadism (from pituitary iron deposition), cardiac dysfunction from cardiomyopathy, skin pigmentation (from melatonin and iron) and arthralgias with arthropathy. The arthropathy may involve the second and third metacarpophalangeal (MCP) joints as well as proximal interphalangeal (PIP) joints, the knees, wrists and hips. The liver is usually the first organ damaged, and patients may present with cirrhosis or hepatocellular carcinoma. However, a diagnosis of haemochromatosis is not excluded by normal liver function test results.

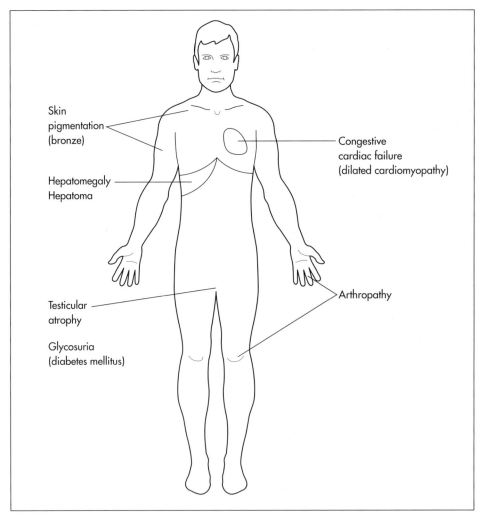

FIGURE 22.9: Clinical features of advanced haemochromatosis.

The defect responsible for iron loading in haemochromatosis appears to lie in deregulation of metabolism and/or intestinal iron absorption. Haemochromatosis is an autosomal recessive condition. The responsible gene (HFE) lies on chromosome 6 near the HLA site. There is approximately 70% linkage with HLA-A3. Approximately 1 in 300 (0.3–1%) Australians of Northern European (including UK) descents are homozygous for the C282Y mutation. People who are homozygous for the C282Y mutation and those with both C282Y and H63D mutations (compound heterozygotes) are at greatest risk of significant iron overload. However, only a limited number of those with these genotypes develop disease. A second defect in iron metabolism may be required to cause pathological iron accumulation. A defect in the hepatic iron-regulatory peptide hepcidin may determine the phenotypic expression of haemochromatosis. Juvenile haemochromatosis has been associated with mutation of the HFE2 (hemojuvelin) gene on chromosome 1.

Iron studies (serum iron, transferrin and ferritin) are used to determine the likelihood of haemochromatosis. In this situation, the transferrin saturation and the serum ferritin concentration are of most value, especially the former. Normal transferrin saturation makes haemochromatosis unlikely.

In males, a transferrin saturation > 62% (in females > 50%) identifies more than 90% of homozygotes. The serum ferritin concentration, a measure of tissue iron stores, predicts approximately 70% of homozygotes. It must be noted that ferritin is an acute-phase reactant and can be non-specifically elevated in many conditions (e.g., alcoholic hepatitis, chronic hepatitis, hepatoma, hyperthyroidism, chronic inflammation, histiocytosis). Moreover, it will be elevated as a direct consequence of hepatocellular injury. As with the transaminases, cytoplasmic ferritin will be lost to the serum when hepatocytes are damaged. Similarly, other components of the iron studies are influenced by many conditions.

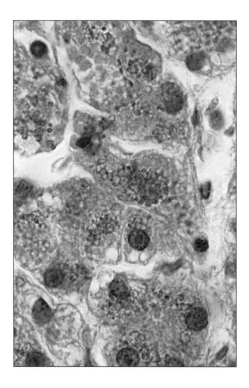

FIGURE 22.10: Haemochromatosis. Abundant haemosiderin pigment is present diffusely throughout the liver.
(From Kanel and Korula, Liver Biopsy Evaluation, 2000, Saunders, with permission.)

The diagnosis of haemochromatosis is established by the measurement of the tissue iron concentration on liver biopsy. The hepatic iron index (HII) is calculated by dividing the liver iron concentration (μmol/g dry weight) by the patient's age in years. An HII > 2 is indicative of haemochromatosis. This is complemented by hepatic histology with staining for iron (Figure 22.10). In haemochromatosis, excess iron occurs predominantly within hepatocytes (as opposed to Kupffer cells in cases of secondary iron overload). A major role of liver biopsy is also to identify the presence of cirrhosis with it implications for long-term prognosis.

Screening of first- and second-degree relatives of patients with haemochromatosis using HFE analysis, fasting serum transferrin saturation and ferritin levels is necessary to identify cases prior to the onset of clinical disease.

Those individuals who are heterozygous for the C282Y mutation may also have abnormal iron test results, especially if they consume excessive amounts of alcohol. In these individuals, iron overload can become significant in the presence of other disorders, such as hereditary spherocytosis, beta-thalassaemia minor, idiopathic sideroblastic anaemia and porphyria cutanea tarda.

The treatment of haemochromatosis is phlebotomy. Venesections may be commenced at weekly intervals and adjusted according to the estimated iron load and the patient's tolerance. Treatment is monitored with serial haemoglobin levels and iron studies. The aim is to achieve and maintain normal iron studies. The haemoglobin level will usually remain stable until the patient is 'de-ironed', then it can fall rapidly. If anaemia becomes problematic before the iron status has been normalised, lower volume or less frequent venesections can be used. Maintenance venesections are started, and continued indefinitely. If the patient is 'de-ironed' within 18 months and there is no end-organ damage, life expectancy is normal.

Haemochromatosis may be complicated by the development of hepatocellular carcinoma, with a 20-fold increased risk. This is more likely in males, in those over the age of 50 years, in the presence of cirrhosis, chronic alcoholism, smoking and past transfusion. It is not related to the amount of iron removed during treatment and only unusually occurs in a non-cirrhotic liver.

Wilson's disease

Wilson's disease occurs in approximately 1 in 40,000 people and is the consequence of mutation of the ATP7B gene on chromosome 13, leading to defective copper trafficking and thereby the progressive accumulation of copper with ongoing liver injury through childhood into adult life. More than 60 polymorphisms have been identified, making genetic testing unhelpful in clinical practice. ATP7B is a trans-Golgi membrane hepatocyte copper-transporting ATPase involved in biliary copper excretion.

Catastrophic haemolysis or an acute hepatic illness are unusual complications. In those who do not succumb to liver disease in early life, neurological abnormalities can evolve in early adulthood (including psychiatric diseases, dysarthria, ataxia, incoordination and tremor). Patients with Wilson's disease may also be at elevated risk of intra-abdominal malignancy.

Low serum caeruloplasmin levels suggest the diagnosis, although this may remain normal in some cases. The presence of Kayser-Fleischer rings (brown deposits around the periphery of the iris which are best seen at slit-lamp examination) suggests this diagnosis. However, Kayser-Fleischer rings are also rarely found in chronic cholestatic liver diseases. Liver biopsy will often demonstrate excessive copper staining, but this occurs in other diseases; chemical analysis of liver tissue copper concentration is

usually a reliable indicator of the diagnosis. Urinary copper excretion and copper dynamic studies may also be needed to establish the diagnosis.

Effective therapy is available for Wilson's disease. D-penicillamine chelates copper and allows its removal from the body. An alternative chelating agent for patients unable to take penicillamine is triethylene tetramine dihydrochloride. Therapy may be supplemented with oral zinc, which leads to inhibition of gastrointestinal copper absorption. Effective chelation therapy early in the disease will stabilise, improve or prevent end-organ injury.

In early, presymptomatic Wilson's disease, zinc (50 mg bd) therapy can prevent progression to clinical disease.

Liver transplantation should be considered when there is liver failure or when chelation therapy fails in the presence of advanced liver disease. Medical therapy is the preferred therapy in those with neurological Wilson's disease, as it is unclear whether transplantation provides any extra benefit in that circumstance.

Alpha-1 antitrypsin deficiency

This autosomal recessive genetic disorder may present in childhood or adult life with features suggestive of chronic hepatitis or with established cirrhosis. This often occurs in the absence of pulmonary disease.

The diagnosis is obtained by measuring the level of alpha-1 antitrypsin in the blood and determining the phenotype. More than 75 variants of the gene have been identified. PiZ and PiS are the most common defective alleles, with the former the most commonly associated with emphysema. Of homozygous deficient (PiZZ) children, approximately 10% will develop significant progressive liver disease. In adults, asymptomatic cirrhosis is a common presentation (Figure 22.11). Serum levels of alpha-1 antitrypsin in homozygotes are often 15% of normal. People who are heterozygous for PiZ may also be predisposed to developing significant liver disease.

Liver biopsy will show the extent of liver injury and the presence of cirrhosis. Histology is characterised by the presence of periodic acid-Schiff (PAS) positive globules within hepatocytes. These globules represent precipitated accumulations of the abnormal alpha-1 antitrypsin protein, which is synthesised but not secreted. Treatment is with liver transplantation.

Heterozygotes may have serum levels of alpha-1 antitrypsin between 40 and 60% of normal and can develop abnormal liver function test profiles without significant liver injury.

Idiopathic, autoimmune chronic hepatitis

Idiopathic, autoimmune chronic hepatitis (IACH) is an uncommon condition predominantly affecting women. It is characterised by the presence of progressive liver disease and a polyclonal hyperglobulinaemia associated with a variety of autoantibodies. Responsiveness to corticosteroid therapy is also typical.

The onset of IACH is usually insidious with progressive fatigue, anorexia and jaundice. Seventy-five per cent of patients are female, mostly between 10 and 40 years of age. In the more aggressive forms, there is progression to cirrhosis and eventually liver failure. Untreated, more than 50% of patients die in 3–5 years.

The aetiology of this condition is unclear, but once established there is progressive cytotoxic T cell-mediated injury of hepatocytes. In certain circumstances, it appears that viral hepatitis could be the initiating event of IACH.

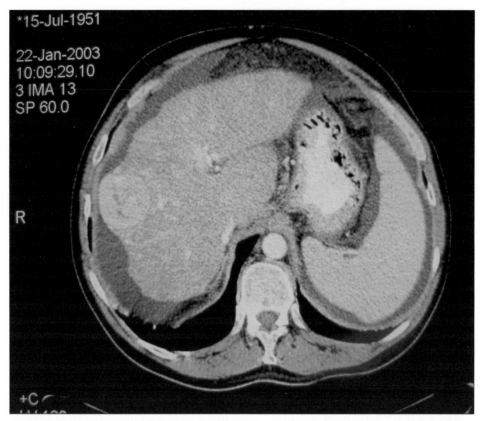

FIGURE 22.11: CT scan showing hepatocellular carcinoma in a patient with cirrhosis secondary to alpha-1 antitrypsin deficiency. Note the tumour enhanced by contrast, the small liver, large spleen and ascites.

Autoantibodies, commonly anti-actin (anti-smooth muscle) and antinuclear antibodies, are present (Type I). There is a prominent polyclonal hypergammaglobulinaemia. In an often aggressive variant (Type II) that usually affects young females, the smooth muscle antibody and antinuclear antibody can be absent while an anti-liver/kidney microsomal antibody (anti-LKM1) is found.

On liver biopsy in aggressive disease, the chronic inflammatory infiltrate, including plasma cells, typically expands the portal areas and extends into the liver lobule, causing erosion of the limiting plate (i.e., interface [or piecemeal] necrosis). Varying degrees of fibrosis may be present. Fibrotic linkage between portal tracts or cirrhosis is a marker of aggressive disease.

Corticosteroid treatment is appropriate when liver biopsy shows more aggressive chronic hepatitis, gammaglobulin levels are greater than twice normal, and ALT levels are greater than five times normal. Corticosteroids with or without azathioprine improve the clinical syndrome and survival. Azathioprine may be used to supplement corticosteroid therapy or to act as a steroid-sparing agent. A positive response to treatment supports the diagnosis. Mortality is reduced, hepatic inflammation and fibrosis are suppressed and symptoms improve on steroids. Sufficient therapy is required to keep the serum transaminase levels below twice the upper limit of normal, preferably normal. Slower progression of the disease may, however, continue. Although some patients can cease therapy after several years, treatment will need to be life-long

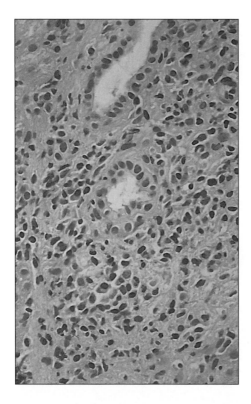

FIGURE 22.12: Autoimmune hepatitis. The portal infiltrate consists of lymphocytes and plasma cells. The interlobar duct is partially infiltrated by lymphocytes.
(From Kanel and Korula, Liver Biopsy Evaluation, *2000, Saunders, with permission.)*

in the majority of cases. If the disease progresses, liver transplantation will eventually need to be considered. The benign, generally non-progressive, chronic persistent hepatitis may not require therapy.

Primary biliary cirrhosis

In primary biliary cirrhosis (PBC) there is an immune-mediated destruction of the small intrahepatic bile ducts. This illness follows a prolonged course with eventual development of cirrhosis and liver failure. Primary biliary cirrhosis typically presents in a middle-aged female with pruritus, a raised ALP level and a positive anti-mitochondrial antibody test.

ALP and, to a lesser extent, serum transaminase levels are usually elevated in patients with primary biliary cirrhosis. The anti-mitochondrial antibody (AMA) is present in the serum in 95% of cases. Its presence is highly suggestive of the diagnosis. IgM levels are often elevated. Differentiation between AMA-negative primary biliary cirrhosis and IACH may be difficult. Smooth muscle and antinuclear antibodies may be present in the former, and low titres of AMA can occur in IACH. A true overlap syndrome can occur, and will present features of both conditions. Furthermore, on liver biopsy, primary biliary cirrhosis can share features with IACH, although differentiation is usually possible (Figure 22.13). If uncertainty remains, a therapeutic trial of corticosteroids is likely to induce an improvement in IACH, but not in primary biliary cirrhosis.

Adverse prognostic signs in primary biliary cirrhosis include a high serum bilirubin concentration (> 100 mmol/L), a low serum albumin concentration, ascites, gastrointestinal bleeding, advanced age, cirrhosis or central cholestasis on liver biopsy and low serum IgM levels.

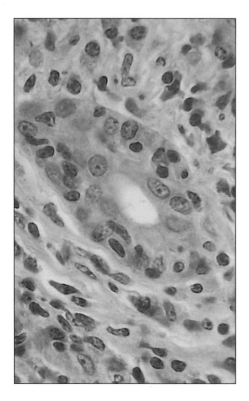

FIGURE 22.13: Primary biliary cirrhosis. This interlobar bile duct is slightly hyperplastic and exhibits lymphocytes within the duct wall.

(From Kanel and Korula, Liver Biopsy Evaluation, *2000, Saunders, with permission.)*

Pruritus is a common clinical feature of primary biliary cirrhosis. This will often respond to ursodeoxycholic acid. Alternative therapy includes cholestyramine. Fat-soluble vitamin deficiency (A, D, E and K), which is secondary to cholestasis, should be sought and treated accordingly. Osteopenia or osteoporosis due to bone mineral density loss may result in disabling fractures. There may be evidence of autoimmune disorders involving other organs such as the eyes, joints and thyroid. Hypercholesterolaemia with xanthelasmas and xanthomas are further features of primary biliary cirrhosis.

Ursodeoxycholic acid is effective therapy for primary biliary cirrhosis, improving survival and delaying the need for transplantation. In the overlap syndrome, a combination of ursodeoxycholic acid and corticosteroids may be required.

End-stage primary biliary cirrhosis is a common indication for liver transplantation in adults, with a success rate of 80% or more. Transplantation should be considered when the serum bilirubin concentration rises progressively above 100 μmol/L, or when there is uncontrolled gastrointestinal bleeding, ascites or intractable pruritus.

Primary sclerosing cholangitis

Primary sclerosing cholangitis (PSC) is characterised by the inflammatory destruction of bile ducts larger than those involved in primary biliary cirrhosis. This condition is considered to be due to an autoimmune process. Approximately 70% of cases of PSC occur in patients with inflammatory bowel disease. Perinuclear anti-neutrophil cytoplasmic antibodies (pANCA) are common, especially in those with associated ulcerative colitis (up to 90% of cases).

The diagnosis of primary sclerosing cholangitis relies on cholangiography identifying focal biliary strictures with associated bead-like dilatations. Liver biopsy is of limited

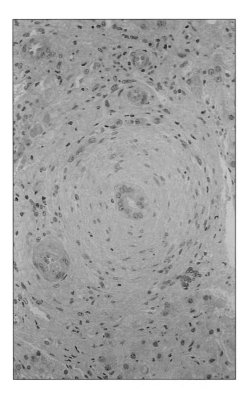

FIGURE 22.14: Primary sclerosing cholangitis. Periductal fibrosis is striking with fibro-obliterative 'onion-skinning' a common feature. Eventually duct depletion occurs.
(From Kanel and Korula, Liver Biopsy Evaluation, *2000, Saunders, with permission.)*

diagnostic value (Figure 22.14). Because of the presence of portal inflammation, there may be difficulty in differentiating primary sclerosing cholangitis from other chronic inflammatory conditions on liver biopsy.

The progression of primary sclerosing cholangitis is difficult to predict. Advanced age, severe changes on liver histology, splenomegaly and high serum bilirubin concentrations are adverse prognostic features.

When localised strictures occur, endoscopic therapy can be considered. Placing stents across strictures or balloon dilation may be of value. The risk of bacterial contamination of the biliary tract needs to be considered, especially if foreign bodies (stents) are left in situ. Recurrent cholangitis is a problem, with and without intervention. Liver transplantation is the only effective treatment for primary sclerosing cholangitis. A successful outcome is expected in more than 70% of well selected cases.

High doses of ursodeoxycholic acid have been reported to be effective in primary sclerosing cholangitis, but that is yet to be confirmed.

Primary cholangiocarcinoma complicates 10–20% of cases of primary sclerosing cholangitis. Sudden rapid progression of pruritus, jaundice and weight loss suggest malignancy. However, this diagnosis can be difficult and may not be made until post mortem. Brush cytology of endoscopic retrograde cholangiopancreatography only provides a positive result in 20% of patients with cholangiocarcinoma. If transplanted, the outcome is poor when primary cholangiocarcinoma is present.

Drugs and the liver

A careful history of medication use is vital in the assessment of the patient with abnormal liver function test results. Toxic or idiosyncratic adverse reactions may occur with many therapeutic agents (Table 22.12). Immune mechanisms are responsible for

many of these reactions. The contraceptive pill may be associated with a number of liver diseases including hepatic adenoma (rare—usually single), hepatocellular carcinoma (very rare), peliosis hepatis (large blood-filled cavities), the Budd-Chiari syndrome (see below), cholestasis and cholesterol gallstones (because of more lithogenic bile).

Paracetamol overdose, deliberate or accidental, is a relatively common cause of severe acute liver disease. In this case toxic metabolites of the drugs are generated by cytochrome P450s, which in turn damage hepatocytes. The induction of these enzymes may enhance paracetamol toxicity.

Polymorphisms of certain P450s may also influence an individual's risk of drug-induced liver injury by affecting the rate of production of toxic metabolites (e.g., nefazodone). The generation of toxic metabolites may also be responsible for liver damage associated with non-steroidal anti-inflammatory drugs.

Liver injury may follow idiosyncratic drug-induced metabolic modification. For example, the statins may induce a mild asymptomatic rise in liver enzymes, but occasionally cause more severe, acute cholestatic hepatitis. This effect seems to be mediated by changes in mevalonic acid metabolism.

Jaundice and other symptoms of drug-induced liver injury generally persist for a limited period after the withdrawal of the offending agent but long-term abnormalities in liver function tests and of hepatic histology may not be as unusual as previously believed. However, late liver failure is not expected. In particular, hepatic injury associated with methyldopa, amiodarone, nitrofurantoin, diclofenac and clavulanic acid/amoxycillin may be followed by chronic, ongoing liver disease.

TABLE 22.12: Drugs and the liver

Liver disease	Clinicopathological features	Drug examples
1. Altered LFTs without liver disease		
Due to microsomal enzyme induction	No clinical features. Raised GGT and ALP. Ground glass cells	Phenytoin, warfarin
Hyperbilirubinaemia	Jaundice rare	Rifampicin
2. Hepatocellular necrosis: hepatocellular necrosis with varying inflammatory change ALT > 5 x normal		
Focal necrosis	Lobular hepatitis, resembles viral hepatitis	Isoniazid, cloxacillin, halothane (mild)
Bridging necrosis	Traces of necrosis connect adjacent portal and/or central veins	Isoniazid, alpha-methyldopa
Zonal necrosis	Well demarcated zone of necrotic hepatocytes; less conspicuous inflammation	Paracetamol, halothane (severe)
Massive necrosis	Entire hepatic acini necrotic. Fulminant hepatic failure	Halothane (fatal), valproic acid, NSAIDs
3. Fatty liver		
Acute fatty change	Usually microvesicular. Clinical features of hepatitis, liver failure	Tetracycline, valproic acid, corticosteroids, NSAIDs, L-asparaginase
Steatohepatitis	Resembles alcoholic hepatitis histologically. Clinical features of chronic liver disease	Perhexiline maleate, amiodarone

(continued)

TABLE 22.12: Drugs and the liver *(continued)*

4. Granulomatous reactions

Non-caseating granulomas	Varying lobular hepatitis, cholestasis or pericholangitis. Usually mixed LFT results, may be hepatocellular	Allopurinol, chlorpromazine, chlorothiazide, isoniazid, phenytoin, sulfonamides

5. Acute cholestasis

Cholestasis without hepatitis	Cholestasis, no inflammation. Pruritus with minimal systemic symptoms. ALP > 2 x normal	OCS, anabolic androgens
Cholestasis with hepatitis	Cholestasis with portal and lobular inflammation. Systemic symptoms. ALT elevated as well as ALP	Chlorpromazine, erythromycin estolate, flucloxacillin
Cholestasis with bile duct injury	Destructive lesions of bile duct epithelium. Clinically similar to acute cholangitis	Flucloxacillin, chlorpromazine

6. Chronic cholestasis: cholestasis > 3 months

Vanishing bile duct syndrome	Paucity of small bile ducts, varying fibrosis. Clinically resembles primary biliary cirrhosis. AMA negative	Chlorpromazine, amitriptyline, flucloxacillin

Liver disease	Clinicopathological features	Drug examples

7. Chronic parenchymal liver disease: abnormalities present > 3 months

Chronic hepatitis	Periportal and/or bridging necrosis, fibrosis or cirrhosis. Clinical and biochemical features of chronic liver disease; liver failure may occur	Alpha-methyldopa, nitrofurantoin, dantrolene
Fibrosis and cirrhosis	Portal hypertension. LFTs often normal	Methotrexate, hypervitaminosis A

8. Vascular disorders

Sinusoidal dilatation	Isolated finding or adjacent to tumours. Hepatomegaly is only clinical feature	OCS
Peliosis hepatis	Destructive lesions of sinusoids resulting in blood-filled lakes	Anabolic androgens
Non-cirrhotic portal hypertension	Portal and perisinusoidal fibrosis. Splenomegaly, oesophageal varices	Vinyl chloride, azathioprine, hypervitaminosis A
Hepatic venous outflow obstruction	Budd-Chiari syndrome, veno-occlusive disease and overlap syndromes	6-thioguanine, OCS, pyrrolizidine alkaloids
Nodular regenerative hyperplasia	Regeneration nodules with minimal fibrosis. Portal hypertension	Azathioprine, dactinomycin

TABLE 22.12: Drugs and the liver		
9. Hepatic tumours		
Focal nodular hyperplasia	Hamartoma, associated vascularity attributable to oestrogens	OCS
Hepatocellular adenoma	Benign neoplasm of hepatocytes	OCS, androgens
Hepatocellular carcinoma	Primary liver cancer (hepatoma)	OCS, androgens
Rarer carcinomas	Fibrolamellar variant, hepatoblastoma, cholangiocarcinoma, cholangiohepatocellular tumours, carcinosarcoma	OCS
Angiosarcoma	Malignant tumour, possibly arises from sinusoidal lining cells	Arsenic, vinyl chloride, thorium dioxide

ALP = alkaline phosphatase; ALT = alanine aminotransferase; AMA = anti-mitochondrial antibody; LFTs = liver function tests; NSAIDs = non-steroidal anti-inflammatory drugs; OCS = oral contraceptive steroids.
(Based on Farrell G, Drug induced liver disease, Edinburgh: Churchill Livingstone, 1994, with permission.)

Vascular and perfusion disorders of the liver

Vasculitis and thrombotic disorders can affect the vessels of the liver. These conditions often produce portal hypertension with varying degrees of hepatocellular dysfunction.

Obstruction of the portal vein may occur in association with sepsis or thrombotic disorders and presents usually with bleeding from varices, or splenomegaly is detected on examination. This results in portal hypertension, often with preservation of hepatocyte function. Portal vein thrombosis can also complicate cirrhosis.

Veno-occlusive disease of the liver is associated with obstruction of the terminal hepatic venules. Precipitating events include exposure to chemotherapeutic agents, bone marrow transplantation and certain plant alkaloids. Clinically, there is right upper quadrant tenderness, hepatomegaly, ascites and jaundice. Progression to liver failure may occur.

The *Budd-Chiari syndrome* involves thrombosis of the hepatic veins. It presents with pain, hepatomegaly and ascites (Chapter 4). There is portal hypertension and loss of hepatocyte function. There are acute and chronic forms of this syndrome. Progression to liver failure is not unusual.

Thrombotic conditions involving the portal and hepatic vessels are associated with hypercoagulable states such as paroxysmal nocturnal haemoglobinuria, polycythaemia rubra vera, pregnancy, the contraceptive pill, lupus anticoagulant, malignancy (e.g., renal, adrenal, testicular, thyroid), a fibrous membrane, amoebic abscess or hydatid cyst and drugs (e.g., azathioprine).

The diagnosis of portal and hepatic vein obstruction can often be established with ultrasonography and Doppler flow studies. Portal venography may be necessary. The diagnosis of veno-occlusive disease requires liver biopsy.

Cardiac disease may cause an abnormal liver function profile. *Hepatic ischaemia* in association with hypotension, as occurs during cardiac arrest, will result in a marked elevation of serum transaminase levels, often to several thousand units per litre. Unlike other conditions, the serum lactate dehydrogenase level is also markedly elevated.

Recovery of the liver is prompt. Liver dysfunction does not interfere with the clinical course of the cause of the hypotension or the prognosis. Moreover, the final prognosis is determined by the underlying illness.

Right-sided heart failure and tricuspid regurgitation cause hepatic congestion, and associated abnormalities in liver function test results are not unusual. Elevations in alkaline phosphatase levels are common and will improve with control of the cardiac failure. Persistent hepatic congestion can eventually lead to fibrosis and cirrhosis.

Hepatocellular carcinoma

It is important to have an understanding of the liver segments. There are eight segments. Each has a separate blood supply from the hepatic artery and portal vein, and a segmental bile duct drains into the right or left hepatic ducts. Removal of separate segments of the liver is feasible and this is important when considering surgical resection of a malignancy.

Cirrhosis is a major predisposing factor in the development of hepatocellular carcinoma. Cirrhosis of any cause may be considered potentially premalignant. However, the most significant aetiological factors include hepatitis B or hepatitis C infection, haemochromatosis and alcohol consumption. Hepatitis B infection and possibly hepatitis C can induce hepatocellular carcinoma without prior cirrhosis.

Symptomatic hepatocellular carcinoma carries a poor prognosis. Effective treatment is not available, but chemotherapy, particularly when delivered via an intra-arterial route, offers some potential benefit. Surgical resection or local ablative therapies (radiofrequency or thermal) is of value for small lesions. Liver transplantation can be considered for lesions up to 3 cm across.

The fibrolamellar variant, usually found in young Caucasian females, responds well to local resection.

Screening of groups at high risk should be considered. Alpha-fetoprotein tests testing every six months has been proposed to be useful. Ultrasonography can identify small, potentially curable lesions.

Benign tumours

Benign hepatic mass lesions are often identified incidentally during investigation (imaging) for unrelated symptoms. Adenomas, focal nodular hyperplasia (FNH) and focal fatty change produce 'masses'. Normal liver function test results are expected. Intervention is not required for focal nodular hyperplasia or fatty change. Hepatic cell adenoma may bleed (50% risk), may be difficult to differentiate from hepatocellular carcinoma and can progress to carcinoma. If an adenoma is suspected, segmental resection is usually indicated (Chapter 23).

Haemangiomas and hepatic cysts are common benign conditions, which are often found incidentally during hepatic imaging. Simple fluid-filled cysts need no further investigation. If a lesion is typical of haemangioma on ultrasound or computer tomography, again no further tests should be necessary. If, however, there remains uncertainty as to the nature of the lesion, a nuclear-labelled red cell scan or MRI can be helpful. Angiography is not usually necessary. Small lesions require no treatment, but large symptomatic lesions may need segmental resection (Chapter 23).

may be prolonged) due to poor absorption of vitamin K, but is rapidly corrected by administering parenteral vitamin K.

There may be constant pain in the right upper quadrant. Severe episodic pain lasting for hours suggests gallstones, possibly in the bile duct. Painless jaundice, on the other hand, is the hallmark of malignant biliary obstruction, as occurs with pancreatic or biliary cancer (Chapter 15; Figure 21.2).

Abdominal ultrasound scans showing dilated extrahepatic and/or intrahepatic ducts indicate the presence of obstruction, while normal duct calibre suggests intrahepatic cholestasis. It should be noted that duct dilatation usually appears 3–5 days after the onset of extrahepatic obstruction and, if the clinical picture is suggestive, a second biliary ultrasound examination may be appropriate.

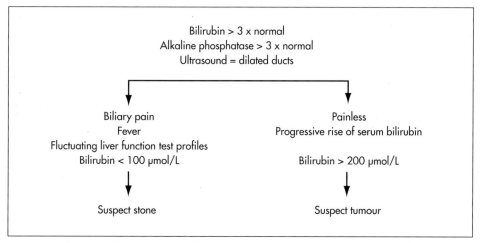

FIGURE 21.2: Typical symptoms and biochemical profiles that help to distinguish biliary obstruction due to stones from malignant biliary obstruction.

Prehepatic jaundice

Unconjugated hyperbilirubinaemia is caused by bilirubin overproduction, impaired uptake by hepatocytes, or impaired delivery to the liver (Table 21.2).

CLINICAL SYNDROMES

Gilbert's disease. Gilbert's disease is the most common cause of an unconjugated hyperbilirubinaemia. Bilirubin conjugation is reduced due to a hereditary deficiency of glucuronyl transferase, which occurs in 5–8% of the population. Bilirubin uptake and transport may also be impaired. Conditions that slow these processes further, such as fasting and febrile illnesses, may produce episodes of frank jaundice. Gilbert's disease is typically identified on routine fasting blood tests in young adults or incidentally in hospitalised patients. There is a mild hyperbilirubinaemia (< 90 µmol/L) and serum transaminases and alkaline phosphatase are normal. Haemolysis is excluded (see below). Patients should be reassured, but counselled that episodic jaundice could occur as the serum bilirubin will fluctuate over time. This condition is completely benign and requires no further investigation.

TABLE 21.2: Mechanisms for the development of unconjugated hyperbilirubinaemia with typical examples

Mechanism	Example
Impaired conjugation	Gilbert's syndrome
Impaired uptake	Drug, e.g., rifampicin
Overproduction: • Red cell destruction • Ineffective erythropoiesis • Red blood cell extravasation	 Haemolysis Severe iron deficiency anaemia Postoperative haematoma
Impaired delivery	Portal-systemic shunt

Bilirubin overproduction. Overproduction arises from accelerated red blood cell destruction as occurs in intravascular and extravascular haemolysis, haematoma resolution or with dyserythropoiesis. This may occur with *chronic haemolysis* as seen in patients with prosthetic heart valves, hereditary spherocytosis, and glucose-6-phosphate dehydrogenase deficiency, or *acute intravascular haemolysis* seen in patients with sickle cell crisis or transfusion reactions. Haemolysis can be diagnosed on the basis of a characteristic blood film, reduced haptoglobin levels and high lactate dehydrogenase levels. In most haemolytic disorders red cell destruction is extravascular (spleen, bone marrow and liver). Bilirubin production is primarily hepatic and renal in intravascular haemolysis.

Ineffective erythropoiesis results in defective red blood cell production in the bone marrow with degradation of unincorporated haemoglobin. This is associated with sideroblastic, megaloblastic and severe iron deficiency anaemia, erythropoietic porphyria and lead poisoning.

Following trauma or surgery, extravasation of blood into tissue or body cavities with reabsorption of the haematoma may also cause a transient rise in unconjugated serum bilirubin as the red blood cells are destroyed.

Impaired delivery to the liver. Impaired delivery of bilirubin to the liver may impede its clearance in those with *portosystemic shunting* or severe congestive heart failure. Decreased flow through the liver reduces the delivery of unconjugated bilirubin to hepatocytes with a resultant rise in serum unconjugated bilirubin.

Certain drugs, such as rifampicin and probenecid, can impair bilirubin uptake by the liver and thereby promote hyperbilirubinaemia.

Crigler-Najjar syndrome. This is a rare hereditary deficiency of UDP glucuronosyl transferase, which causes an unconjugated hyperbilirubinaemia. In Type 1 there is complete absence of the enzyme leading to kernicterus in infancy and early death; children rarely reach adolescence. In Type 2 there is a moderate deficiency and a good prognosis.

Hepatic jaundice
This is discussed in Chapter 22.

Cholestatic and obstructive jaundice
Intrahepatic cholestasis
Drug reactions. Idiosyncratic drug reactions are a relatively common cause of intrahepatic cholestasis. Certain drugs can inhibit hepatobiliary transport systems. Moreover, genetic polymorphisms of biliary transporters may predispose individuals

to drug-induced cholestasis. Offending agents include amoxycillin, flucloxacillin, macrolide antibiotics, non-steroidal anti-inflammatory drugs, oral contraceptives, oral hypoglycaemics, statins, chlorpromazine, and captopril. Jaundice is more frequent after prolonged exposure and in elderly patients.

Thiazolidinediones (e.g., rosiglitazone) have also been found to induce severe, reversible cholestatic hepatitis. Symptoms typically appear some weeks after the onset of treatment, and usually resolve when the medication is withdrawn. However, recovery may take several months.

Drugs such as methyltestosterone and ethinyloestradiol can induce cholestasis which is dose related, in some individuals.

The diagnosis of drug-induced cholestasis is presumed if jaundice occurs shortly after a course of medication and resolves on withdrawal of the drug and other causes been excluded. When the clinical features are atypical, a liver biopsy may be useful. Rechallenge with the offending drug carries risk and is rarely done.

Viral infection. Viral hepatitis, particularly hepatitis A, can occasionally cause intrahepatic cholestasis. Acute hepatitis A can cause a cholestatic hepatitis with an elevated alkaline phosphatase level, fever, arthralgia, and jaundice lasting 2–8 months. Severe alcoholic liver disease can, on occasion, also be associated with a cholestatic picture.

Immune-mediated diseases. Primary biliary cirrhosis and primary sclerosing cholangitis may present as cholestatic jaundice or chronic liver disease or as a combination of both. These diseases are discussed in Chapter 22.

Other. HIV and post surgical or critically ill patients can develop cholestatic jaundice and these are discussed later in this chapter.

Extrahepatic obstructive jaundice

Gallstone/tumour. Extrahepatic biliary obstruction is usually caused by either gallstones (Figures 21.3 and 21.4) or tumours involving the major biliary structures. Approximately 80% of patients with choledocolithiasis have biliary pain (Chapter 4). This is severe abdominal pain that is constant in nature rather than colicky, localises to the epigastrium (or right upper quadrant if cholecystitis is present), and may radiate to the back. The pain lasts from 30 minutes to several hours and occurs episodically. As the bile duct obstruction due to stones is often intermittent, the level of jaundice may fluctuate. However, with stones the obstruction is less complete than that usually seen with malignancy and the serum bilirubin level usually does not exceed 100 µmol/L. Furthermore, with gallstones there is often an abrupt rise and fall of serum transaminase levels over 48 hours coinciding with the pain.

On the other hand, obstructing tumours usually cause painless jaundice. There may be associated weight loss, while fever is unusual and suggests the development of cholangitis. As the obstruction becomes more complete, the level of serum bilirubin increases steadily and is often greater than 150 µmol/L at presentation.

An abdominal ultrasound scan performed to differentiate between the two causes of obstructive jaundice may identify stones within the ducts or a tumour mass. However, equivocal results are not uncommon.

Gallstones (choledocholithiasis) found in the bile duct are usually passed down from the gall bladder through the cystic duct into the common bile duct. Gallstones may also form de novo in the common bile duct. These primary duct stones are uncommon in Western societies. They are more common in Japan and Hong Kong where chronic parasitic infections predispose to their formation. In Western societies, primary duct stones are associated with biliary strictures and may also be found in the common bile duct after a cholecystectomy has been performed. The latter may be retained stones or primary duct stones. Retained stones, left behind at the time of surgery, usually present within three months to two years of the original operation with similar symptoms to those noted before surgery. Primary duct stones may present up to 20–30 years following the original operation.

Tumours causing obstruction of the bile duct include carcinoma of the pancreas or gall bladder, cholangiocarcinoma and metastases to the hepatic hilar lymph nodes. Carcinoma of the pancreas is the most common and causes obstruction of the distal bile duct where it passes in a groove behind the head of the pancreas before entering the duodenum. It is an aggressive tumour that locally invades or obstructs the major vessels which traverse the pancreas, and metastasises early to the lymph nodes and liver (Chapter 15; Figure 21.5). Carcinoma of the ampulla of Vater is an uncommon tumour that may present with progressive obstructive jaundice but can also mimic choledocholithiasis and present with cholangitis or pancreatitis. It is important to distinguish ampullary carcinoma from carcinoma of the pancreas, as it is a relatively slow growing tumour and surgical resection produces a cure in more than 40% of patients.

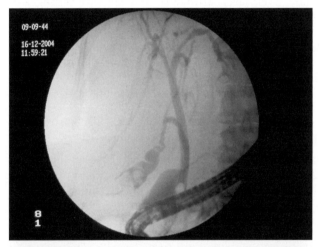

FIGURE 21.3: Endoscopic retrograde cholangiopancreatography demonstrating gallstones within the gall bladder and common bile duct.

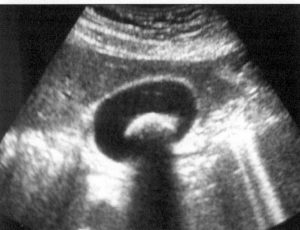

FIGURE 21.4: Ultrasound demonstrating a single large gallstone within the gall bladder. Note the typical shadowing below the stone.

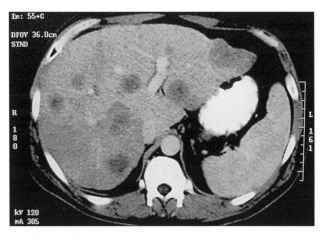

FIGURE 21.5: CT scan showing multiple hepatic metastatic lesions in a patient with colorectal carcinoma.

Benign strictures of the bile duct. These may present with progressive jaundice mimicking a malignant stricture, with cholangitis and pain mimicking choledocholithiasis, or occasionally with the insidious onset of secondary biliary cirrhosis. The most common causes are an ischaemic or traumatic injury following cholecystectomy. These injuries may be due to a suture or clip occluding the bile duct, in which case they present shortly after the operation with cholangitis, a bile leak or increasing jaundice. Interruption of the blood supply to the bile duct leads to slow development of fibrotic strictures, which present at least three months after the original operation and may not become clinically apparent for up to 5–10 years.

Chronic pancreatitis. This condition may also cause stricturing, with obstruction of the lower common bile duct where it passes behind the head of the pancreas. The duct is compressed by fibrosis and oedema within the pancreas (Chapter 5).

There is usually a long history of chronic alcoholic pancreatitis and care needs to be taken to distinguish any change in the liver function test profile due to alcoholic liver disease from that of biliary obstruction.

Infections. Chronic parasitic infestation can lead to episodes of recurrent cholangitis, stricture formation and biliary cirrhosis. These are most common in developing countries in South East Asia, China, India and South America. The major parasites are *Ascaris lumbricoides* and the liver fluke *Clonorchis sinensis.* Diagnosis is made by noting fluctuating alkaline phosphatase and bilirubin levels, recurrent episodes of cholangitis (see 'Cholangitis' below), and demonstrating the worm on cholangiogram. Biliary infection in patients with AIDS may cause jaundice.

DIAGNOSTIC TESTS

Laboratory evaluation

A detailed history, thorough physical examination, combined with appropriate laboratory evaluation yields the diagnosis in most cases of cholestasis. Clues to the diagnosis of various diseases have been mentioned in previous sections. The assessment of this clinical picture then leads to more definitive investigations to establish the diagnosis and treatment plan.

Organ imaging

The results of imaging must be interpreted together with the clinical history and laboratory investigations. If an imaging study is not consistent with the clinical impression, then consideration should be given to further investigation. A comparison of the various imaging modalities is shown in Table 21.3.

Ultrasonography. An abdominal ultrasound scan is simple, widely available and is the *initial test of choice* in suspected obstructive jaundice. It accurately identifies the bile duct diameter (Chapter 23), although it should be noted that the bile duct diameter may be normal shortly after the onset of obstruction. This problem is avoided by repeating the ultrasound scan 5–7 days after the onset of jaundice. Stones in the gall bladder are readily identified, with a false negative rate of only 5%. Bile duct stones are more difficult to identify because the duct passes behind the air-filled duodenum. The false negative rate in this instance approaches 70%. Ultrasound examination may also identify primary tumours in the pancreas, gall bladder and bile duct, and liver metastases. Real-time ultrasound with Doppler flow studies has an advantage over computerised tomography in that it can assess the patency of the portal vein, hepatic artery, inferior vena cava, and splenic vein. This is useful in staging tumours, identifying portal hypertension and identifying vascular thrombosis. Obesity, distortion of the normal anatomy by previous surgery and the presence of intestinal gas obscuring the area of interest can detract from the accuracy of this examination.

Computerised tomography (CT). CT complements ultrasound scanning in the assessment of biliary disease. Where ultrasound scanning has not provided satisfactory images for technical reasons, CT can provide good views of the pancreas, bile ducts

TABLE 21.3: Imaging in jaundice

Test	Advantage	Disadvantage
Ultrasound	Detects dilated ducts Best test for stones in gall bladder Detects small liver masses	Misses ~70% of common bile duct stones Pancreas visualisation may be inadequate
Computerised tomography (CT)	Visualisation of pancreas Detects nodes or metastases Differentiates types of liver masses	Expensive Radiation exposure
Magnetic resonance imaging (MRI)	Similar to CT	Expensive Not as widely available
Endoscopic retrograde cholangiopancreatography (ERCP)	Identifies cause of biliary obstruction in 95% of cases Diagnostic and therapeutic	Invasive
Magnetic resonance cholangiopancreatography (MRCP)	Diagnostic alternative to ERCP	Non-therapeutic
Percutaneous transhepatic cholangiography (PTC)	Alternative to ERCP Diagnostic and therapeutic	Invasive More uncomfortable for the patient
Liver biopsy	Helpful in obscure causes of hepatitis/cholestasis	Invasive May miss diseased tissue
Endoscopic ultrasound	Good for common duct stones and pancreatic masses	Invasive Not widely available

and liver. It is useful in staging malignancy and assessing the extent of local and distant spread. The presence of obesity or overlying bowel gas does not interfere with this examination. CT cholangiography can provide even more detailed information in relation to biliary anatomy and pathology.

Percutaneous transhepatic cholangiography (PTC). PTC is performed by passing a long 22-gauge needle into the liver under radiographic guidance and injecting a radiocontrast agent into the biliary system. The success rate is about 70% in non-dilated ducts and approaches 100% in patients with dilated ducts. PTC enables accurate determination of the level of biliary obstruction in up to 95% of cases and can identify the specific lesion in 75–90% of cases. The rate of complications with PTC is approximately 5%, with the most serious and frequent complications being bile peritonitis, haemorrhage and sepsis. Overall mortality is 0.2–1%.

PTC is more invasive and slightly more uncomfortable for the patient than endoscopic retrograde cholangiopancreatography. Therefore, this procedure is usually performed if a cholangiogram is required and an endoscopic retrograde cholangiopancreatography has been unsuccessful.

Endoscopic retrograde cholangiopancreatography (ERCP). This examination is performed by placing a side-viewing endoscope into the second part of the duodenum and then inserting a small catheter into the bile duct through which a contrast agent can be injected. The advantages this process has over PTC include visualisation of the stomach, duodenum and ampulla, visualisation of the pancreatic duct, and direct viewing of the papilla which can sometimes be involved with cancer. In addition, biopsies and brushings of any lesion can be taken, stones can be removed and stents can be placed to relieve obstruction.

The bile ducts can be successfully cannulated in 90–95% of cases by an experienced operator. The overall complications rate is 5%. The most common and important complications are pancreatitis, cholangitis, bleeding and duodenal perforation, most of which settle with conservative management. Mortality for diagnostic ERCPs is 0.1%, rising to 0.5–1.0% if a sphincterotomy is performed.

Liver biopsy. Biopsies are not typically required for the evaluation of jaundice (Chapter 22). They are usually reserved for the evaluation of suspected hepatocellular or infiltrative liver disease.

Endoscopic ultrasound (EUS). EUS shows promise as a means to evaluate jaundiced patients where ultrasound and CT scanning have not revealed the cause of obstruction. It is useful in evaluating small pancreatic masses, common bile duct stones, and masses in the hilum of the liver.

Magnetic resonance imaging (MRI). MRI yields good images, but this test is more costly and less available than CT. It offers no definite advantage over CT in the evaluation of jaundice.

Magnetic resonance cholangiopancreatography (MRCP). This is non-invasive and may be used to replace diagnostic ERCP. Indications currently include failed ERCP, suspected pancreas divisum and incomplete imaging of the pancreatic duct (e.g., obstructed by tumour).

Scintigraphy (HIDA scanning). Hepatobiliary scintigraphy plays little part in the evaluation of jaundice. The examination is performed by injecting a radiolabelled organic anion (HIDA), which is taken up by the hepatocytes and excreted into the biliary system. The liver and biliary system are then scanned by a gamma camera. The main role for scintigraphy is in evaluating the patency of the cystic duct when cholecystitis is suspected. It is sensitive in detecting the presence of complete bile duct obstruction but it yields false positive results in up to 30% of cases. It is also used to evaluate drainage of the biliary tree non-invasively after biliary surgery.

Intravenous cholangiogram. X-ray tomography of the bile duct is performed following the administration of an intravenous contrast agent, which is excreted by the liver into the bile ducts. Significant elevation of serum bilirubin is associated with failure of uptake of the contrast agent by the liver so the test is only useful for identifying stones in non-obstructed ducts. In the past, intravenous cholangiography has not often been used because of allergic reactions to the contrast agent and poor accuracy. The recent development of new contrast agents with fewer adverse reactions and the use of CT scanning has improved the accuracy.

MANAGEMENT OF SUSPECTED OBSTRUCTIVE JAUNDICE

Bile duct obstruction

Patients with suspected obstructive jaundice should be initially investigated by ultrasonography. If the bile ducts are *not* dilated, the causes of intrahepatic cholestasis need to be considered (Chapter 22); for example, re-examine the patient's drug history, check viral serology (e.g., hepatitis B and C, Epstein-Barr virus and cytomegalovirus), check for autoantibodies (for autoimmune hepatitis) and anti-mitochondrial antibody (for primary biliary cirrhosis). Liver biopsy may sometimes be needed for a definitive diagnosis. Treatment must be directed at the underlying cause and, where necessary, managing the complications of irreversible liver disease.

Patients with *dilated ducts* usually have stones or a tumour.

Tumour

Carcinoma of the pancreas is the most common tumour that causes biliary obstruction (50–60% of tertiary referrals; Chapter 15). The principles of management are similar for other tumours such as cholangiocarcinoma and gall bladder carcinoma (Figure 21.6). An abdominal ultrasound examination will usually identify the tumour mass and the site of obstruction in addition to any liver metastases. If the ultrasound results are equivocal and clinical suspicion is high, then a CT scan may provide more information. Occasionally, cholangiography by ERCP or MRCP is required to define a small pancreatic or bile duct lesion.

Once the diagnosis has been established, the patient should be assessed to determine his or her risks for a surgical resection. For a pancreaticoduodenectomy (Whipple's procedure) or hepatobiliary resection, the morbidity and mortality increase for patients over the age of 70 years. Patients with cardiovascular and pulmonary diseases or diabetes have higher complication rates.

If the patient is fit for surgery, and does not have evidence of tumour spread to lymph nodes or liver, then further assessment for surgical resection may be worth undertaking, although this is not routine. Useful investigations may include:

- angio CT of the liver and pancreas looking for previously undetected liver metastases, and invasion or encasement or involvement of vascular structures such as the portal vein, the superior mesenteric vein and the hepatic artery and its branches, which may preclude the possibility of resection for cure if finding is confirmed;
- duplex scanning of the superior mesenteric and portal veins looking at possible local involvement; and
- laparoscopy looking for small peritoneal seedings or small liver metastases not detected by previous imaging.

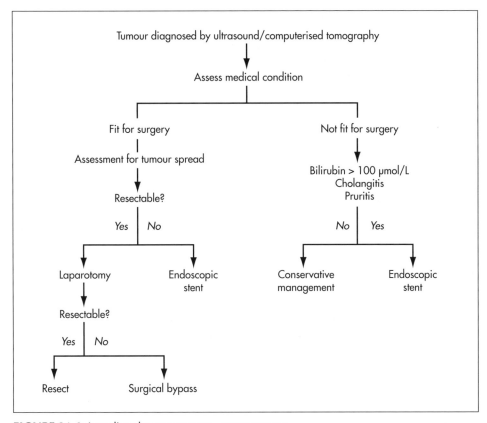

FIGURE 21.6: Jaundice due to tumours—management.

Large tumours of the pancreas (> 4 cm) tend to be unsuitable for resection either because of local involvement or distant metastases. Cholangiocarcinoma of the biliary tree below the confluence and ampullary carcinoma tend to present earlier and are more likely to be resectable. Jaundice caused by carcinoma of the gall bladder, like carcinoma of the pancreas, tends to present late, making resection for cure uncommon.

The optimum management of jaundice in patients with non-resectable disease remains controversial. Prior to the development of endoscopically placed biliary stents, most patients underwent surgical biliary bypass. Surgical bypass, usually with a choledochojejunostomy, is presently restricted to younger and fitter patients who are thought likely to survive for more than six months. In older, frailer patients with a worse prognosis, the morbidity and mortality of endoscopic stenting is less than with surgical bypass.

The other consideration is pancreatic carcinoma causing duodenal obstruction. This occurs in 10% of these patients. Patients with evidence of gastric outlet obstruction should have a biliary bypass and gastroenterostomy.

Stones

Patients with choledocholithiasis can usually be identified by their history of biliary pain, fluctuating jaundice, and their obstructive liver function test profiles. Abdominal ultrasound scans usually demonstrate a dilated bile duct. It should be noted that ultrasound scans are very accurate in identifying stones in the gall bladder; however, the bile duct is more difficult to image as it passes behind the air-filled duodenum and ultrasonography may miss bile duct stones in up to 70% of patients. A high index of suspicion in a patient with a negative or equivocal ultrasound result should prompt further investigation with an ERCP or MRCP to obtain a cholangiogram.

For the purpose of planning management, patients with stones in the common bile duct can be divided into those with and those without a gall bladder (Figure 21.7). In patients who have had a cholecystectomy, ERCP with sphincterotomy and stone extraction is the treatment of choice. Patients with their gall bladder in place have several treatment options. Those who are at high risk for surgery, have severe cholangitis, or have severe gallstone pancreatitis should be treated with ERCP, sphincterotomy and stone extraction. Cholecystectomy can be considered after their other medical conditions have stabilised. In young, fit patients with choledocholithiasis and the gall bladder in situ, laparoscopic cholecystectomy has largely replaced open cholecystectomy. Some surgeons currently favour endoscopic removal of the bile duct stones followed by an elective laparoscopic cholecystectomy. Others reserve endoscopic removal for patients in whom laparoscopic clearance of the common bile duct has been unsuccessful.

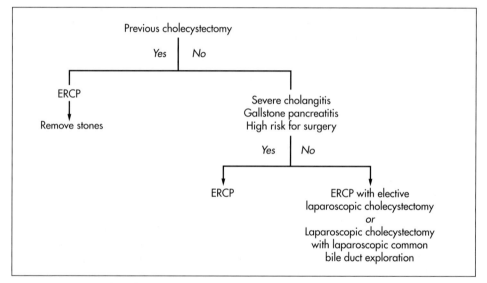

FIGURE 21.7: Jaundice due to stones—management.
ERCP = endoscopic retrograde cholangiopancreatography.

Successful drainage of an obstructed biliary tree is signalled by a gradual fall in serum bilirubin, relief of pruritus over 3–5 days, return of appetite, and improved sense of well-being. These patients have a conjugated hyperbilirubinaemia; 60% of conjugated bilirubin is irreversibly bound to albumin and this limits the rate of fall in serum bilirubin. Albumin is not filtered by the kidneys, and its half-life in serum ranges from 17 days to greater than 20 days. Therefore, serum bilirubin will demonstrate an initial fall of 20–40% as unbound bilirubin is quickly cleared, followed by a gradual fall to normal as the albumin is metabolised.

Cholangitis

Obstruction of the bile duct due to stones and occasionally malignancy allows bacterial overgrowth in the bile. An increase in biliary pressure may disrupt liver defence mechanisms and allow bacteria to invade into the liver parenchyma and blood stream (cholangitis). *Fever, abdominal pain,* and *jaundice* follow (*Charcot's triad*). There may also be changes in mental status and shock. The mortality is 80% if pus is left undrained in the bile ducts. The treatment has two objectives: 1) relief of biliary obstruction; and 2) appropriate antibiotic coverage and fluid resuscitation.

Most cholangitis is mild and responds to appropriate antibiotics so that drainage can be performed electively. However, in about 15% of patients cholangitis is severe and life-threatening. Old age, concomitant medical conditions, a low platelet count, a markedly elevated bilirubin level, and renal failure are markers of severity. If three or more of these factors are present, the cholangitis is severe and requires urgent drainage. Clinical trials have shown that ERCP with sphincterotomy is preferable to open surgical drainage in acute, severe cholangitis.

The main bacterial pathogens are *Escherichia coli, Klebsiella* and *Streptococcus faecalis. Pseudomonas* should also be considered if there has been a previous endoscopic or surgical manipulation of the bile duct. Ampicillin and gentamicin have been recommended for treatment of cholangitis in the past. However, gentamicin does not achieve therapeutic concentrations in the bile and its toxicity is increased in the presence of jaundice, renal impairment and increased age. More recently, a combination of ceftriaxone plus ampicillin, or a ureido-penicillin combined with a betalactam inhibitor such as pipercillin plus tazobactam have been used.

PRURITUS

Pruritus is a common, unpleasant feature of cholestatic syndromes. The exact cause of pruritus is unknown. In cholestatic conditions, pruritus appears to be associated with increased central opioidergic activity.

Pruritus is often worse at bedtime and resolves or improves by morning. Pruritus will occur in 75% of patients with malignant biliary obstruction. Pruritus due to biliary obstruction improves over 3–5 days following relief of the obstruction.

In patients with intrahepatic cholestasis, a variety of medical regimens have been used. Treatment is largely empirical and responses are variable. Bile acid binding resins such as cholestyramine, one 4 g packet four times a day, is reasonable initial therapy, however some patients find its taste unpalatable. Ursodeoxycholic acid is often useful. It is a choleretic agent which replaces the more toxic endogenous bile salts. Rifampicin is effective and may work by inducing P4503A, which, in turn, modifies bile acids, making them less pruritogenic. Antihistamines and topical agents are usually ineffective but may help with mild itching at bedtime. Other drugs with demonstrable benefit are phenobarbitone, H_2-receptor antagonists, methyltestosterone, corticosteroids, and opioid antagonists. In extreme cases charcoal haemofiltration and plasmapheresis have been used with success.

THE POST-SURGICAL AND CRITICALLY ILL, JAUNDICED PATIENT

The evaluation of a post-surgical patient with jaundice is a challenging exercise. The cause is often multifactorial and may include increased bilirubin production from reabsorption of a haematoma, impaired hepatocellular function from decreased blood flow, total parental nutrition (TPN), sepsis and occasionally extrahepatic biliary obstruction (Table 21.4). Therefore, information on the pattern of development, review of the operative and anaesthesia reports, pre- and postoperative drug use, haemodynamic changes and fluid management, and any history of hypovolaemia or hypotension are required.

TABLE 21.4: Distinguishing features that help to determine the cause of postoperative jaundice	
Aetiology	**Feature**
Hypotension	ALT > 1000 U/L, LDH elevated
Drugs, e.g., halothane	None
Infection	Increased white cell count, fever
Total parenteral nutrition (TPN)	Liver function test profiles rise 1–4 weeks after TPN commencement
Haematoma resorption	↑Unconjugated bilirubin
Cardiac failure	Elevated jugular venous pressure, enlarged pulsatile liver
Haemolysis	↑Unconjugated bilirubin, ↑LDH, ↓haptoglobin, abnormal blood smear
Renal failure	↑Creatinine
ALT = alanine aminotransferase; LDH = lactate dehydrogenase.	

Increased bilirubin production can occur from rapid destruction of transfused red cells (20% of administered blood stored for 21 days is destroyed within 24 hours). Other causes of red blood cell destruction include breakdown of red blood cells damaged by cell-savers, reabsorption from haematomas, or haemolysis from heart valves or genetic diseases (e.g., sickle cell anaemia). In these cases, an unconjugated hyperbilirubinaemia develops. The level may be greater than 90 µmol/L if concurrent liver dysfunction is present.

Hypotension causing hepatic ischaemia can occur intra-operatively, in recovery, or postoperatively. The precipitating event may not be obvious and careful review of nursing records and anaesthesia charts is essential. Typically, ischaemic hepatitis presents as a rapid rise of transaminase levels to 1000–10,000 U/L with hyperbilirubinaemia and a rapid fall within 24–48 hours, if blood flow is normalised. The prognosis is related to that of the underlying event, e.g., myocardial infarction, not the hepatic injury.

Systemic infections can cause cholestasis. Up to one-third of septic patients have been found to have elevated serum bilirubin levels. In this circumstance, jaundice most often reflects Gram-negative infections, although Gram-positive organisms have also been implicated. The pathogenesis is unclear, but circulating endotoxins probably cause a reduction in excretion of conjugated bilirubin into the biliary system, but do not affect conjugation.

One of the most difficult aetiologies to identify is that due to drug toxicity, as it is a diagnosis of exclusion. Antibiotics are most often the culprit (e.g., ampicillin), although occasionally an anaesthetic agent (e.g., halothane) is the cause.

Total parenteral nutrition (TPN) causes many liver abnormalities including fatty liver, cholestasis, portal inflammation, gallstone formation and occasionally steatohepatitis and micronodular cirrhosis (Chapter 15). Liver function abnormalities usually occur 1–4 weeks after the initiation of TPN and resolve on discontinuing therapy. Transaminase levels can become elevated within one week, and alkaline phosphatase and gamma-glutamyl transpeptidase (GGT) levels often begin to rise after 3–4 weeks. Increases in serum bilirubin levels can occur but are unusual. The causes are commonly multifactorial. The transaminase rise is most likely due to glucose intolerance, while cholestasis is considered to be the result of abnormal lipid metabolism. Often small adjustments in TPN composition can correct the liver dysfunction and discontinuing the TPN usually leads to regression of dysfunction.

Renal failure will lead to decreased excretion of bilirubin and may cause a mild case of hyperbilirubinaemia to manifest itself as jaundice following surgery.

THE IMMUNOCOMPROMISED PATIENT WHO IS JAUNDICED

Patients who are immunocompromised by infection with HIV or who are receiving immunosuppressive therapy may develop hepatobiliary infections not usually found in the immunocompetent patient. Biliary tract infections can produce marked jaundice and right upper quadrant pain. Other causes of jaundice in these patients include neoplasms and drug reactions (Table 21.5).

TABLE 21.5: Common causes of jaundice in immunosuppressed patients	
Aetiology	**Examples**
Hepatitis—infectious	*Mycobacterium avium intracellulare*, tuberculosis, cytomegalovirus
Hepatitis—drugs	Isoniazid, AZT, sulfonamides
AIDS cholangiopathy	Cytomegalovirus, cryptosporidia
Veno-occlusive disease	Antineoplastic drugs (e.g., busulfan)
Neoplasm	Lymphoma, Kaposi's sarcoma

Human immunodeficiency virus (HIV)

Hepatomegaly is present in 60–80% of patients with AIDS. Jaundice is uncommon but elevation in liver enzyme levels may occur in two-thirds of patients with abnormal histological findings in 85% of patients.

The most common causes of hepatocellular disease in these patients, in order of decreasing frequency, are *Mycobacterium avium intracellulare* (MAI), drugs, cytomegalovirus (CMV), bacillary peliosis hepatis, lymphoma, and *Mycobacterium tuberculosis*. Kaposi's sarcoma, hepatitis C and B and cryptococcal infection are other causes of jaundice. Drugs such as sulfonamides, isoniazid, phenytoin and AZT may cause cholestatic jaundice.

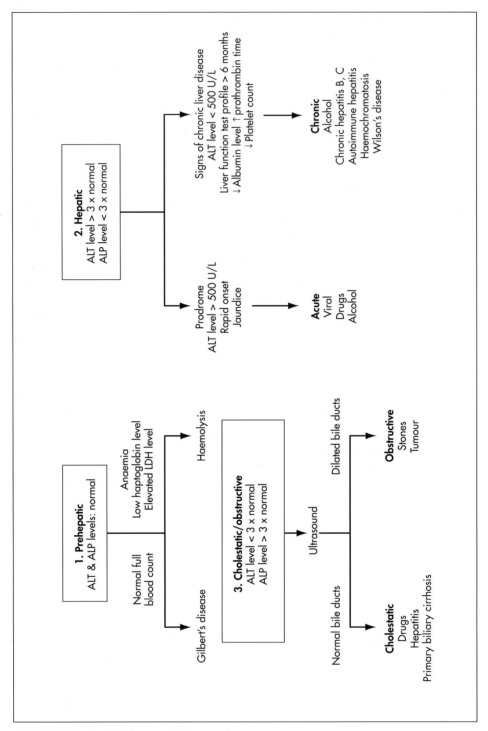

FIGURE 21.8: A clinical approach to jaundice.
AL P= alkaline phosphatase; ALT = alanine aminotransferase; LDH = lactate dehydrogenase.

There is also a syndrome of biliary pain and fever termed AIDS cholangiopathy. However, clinical jaundice is unusual. There are different types: sclerosing cholangitis (focal strictures and dilatations of intrahepatic and extrahepatic bile ducts), papillary stenosis (causing a dilated bile duct) and extrahepatic biliary strictures. The syndrome can be caused by biliary infection with CMV, *Cryptosporidium,* or microsporidia. ERCP with sphincterotomy leads to rapid relief of pain in 80% of patients with sclerosing cholangitis or papillary stenosis.

Acalculous cholecystitis is more common in this group of patients and can be caused by CMV, *Cryptosporidium* and *Campylobacter.* Bile duct obstruction can also occur as a result of primary duct lymphoma, nodal metastases or Kaposi's sarcoma.

Organ transplantation

Patients receiving transplanted organs may develop complications from their immunosuppressive therapy or the transplanted organ. Bone marrow transplantation recipients seem particularly susceptible to developing hepatobiliary dysfunction.

Hepatic graft versus host disease (GVHD). Hepatic GVHD following bone marrow transplant causes cholestasis and jaundice, typically with an erythrodermatous skin rash and diarrhoea. It usually responds to immunosuppression, and progression to cirrhosis occurs rarely.

Veno-occlusive disease. This is the most common cause of jaundice in the first few weeks after bone marrow transplant. Diffuse venous occlusion within the liver leads to rapid onset of ascites, hepatomegaly and jaundice. Up to 75% of patients recover spontaneously; 25% develop multi-organ failure and die.

Viral hepatitis. This may develop following transplantation of any organ. Hepatic CMV infection presents as an acute hepatitis often with extrahepatic disease, and responds to treatment with ganciclovir. Immune suppression may cause an exacerbation of chronic hepatitis B infection leading to acute hepatitis with jaundice. Hepatic abscesses can develop following the use of immunosuppression or transplantation; these are usually diffuse fungal microabscesses.

Drug-induced liver disease. This is common but jaundice is not. Cyclosporin does cause a conjugated hyperbilirubinaemia and jaundice, but other signs of cyclosporin toxicity such as hypertension, renal dysfunction and oedema are also usually present.

Orthotopic liver transplantation. Cholestasis following liver transplantation may reflect an operative complication (e.g., bile duct stricture) or chronic graft rejection (vanishing bile duct syndrome).

Summary

An overview of the approach to jaundice is shown in Figure 21.8.

Further reading

Anonymous. The familial unconjugated hyperbilirubinemias. *Sem Liv Dis* 1994; 14: 356–85.
Bergasa NV. An approach to the management of the pruritus of cholestasis. *Clin Liver Dis* 2004; 8: 55–66, vi.
Cappell MS. Hepatobiliary manifestations of the acquired immune deficiency syndrome. *Am J Gastroenterol* 1991; 86: 1–15.
Faust TW, Reddy KR. Post operative jaundice. *Clin Liver Dis* 2004; 8: 151–66.
Freeman ML, Sielaff TD. A modern approach to malignant hilar biliary obstruction. *Rev Gastroenterol Disord* 2003; 3: 187–201.
Heneghan MA, Lara L. Fulminant hepatic failure. *Semin Gastrointest Dis* 2003; 14: 87–100.

Kraft M, Lerch MM. Gallstone pancreatitis: when is endoscopic retrograde cholangiopancreatography truly necessary? *Curr Gastroenterol Rep* 2003; 5: 125–32.

Mohi-ud-din R, Lewis JH. Drug- and chemical-induced cholestasis. *Clin Liver Dis* 2004; 8: 95–132, vii.

NIH state-of-the-science statement on endoscopic retrograde cholangiopancreatography (ERCP) for diagnosis and therapy. *NIH Consens State Sci Statements* 2002; 19: 1–26.

O'Regan D, Tait P. Imaging of the jaundiced patient. *Hosp Med* 2005; 66: 17–22.

Roche SP, Kobos R. Jaundice in the adult patient. *Am Fam Physician* 2004; 69: 299–304.

Sgro C, Clinard F, Ouazir K *et al.* Incidence of drug-induced hepatic injuries: a French population-based study. *Hepatology* 2002; 36: 451–5.

Tomer G, Shneider BL. Disorders of bile formation and biliary transport. *Gastroenterol Clin North Am* 2003; 32: 839–55, vi.

Trauner M, Wagner M, Fickert P, Zollner G. Molecular regulation of hepatobiliary transport systems: clinical implications for understanding and treating cholestasis. *J Clin Gastroenterol* 2005; 39: S111–24.

chapter **22**

ABNORMAL LIVER FUNCTION TEST RESULTS

AN APPROACH TO THE PATIENT WITH LIVER DISEASE

The liver is a remarkable organ with substantial functional reserve and impressive regenerative capacity. The presence of abnormal liver function profiles, therefore, may not be apparent at the bedside. However, when abnormal liver function test results are found, their significance needs to be assessed in the light of clinical (bedside) findings. The pattern of liver function test abnormalities can be subdivided into either a hepatocellular or cholestatic disease category as discussed below. Organ imaging is an important complementary tool in the assessment of abnormal liver function profiles. The presence of normal liver function profiles makes hepatic disease unlikely, although there are many exceptions, including well-compensated cirrhosis, some cases of chronic hepatitis C, and those with certain space-occupying lesions of the liver.

Liver disease will present as one of a limited number of clinical syndromes. Each syndrome may be caused by a number of specific disease processes. A diagnosis is achieved by paying attention to historical features and physical findings (Table 22.1) and the results of laboratory and other investigations. Only then can specific treatment for the cause of the liver abnormality be planned. Therapy, in many instances, is directed to the management of the clinical problem in addition to treatment of the underlying condition.

In this chapter, liver function tests and their clinical relevance are first discussed because abnormalities are commonly detected in asymptomatic individuals. Next, the common clinical presentations of liver disease are covered. Finally, important liver diseases are described.

TABLE 22.1: Symptoms and signs of liver disease

Symptoms

Fatigue, pruritus, bleeding, abdominal pain, nausea, anorexia, myalgia, jaundice, dark urine, pale stools, fever, weight loss; may be no symptoms

Peripheral signs of chronic liver disease, hepatocellular dysfunction

Spider naevi, palmar erythema, white nails, gynaecomastia, body hair loss, testicular atrophy, hepatomegaly

Signs of portal hypertension

Splenomegaly, ascites, peripheral oedema

Signs of poor hepatocellular synthetic function

Bruising, peripheral oedema (reflecting depleted coagulation factors and albumin levels)

Signs of end-stage liver disease

Wasting, progressive severe fatigue, encephalopathy (asterixis, fetor, coma)

Other signs

Hepatic rub—peritoneal inflammation from underlying infarction or malignancy
Right upper quadrant bruit—intrahepatic shunting, alcoholic hepatitis, malignancy, large haemangioma

LIVER FUNCTION TEST INTERPRETATION

In the initial assessment of a patient with abnormal liver function test results, a number of questions need to be considered:

- Is the illness a primary liver disorder, or is it secondary to some other condition (which could be more clinically important)?

- Is the source of the abnormal test levels extrahepatic? An abnormality in a single 'liver function test' may be due to a non-hepatic cause. Evidence of disease processes involving other organs should be sought.

- Do the liver function test abnormalities signify a serious illness? What is the severity of the illness, i.e., is the cause of the abnormality a threat to the patient's well-being now or in the future? What is the diagnosis and, more importantly, what is the prognosis?

- Is this an acute illness or a chronic one? If chronic, is it compensated or decompensated?

Routine liver function tests usually include serum bilirubin, albumin, international normalised ratio (or prothrombin time), transaminases, alkaline phosphatase, gamma-glutamyl transpeptidase and, in some laboratories, lactate dehydrogenase. Other tests should only be ordered for specific indications.

Bilirubin

Elevated serum bilirubin levels may occur in all forms of liver disease. However, it must be remembered that a jaundiced patient does not necessarily have significant hepatic disease. Serum levels of bilirubin reflect production, hepatic uptake, processing (conjugation) and secretion. The physiology of bilirubin and an approach to diagnosis and management of jaundice is described in Chapter 21.

The value of the ratio between conjugated and unconjugated bilirubin in distinguishing the nature of a liver disorder is limited. Conjugated bilirubin levels are highest in cholestatic disease and in fulminant hepatic failure. Unconjugated hyperbilirubinaemia may reflect haemolysis, neonatal physiological jaundice or genetic defects in bilirubin transport and conjugation (Gilbert's and Crigler-Najjar syndromes). Haemolysis rarely produces total bilirubin levels greater than 50–90 µmol/L.

In acute liver disease, the bilirubin level is of little prognostic significance. On the other hand, rising serum bilirubin levels reflect the approach of end-stage disease in many chronic liver diseases. For example, in primary biliary cirrhosis this signals the need to consider liver transplantation. In secondary malignancy it is often a signal of a preterminal event.

In the presence of chronic liver disease, when hepatic reserve is limited, relatively small increases in bilirubin production (as with haemolysis) can produce a disproportionate increase in serum bilirubin. When there is cholestasis, renal failure will reduce the clearance of conjugated bilirubin sufficiently to increase serum levels. Furthermore, conjugated bilirubin binds irreversibly to albumin such that bound bilirubin will not be cleared until the albumin to which it is bound is catabolised.

Tests reflecting hepatic function

Serum albumin. This protein is a major synthetic product of the liver. Its concentration in the serum is dependent on nutrition, hepatic synthesis and losses (e.g., nephrotic syndrome, protein-losing enteropathy).

In chronic liver disease, low serum albumin concentrations represent a major prognostic indicator (see Child-Pugh score). This can reflect the absence of sufficient functioning hepatocytes to maintain albumin production. Furthermore, malnutrition can be a major contributor to hypoalbuminaemia in patients with chronic liver disease. Alcohol consumption can reduce albumin synthesis. Serum albumin concentrations may also fall without a reduction in hepatic synthesis when the volume of distribution of albumin is expanded by ascites and oedema. As albumin has a half-life of 17–26 days, low levels usually reflect chronic rather than acute hepatic dysfunction.

Prothrombin time or international normalised ratio (INR). As with albumin, the vitamin-K-dependent clotting factors are synthesised by the liver. The plasma concentrations of prothrombin (II) and factors VII, IX and X often fall in the presence of significant liver disease. The prothrombin time assesses the activity of these coagulation factors. The INR is the ratio between the clotting time (in seconds) using the patient's plasma divided by that of a control sample using standardised reagents (normal range: 0.8–1.2).

Because of the relatively short half-life of some of these proteins, abnormalities can develop quickly following the onset of hepatic decompensation. In certain circumstances, this may occur within hours (e.g., fatty liver of pregnancy).

Cholestasis can result in vitamin K malabsorption and, in so doing, lead to a raised INR. In that situation, parenteral vitamin K promptly reverses the abnormality. On the other hand, a raised INR that is unresponsive to vitamin K often suggests significant hepatocellular dysfunction.

In a patient with liver disease who is bleeding, the abnormal clotting may represent direct losses and consumption of clotting factors. Stored blood has no effective clotting factors, and contains anticoagulant. After a large transfusion, the clotting factors must therefore also be replaced by giving fresh frozen plasma.

It should be noted that the INR does not necessarily reflect the severity of chronic liver disease. It may be normal or near normal in the presence of advanced cirrhosis. In fulminant hepatic failure, serial INR measurements are of prognostic value with recovery being more likely if the INR decreases. Prognosis is poor when the INR is greater than 3.

Tests of liver injury

Transaminases. The serum transaminases are best considered as tests of hepatocyte damage or injury. They do not reflect the functional capacity of the liver. Transaminases enter the circulation following hepatocellular lysis. However, sublethal hepatocyte injury can also release these enzymes. Budding of cytoplasm or leakage from breaches in the plasma membrane may occur.

Marked elevations in serum transaminase levels (> 1000 U/L) often reflect acute viral hepatitis. Drug reactions and acute exacerbations of chronic autoimmune hepatitis can produce similar levels. Non-hepatocellular disease, including acute cholestasis, shock and cardiac failure, can also produce substantial rises. Lesser rises in serum transaminases do not, however, exclude the diagnosis of these conditions.

Persistent elevation of serum transaminase levels may indicate significant chronic liver disease, such as chronic viral or autoimmune hepatitis, and require investigation. Thus, treatable diseases can be identified and managed prior to the onset of symptomatic (often end-stage) liver disease.

In the presence of malignant disease, increases in transaminases often indicate hepatic metastases.

Alanine aminotransferase (ALT). ALT is a liver-specific enzyme; thus, an isolated elevation of ALT is highly suggestive of liver disease. Persisting abnormalities should precipitate a search for the cause.

Aspartate aminotransferase (AST). This enzyme is found in liver, skeletal muscle, myocardium, kidney, pancreas and erythrocytes. Damage to any of these cell types will result in an elevation of serum AST. ALT levels are usually higher than AST levels in viral liver injury. When liver disease is present, and the AST level is more than twice that of ALT, alcoholic liver disease must be considered (see later). In the presence of cirrhosis, the diagnostic value of the AST/ALT ratio is lost. The mitochondrial isoenzyme of AST is especially elevated in the presence of alcoholic liver injury.

Alkaline phosphatase (ALP). This enzyme is localised to the biliary membrane of hepatocytes. An elevation of the serum ALP level is a marker of biliary disease or a hepatic infiltrative disorder.

Although cholestasis may be present with a normal ALP level, in three-quarters of patients with cholestasis, serum ALP levels will be three or more times greater than the upper limit of normal (Chapter 21). Mild elevations of hepatic ALP levels are often seen in hepatocellular injury. Serum ALP levels may also be elevated, at times in isolation, in other disorders affecting the liver, including congestive cardiac failure and lymphoma. A mild elevation is often seen in patients with a non-hepatic illness; this returns to normal over a period of weeks to months, after the underlying condition is treated.

ALP is also found in bone, intestine, kidney and placenta. Consequently, damage to these organs will elevate the serum ALP level. Furthermore, during pregnancy and periods of rapid growth (neonatal and adolescent periods), serum levels of this enzyme are higher. When the serum ALP level is elevated in the absence of other abnormalities in the liver function tests, consider a non-hepatic cause, such as Paget's disease, tumour involving bone, acromegaly and fractures. Milder rises in ALP may occur following infarction involving the heart, lung, gastrointestinal tract or kidneys.

5'-Nucleotidase, a membrane-associated enzyme, is elevated in the plasma primarily in cholestatic liver disease. Although present in pancreas, brain, intestine and heart, this enzyme is more specific for liver disorders than is alkaline phosphatase.

Gamma-glutamyl transpeptidase (GGT). This membrane-bound enzyme is present in the liver, pancreas, kidney, intestine and prostate. GGT levels increase with any liver disease. Its greatest value is its association with alkaline phosphatase in cholestatic disorders (Chapter 21). An elevated serum GGT level supports a hepatic origin of an elevated alkaline phosphatase, as serum GGT is not raised in pregnancy or bone disease.

Although a marker of prognostic significance in alcoholic liver disease, not all heavy drinkers will display elevated serum GGT levels. Elevations of the serum levels of this enzyme are associated with biliary disease, pancreatitis, obesity, hyper-lipidaemia, anorexia nervosa, diabetes mellitus, hyperthyroidism, porphyria, myocardial infarction and liver disease in general. Enzyme-inducing drugs, such as barbiturates, tricyclic antidepressants and anticonvulsants, are also associated with elevated serum GGT activity.

The serum levels of this enzyme can be raised in the absence of other liver function test abnormalities in obese individuals, with excessive alcohol consumption and following the use of enzyme-inducing medications.

Lactate dehydrogenase (LDH). This glycolytic enzyme is present in all cells. Different isoenzymes occur with limited tissue specificity, and their measurement is of limited clinical value. However, when the LDH level is elevated out of proportion to the transaminases, ischaemic liver injury and secondary malignancy need to be considered.

Cholestasis versus hepatocellular disease

Liver function test patterns may be used to guide the discrimination between cholestasis (e.g., due to stones or tumour obstructing the large bile ducts) and hepatocellular disease (e.g., cirrhosis or chronic hepatitis). These patterns can only be used as a broad guide and should not be relied on alone (see Figure 21.8 in Chapter 21). However, if cholestasis is suspected, then looking for evidence of duct obstruction (e.g., by ultrasound) is the next step, while if hepatocellular disease is suspected, then a search for liver disease markers (e.g., virology, immunological tests) is the next step.

Other tests useful in hepatic assessment

Alpha-fetoprotein. A marked elevation (> 1000 U/L) of alpha-fetoprotein is most often due to hepatocellular carcinoma. This test is useful in screening an individual with chronic hepatitis B for the development of hepatocellular carcinoma, having a sensitivity of 70%. It is of limited value, however, because the sensitivity falls to 30% in non-hepatitis B hepatocellular carcinoma. Milder elevations occur in both acute and chronic liver disease of many causes.

Autoimmune, metabolic and viral markers. Autoantibodies are helpful in diagnosing certain forms of liver disease (Table 22.2). Serum concentration of caeruloplasmin and iron studies are important tools in the diagnosis of Wilson's disease and haemochromatosis, respectively (Table 22.3), but are also altered by liver injury unrelated to either of these conditions. Tests for viral hepatitis are also important (Table 22.4).

TABLE 22.2: Tests for autoimmune liver disease

Test	Condition	Comment
Antinuclear antibody (ANA)	Autoimmune chronic hepatitis	Diagnosis requires liver biopsy
Smooth muscle antibody (SMA) (anti-actin)	Autoimmune chronic hepatitis	Diagnosis requires liver biopsy
Anti-liver kidney microsomal antibody (anti-LKM1)	Autoimmune chronic hepatitis	Diagnosis requires liver biopsy
Antimitochondrial antibody (AMA)	Primary biliary cirrhosis (95%)	Diagnosis requires liver biopsy
Antineutrophil cytoplasmic antibody (pANCA)	Primary sclerosing cholangitis	Diagnosis requires endoscopic retrograde cholangiopancreatography magnetic resonance or cholangiopancreatography

TABLE 22.3: Tests for metabolic disorders affecting the liver

Test	Condition	Comment
Iron studies	Haemochromatosis	See text
Copper and caeruloplasmin	Wilson's disease	See text
Alpha-1 antitrypsin level and phenotype	Alpha-1 antitrypsin deficiency	Heterozygotes may have abnormal LFTs without significant liver disease
Thyroid function tests	Hypothyroidism	Fatty liver
Blood glucose level	Diabetes mellitus	Fatty liver, haemochromatosis
Insulin / C-peptide	Insulin resistance	Fatty liver, metabolic syndrome
Cholesterol and triglycerides	Primary and secondary hyperlipidaemia	Fatty liver, alcoholic liver disease
LFTs = liver function tests.		

TABLE 22.4: Tests for viral hepatitis

Test	Meaning of a positive result	Comment
1. Tests for hepatitis A virus (HAV)		
Anti-HAV IgM	Recent acquisition of HAV	Acute hepatic illness likely to be HAV
Anti-HAV IgG	Past infection/vaccination	Immunity
2. Tests for hepatitis B virus (HBV)		
HBsAG (surface ag)	Present/chronic infection	Structural component of virus
Anti-HBsAg (surface ab)	Past infection/vaccination	Immunity
Anti-HBc IgM (core ab)	Recent acquisition of HBV	The test for acute HBV infection
HBeAg (e ag)	Marker of viral replication	High risk of infectivity
Anti-HBeAg (e ab)	Suggests no viral replication	Unlikely to be infectious
HBV DNA	Presence of complete virus	High risk of infectivity
3. Tests for hepatitis C virus (HCV)		
Anti-HCV	Exposure to HCV	Interpret in conjunction with other clinical and laboratory data
HCV RNA by PCR	Presence of virus	—
HCV genotyping		Treatment planning and response
4. Tests for hepatitis D virus (HDV)		
Anti-HDV IgG/IgM	Exposure to HDV	Acute or chronic HDV
Delta antigen	HDV present	Acute or chronic HDV
5. Tests for hepatitis E virus (HEV)		
Anti-HEV IgM	Recent acquisition of HEV	Acute hepatitic illness likely to be HEV
6. Tests for other organisms		
Cytomegalovirus (CMV) IgM	Recent acquisition of CMV	Acute hepatitic illness likely to be CMV
Epstein-Barr virus (EBV) IgM	Recent acquisition of EBV	Acute hepatitic illness likely to be EBV
Anti-HIV	HIV-AIDS	Opportunistic hepatobiliary infections
Toxoplasmosis serology	—	Consider toxoplasmosis
Q fever serology	—	Consider Q fever

ag = antigen; ab = antibody; PCR = polymerase chain reaction.

Liver biopsy

Histological and, on occasion, chemical analysis and microbiological examination of the liver are essential in the diagnosis of many hepatic disorders. The usual technique for obtaining a liver biopsy involves a percutaneous approach through a lower intercostal space in the right mid-axillary line. Ultrasound scanning or CT can be used to optimise the needle entry point or target specific abnormalities. Haemorrhage from the biopsy wound to the liver or injury to adjacent organs are the major risks. These may be significant in approximately 1% of biopsies. The risk of haemorrhage is minimised by ensuring a platelet count greater than 80×10^9/L (80,000/mm^3) and an INR less than 1.2. When coagulopathy or gross ascites prevents a percutaneous biopsy, a transjugular approach can be used.

The decision to proceed to liver biopsy is reached when the potential information gained outweighs the risks of the procedure. In particular, obtaining information about the patient's prognosis or diagnostic information that might alter therapy is the important consideration. Although it is not always appropriate to perform a liver biopsy to only achieve a diagnosis, it is not unusual for the clinical diagnosis to be altered by the information gained at biopsy. The clinical course of the illness should also be considered. The patient with improving liver function test profiles and resolving symptoms is probably best observed rather than biopsied early. It should be noted, however, that in certain conditions such as chronic hepatitis C and haemochromatosis and in some alcoholic patients, hepatic fibrosis can progress to cirrhosis with little clinical or laboratory evidence of aggressive liver disease.

The significance of liver biopsy features is considered in relation to specific disorders later in this chapter. The extent, nature and activity of inflammatory and fibrotic processes are of particular concern. The presence of fibro-inflammatory changes is more likely to be related to a progression to cirrhosis. The absence of such changes carries a better prognosis.

THE WELL PATIENT WITH ABNORMAL LIVER FUNCTION PROFILE

Many patients now present to their practitioner apparently in good health but with an abnormal set of liver function test results, often found at routine insurance medical examination. These patients raise a whole range of diagnostic possibilities and, in evaluating them, a full history and examination is required. The most common causes of abnormal liver function test results in otherwise well individuals are non-alcoholic fatty disease (which may or may not be associated with significant inflammation) and alcohol-related liver damage. Another common cause will be the ingestion of medications. However, the presence of other serious, progressive and eventually potentially life-threatening conditions needs to be considered.

History

All patients with abnormal liver function test results need to be questioned about their family history of liver disease, and their ingestion currently or in the past of alcohol and medications.

A history of diabetes mellitus, thyroid disease and high lipid levels should be sought; these together with obesity are associated with hepatic steatosis. The features of the metabolic syndrome with rising body weight and reduced physical activity are common in those with non-alcoholic fatty liver disease, especially when there is a family history of Type 2 diabetes.

A history of overseas travel and exposure to blood products from transfusions or injection of drugs, legally or illegally, needs to be sought (e.g., hepatitis B or C). A history of known exposure to patients with infectious liver diseases should be asked about. A sexual history must be obtained because exposure to some viruses is much more common in individuals with multiple sexual partners (e.g., hepatitis B, HIV).

When there is a family history of liver disease, social background requires close review. 'Learned' excessive alcohol consumption can lead to liver disease without the patient being aware that their intake is potentially dangerous. The amount of alcohol the 'social drinker' consumes varies according to his or her background. There is a possibility of genetic predisposition to alcoholic liver disease.

Migration from areas of high prevalence of hepatitis B or C (e.g., South East Asia) should be noted. These viruses, acquired at birth or in early childhood, may not generate symptoms for many years.

Haemochromatosis is preferably diagnosed prior to the onset of symptoms; abnormalities of liver function tests and abnormal iron study findings are clues. However, a history of joint pains, diabetes mellitus, cardiac disease or impotence in the patient or the existence of an affected relative suggests the possibility of haemochromatosis.

Wilson's disease is likely to be asymptomatic only in younger children. At older ages, features of cirrhosis or neurological abnormalities are likely. A homozygote or heterozygote for alpha-1 antitrypsin deficiency may present with the incidental finding of abnormal liver function profiles in an otherwise well patient.

In the otherwise well patient, a history of abdominal pain (e.g., biliary pain; Chapter 21), loss of appetite or weight (Chapter 15), or a change in the colour of stools or urine (Chapter 21) needs to be sought, but is almost invariably absent.

Examination

Patients with abnormal liver test results must be regarded as having a liver disorder and thus signs of chronic liver disease should be sought because cirrhosis may be completely asymptomatic (Figure 22.1). The patient's weight and height should be measured during the examination to allow evaluation of the body mass index (weight in kilograms divided by the square of the height in metres: kg/m^2). Truncal obesity is common and waist measurement should be taken.

There should be an examination for signs of acute liver disease because the patient may be in the prodromal phase of a viral hepatitis (e.g., jaundice, encephalopathy).

In the usual patient presenting with no history of symptoms and no awareness of liver problems, it is likely that there will be no signs of liver disease. A minor degree of hepatomegaly should be expected in patients with alcohol-related fatty liver or non-alcoholic fatty liver disease. Mild splenomegaly may also be seen.

Investigation

The approach to investigations is guided by the history, examination and liver function test pattern. Further testing is based on the provisional diagnosis and likely prognosis. When no hints as to the diagnosis have been found, a systematic investigation for potentially dangerous causes of liver disease needs to be considered. This would normally be done after a period of observation with serial liver function tests to determine whether there is a spontaneous recovery, a stable abnormality or deterioration.

Liver imaging is of value (Chapters 21 and 23). Abdominal ultrasound scans can provide information about the size and shape of the liver and spleen. Often any mass lesions present can also be identified. Ultrasonography will often detect fatty liver. Abdominal CT will provide information on the presence or absence of space-occupying lesions while, in addition, providing insight into liver density, which may be increased in haemochromatosis.

Tests for evidence of viral hepatitis (Table 22.4), autoimmune liver disease (Table 22.2) and other causes of chronic liver disease (iron or copper overload, and other inherited liver diseases) (Table 22.3) should be done if hepatocellular disease is possible. A liver biopsy is required if the diagnosis remains unclear and the prognosis is of concern.

Chronic hepatitis is an ongoing inflammatory process. The causes are listed in Table 22.5. If fibrosis follows as part of the healing process consequent to this inflammation, progression to cirrhosis and eventual liver failure is possible. For this reason, potentially controllable chronic hepatitis needs to be identified and treated before irreversible injury has occurred.

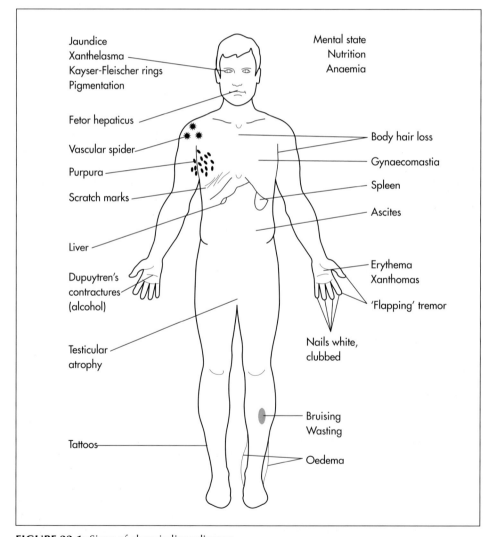

FIGURE 22.1: Signs of chronic liver disease.

(Based on Sherlock S & Dooley J, Diseases of the liver and biliary system, 11th edn, Oxford: Blackwell, 2002, with permission.)

In each of the conditions generating chronic hepatitis there is an ongoing inflammatory attack directed towards the hepatocyte. This can be the result of direct hepatocyte injury, as is the case in hepatitis C infection, the most common cause of chronic hepatitis in Australia, and Wilson's disease, which is rare. On the other hand, liver cell injury may be immune-mediated, as occurs with hepatitis B infection, autoimmune chronic hepatitis and certain drug reactions.

TABLE 22.5: Important causes of chronic hepatitis and cirrhosis	
Chronic hepatitis	**Cirrhosis**
• Hepatitis C virus	• Alcohol
• Hepatitis B virus	• Hepatitis C and B
• Autoimmune	• Drugs (as for chronic hepatitis)
• Drug induced	• Non-alcoholic steatohepatitis (fatty liver disease)
• Wilson's disease	• Primary sclerosing cholangitis
• Alpha-1 antitrypsin deficiency	• Primary biliary cirrhosis
	• Haemochromatosis
	• Wilson's disease
	• Chronic constrictive pericarditis
	• Alpha-1 antitrypsin deficiency
	• Idiopathic (cryptogenic)

Evidence of continuing hepatic inflammation based on a persistent elevation of serum transaminases ($\geq$ 6 months) is usually required to entertain the diagnosis of chronic hepatitis. However, it can take many months for serum transaminases to return to normal levels following some acute hepatic illnesses. Once the presence of chronic hepatitis is considered likely, establish the aetiology of the illness, the extent of liver damage and the activity of the inflammatory process. These latter two features can only be assessed by histological examination of a liver biopsy.

THE SICK PATIENT WITH JAUNDICE: ACUTE LIVER DISEASE

Acute hepatitis

History

Acute hepatitis of any cause can present with similar clinical features. Typically there is nausea with or without vomiting, right upper quadrant pain, weakness, fever, fatigue, itching and jaundice. An acute icteric illness may follow infection with one of the hepatitis viruses (see below). A similar clinical picture may be seen in Epstein-Barr virus (EBV) and cytomegalovirus (CMV) infections, in toxoplasmosis and occasionally in other viral infections. Viral exposure is suggested by parenteral risk factors such as intravenous drug use, tattooing, intimate contacts with hepatitic patients, blood transfusion, travel to endemic areas and during local epidemics. Acute autoimmune disease is suggested by the presence of other autoimmune disorders (e.g., thyroid disease). A careful and complete drug history is vital. Both recently commenced drugs and those taken for prolonged periods should be considered. In patients showing evidence of depressive behaviour, drug overdose must be considered. If paracetamol (acetaminophen) has been used, then a careful ethanol consumption history is vital. Normally safe, therapeutic doses of paracetamol may produce significant liver injury in those chronically consuming excessive amounts of ethanol. Excessive ethanol consumption, especially recent bingeing, could indicate acute alcoholic hepatitis. Gallstone disease can occasionally present as an acute hepatic illness that can be difficult to differentiate clinically. A family history of liver disease should be noted. Wilson's disease may present as an acute illness, usually in childhood.

Acute hepatitis may occur in a previously well person or in the presence of underlying chronic liver disease. In the latter case, the result can be devastating when pre-existing liver disease results in little functional hepatic reserve. In pregnancy, acute viral hepatitis is the most common cause of this syndrome, but consideration should be given to pregnancy-related liver disease (see *Liver disease in pregnancy*).

Examination

The patient can appear relatively well or profoundly ill. Jaundice may or may not be present. The liver size is noted. It will often be enlarged and tender. There may be splenomegaly. Look for evidence of an underlying condition (e.g., signs of alcohol excess). Complications (e.g., hepatic encephalopathy) may supervene. Look for signs of chronic liver disease (Figure 22.1).

Investigation

Serum transaminase levels are elevated, usually more than five times the upper limit of normal. In viral hepatitis, transaminase levels ≥ 1000 U/L are not unusual. Moderate elevations of alkaline phosphatase also occur. Serum albumin and INR usually remain normal. Specific blood tests are required to diagnose viral illnesses, including viral hepatitis (A, B, C, D, E; Table 22.4), cytomegalovirus and Epstein-Barr virus, toxoplasmosis, Q fever and autoimmune disease (Table 22.4). Paracetamol levels should be determined and laboratory evidence of alcohol excess sought. Abdominal ultrasound scans are useful to document the size of the liver and spleen and to exclude biliary disease.

Management

Treatment of viral hepatitis is supportive. Patients should be observed to ensure that fulminant hepatic failure (see below) or, with hepatitis C or B, chronic disease does not develop. It may take months for liver function profiles to normalise and liver biopsy should be considered if this does not occur. Absolute exclusion of ethanol is not necessary in the recovery phase.

Offending drugs must be withdrawn. In the case of paracetamol, N-acetylcysteine is administered and close observation maintained over several days, with the patient's clinical status, INR and transaminase levels monitored regularly.

Alcoholic hepatitis is managed supportively although, in certain circumstances, specific interventions may be of value. Alcohol is withdrawn, and vitamin (especially thiamine) and nutritional supplementation should be given (enteral feeding may provide a survival benefit). Corticosteroids (prednisone, 40 mg daily for 28 days) may provide a survival benefit when there is encephalopathy (see below) and no gastrointestinal haemorrhage. Abstinence remains the mainstay of therapy. Propylthiouracil may be of benefit in less severe cases of alcoholic hepatitis, but is rarely used.

When gallstone disease is found to be the cause of an acute hepatitic illness, cholecystectomy may be indicated. Choledocholithiasis may require endoscopic clearance of the bile duct (Chapter 21). Acute autoimmune hepatitis is managed with corticosteroids (e.g., prednisone, 30–60 mg daily, then taper).

FULMINANT HEPATIC FAILURE

Definition

Liver failure occurring in a previously well patient is termed fulminant hepatic failure; hepatic encephalopathy (an organic neurological syndrome) evolves within eight weeks of the onset of the illness. Subfulminant or subacute hepatic failure is used to describe the onset of hepatic decompensation up to 26 weeks after the initial illness. These need to be differentiated from acute hepatic failure evolving in the presence of established chronic liver disease.

History

Enquire about the historical features of acute hepatitis. However, details will need to be obtained from others when the patient has established encephalopathy. Acute infection with the hepatotropic viruses A, B, D or E (and very rarely C) can cause fulminant hepatic failure. In late pregnancy, acute fatty liver should be considered. Ask about drugs, which may cause direct toxic effects (e.g., following overdose of paracetamol) or cause idiosyncratic reactions (e.g., halothane, sulfonamides).

Following an acute overdose of 140 mg/kg or more of paracetamol, the glucuronide and sulfate pathways in the liver become saturated and hepatic glutathione becomes depleted, leading to reactive metabolites covalently binding to liver cells causing lysis. Hepatotoxicity manifests 24–48 hours after ingestion. The early identification of *paracetamol overdose* is crucial. Serum levels should be measured 4 and 24 hours after suspected ingestion; the administration of N-acetylcysteine will prevent progression to hepatic failure. It gives maximal benefit if instituted within 8–10 hours of ingestion (but is indicated for up to 24 hours). An intake of a normally subtoxic dose of paracetamol in the presence of chronic alcohol abuse may lead to acute hepatic failure.

Fluorinated hydrocarbon solvents (from glue sniffing) and mushroom poisoning have also been linked to acute hepatic failure. Wilson's disease may rarely present in acute liver failure, and death usually follows without liver transplantation.

In fulminant hepatic failure there is a sudden loss of functional hepatocyte mass, often associated with portal hypertension. The associated complications of encephalopathy, coagulopathy, renal failure and sepsis evolve. Multi-organ failure often results in the patient's death.

Assessment and management

Examination is directed towards assessing the possible aetiology and evolving complications of hepatic failure (outlined below). Serial liver function tests can be useful, but a falling ALT level may reflect either recovery or progression to massive hepatic necrosis.

Hepatic encephalopathy. This may develop rapidly and may precede the onset of jaundice. The deeper grades (described later) of encephalopathy are associated with a worse prognosis. Unlike the encephalopathy of chronic liver disease, there is often early agitation and delusional ideation. Cerebral oedema, present in up to 80% of those in grade IV encephalopathy, is a major cause of death. Clinically, this is reflected by systemic hypertension, bradycardia with progressive rigidity and decerebrate posturing. Direct pressure monitoring with a subdural or epidural transducer is the only reliable means of assessing cerebral pressure. Cerebral oedema is managed with intravenous mannitol. Prognosis is poor and liver transplantation inappropriate when the cerebral perfusion pressure is less than 50 mmHg, and is refractory to mannitol therapy.

Coagulopathy. Coagulopathy of acute hepatic failure occurs as the result of loss of hepatic synthetic function, sepsis, bleeding and intravascular coagulation. Platelet levels decrease and their function is impaired. Platelet transfusion and fresh frozen plasma can be of value when there is active haemorrhage. The value of these measures in the absence of bleeding is not established.

Hypotension, renal failure and hypoglycaemia. Hypotension is common and renal failure is not unusual. The latter is usually associated with the hepatorenal syndrome. This syndrome represents a functional renal impairment and carries a poor prognosis. Normal renal function returns with recovery or liver transplantation. Acute tubular necrosis secondary to hypotension may also occur in acute hepatic failure. When renal failure does occur, therapy is supportive; dialysis is problematic because of the associated coagulopathy, hypotension and cerebral oedema. N-acetylcysteine may improve oxygen delivery.

In acute liver failure, peripheral circulatory changes lead to impaired oxygen delivery, tissue hypoxia and lactic acidosis (a poor prognostic sign). As the functional hepatocyte mass decreases, the liver is unable to sustain gluconeogenesis, and life-threatening hypoglycaemia follows. Blood sugar levels require close monitoring and are a measure of remaining hepatic function. Ten per cent glucose infusions are usually required. Hypokalaemia (with respiratory alkalosis) and dilutional hyponatraemia may also occur.

Infection. Evidence of infection must be actively sought in any episode of hepatic failure. Multifactorial mechanisms leave these patients prone to severe bacterial and fungal infections. Death will rapidly follow unless aggressive antibiotic therapy, or drainage of pus, if possible, is instituted once the possibility of infection is considered.

The patient with fulminant hepatic failure needs to be admitted directly to a unit capable of offering liver transplantation. Admission to intensive care is required with careful management of cerebral oedema, gastrointestinal bleeding, infection and renal failure.

The prognosis of acute hepatic failure related to paracetamol overdose, hepatitis A viral infection and fatty liver of pregnancy (if there has been prompt delivery) tends to be better than that of other causes. The outcomes appear worst in those in whom the cause is unclear.

Liver transplantation is a therapeutic option. The decision to transplant and the timing of transplantation are difficult. However, survival rates of approximately 60% can be achieved. This compares favourably with mortality rates from fulminant hepatic failure without transplantation of up to 90%.

PATIENTS PRESENTING WITH CIRRHOSIS AND ITS COMPLICATIONS

Cirrhosis represents the non-specific end stage of hepatic disease that has disrupted the structural organisation of the liver. The presence of cirrhosis is established on a liver biopsy. Fibrosis or scarring surrounding regenerative nodules of hepatocytes is its hallmark. Although cirrhosis is a histological diagnosis, its presence is clinically suspected by finding signs of chronic liver disease and portal hypertension (Table 22.1) or on high quality imaging. Symptomatic liver disease and, eventually, liver failure occur as the result of impaired hepatocellular function within the distorted architecture of the regenerative nodules and, with progression, eventual loss of an effective liver cell mass. Distortion of the hepatic circulation contributes to portal hypertension and inefficient/ineffective perfusion of parenchymal cells. Portosystemic shunts may develop allowing blood from the gastrointestinal tract to flow directly to the systemic circulation.

Cirrhosis should be considered as either *compensated,* with no signs of complications and a relatively good prognosis, or *decompensated.* Those with compensated cirrhosis are likely to be asymptomatic and the diagnosis may be made incidentally during the investigation of an unrelated condition. In this situation, counselling regarding diet, alcohol consumption and the identification and management of any underlying treatable condition are warranted (see *The well patient with abnormal liver function profile*). Recent data has indicated that the removal/cure of the underlying disease process can be followed by a reduction in hepatic fibrosis (e.g., after cure of hepatitis C).

The serum levels of liver enzymes (ALT, AST and ALP) can be mildly abnormal or even normal in compensated cirrhosis. However, because of reduced hepatic synthetic function or poor nutrition, the serum albumin concentration is often reduced, and the INR may be increased. There may be thrombocytopaenia related to splenomegaly from portal hypertension. Anaemia can be multifactorial but is often related to gastrointestinal blood loss, poor nutrition (e.g., in alcoholics), chronic disease and hypersplenism.

The Child-Pugh score (Table 22.6) provides a useful means of assessing the severity of cirrhosis and the prognosis. A Child-Pugh 'A' classification applies to a score of less than 7; 'B', a score between 7 and 9; and 'C', greater than 9. The one-year survival of these classification groups is 100%, 80% and 45%, respectively. A higher score also indicates those more likely to succumb to complications during hepatic and non-hepatic surgical procedures.

	TABLE 22.6: Child-Pugh score				
Score	**Serum albumin (g/L)**	**Serum bilirubin (µmol/L)**	**Prothrombin time (seconds prolonged)**	**Ascites**	**Encephalopathy**
1	> 35	< 35	1–3	Nil	Nil
2	28–35	35–51	4–6	Slight	Grade 1–2
3	< 28	> 51	> 6	Moderate	Grade 3–4

An alternative chronic liver disease severity score (called the model for end-stage liver disease, or MELD) has been developed.

MELD = 3.8 [$\log_e$ serum bilirubin (mg/dL)] + 11.2 [$\log_e$ INR] + 9.6 [$\log_e$ serum creatinine (mg/dL)] + 6.4.

The higher the score, the worse the prognosis. The MELD score is used to help priortise allocation of liver transplantation, for predicting mortality in chronic liver disease and alcoholic hepatitis, and for those being considered for transjugular intrahepatic partosystemic shunting (TIPS).

THE WELL PATIENT WITH CIRRHOSIS

History

Patients with cirrhosis may be asymptomatic, coming to medical attention following an incidental finding of abnormal laboratory tests or physical findings suggestive of chronic liver disease.

Such patients should be assessed to determine the likely aetiology as outlined in *The well patient with abnormal liver function profile*. Attention should be directed to identifying evidence of ongoing hepatic injury that may be modified by therapeutic intervention. A careful history of exposure to alcohol, drugs and potential hepatotropic agents (e.g., solvents) is required. Restricting exposure may help slow progression. Risk factors for exposure to hepatitis B and C viruses and family history of liver disease should be assessed.

Examination

Physical examination includes a search for signs of chronic liver disease (Table 22.1) and evidence of extrahepatic features of possible aetiological factors.

Investigation

Investigations are directed to determining the aetiology of the cirrhosis (Table 22.5) and assessing the severity of hepatic injury. When physical findings and investigations suggest cirrhosis, liver biopsy should be considered to establish its presence, to assess the activity of the fibroinflammatory process and to seek evidence of the aetiology. A past history of excessive alcohol consumption is often identified. In other cases, a specific aetiology can often be established by using special tests for autoantibodies, viral serology and metabolic disorders (Tables 22.2, 22.3 and 22.4). Elevations in serum transaminase levels imply ongoing hepatocellular injury. Prolonged prothrombin time and hypoalbuminaemia suggest reduced hepatocellular synthetic function. Abdominal ultrasound scans with Doppler studies will provide evidence of portal hypertension (splenomegaly, portal flow and wave pattern), ascites, and liver size (reflecting remaining liver cell mass).

Management

The management of the well cirrhotic patient depends on the underlying cause. The patient with alcoholic cirrhosis should cease drinking completely. Failure to do so is likely to cause progression and early death. Abstinence, on the other hand, can allow a long and productive life, despite the cirrhosis. Cirrhotic patients with autoimmune chronic hepatitis and significant inflammation on biopsy could benefit from corticosteroid therapy. Interferon is of limited benefit, and potentially dangerous in those with cirrhosis due to chronic hepatitis B. Lamivudine, on the other hand, may be of value. Counselling of the patient and, if necessary, family members is required when infectious or genetic conditions are identified. Regular screening for hepatocellular carcinoma should be considered.

Apart from any treatment associated with the underlying cause, the asymptomatic patient with cirrhosis needs to maintain an adequate diet. Sufficient kilojoules, protein and micronutrients should be ingested. A complex carbohydrate snack before retiring in the evenings could help prevent the patient from becoming catabolic overnight as the hepatic glycogen stores become depleted. Regular follow-up is necessary, specifically seeking evidence of evolving complications of cirrhosis (namely, portal hypertension and ascites, portal vein thrombosis, spontaneous bacterial peritonitis, hepatic encephalopathy, hepatorenal syndrome and hepatocellular carcinoma).

COMPLICATIONS OF PORTAL HYPERTENSION IN THE PATIENT WITH CHRONIC LIVER DISEASE

Portal hypertension

In cirrhosis, the disturbed architecture of the liver and perivascular fibrosis increase the resistance of portal blood flow. Portal pressure is also increased due to sodium retention and expansion of the blood volume that follows the peripheral vasodilatation of cirrhosis. Cirrhotic patients suffer the combined effects of hepatocellular dysfunction and portal hypertension. Although cirrhosis is the most common cause, primary liver disease is not the only basis for portal hypertension.

Portal and hepatic vascular disorders can also cause portal hypertension while leaving hepatocyte function relatively intact (Table 22.7). In these situations when liver cell function is maintained, portosystemic shunt surgery, rather than transplantation, may be appropriate for severe disease (Figures 22.2A and 22.2B). When vascular or thrombotic processes are found, an underlying cause for these should be sought and managed accordingly.

TABLE 22.7: Classification of causes of portal hypertension

---

1. Intrahepatic sinusoidal—cirrhosis
2. Presinusoidal (the portal vein end: liver function is largely unimpaired):
   a. Extrahepatic, e.g., neonatal sepsis, hypercoagulable blood disease
   b. Intrahepatic, e.g., lymphoma, schistosomiasis
3. Postsinusoidal (the hepatic vein end):
   a. Budd-Chiari syndrome and inferior vena cava obstruction
   b. Veno-occlusive disease (small hepatic veins injured by bush teas, drugs, e.g., azathioprine)

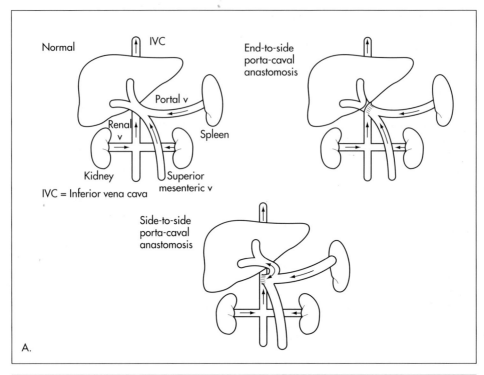

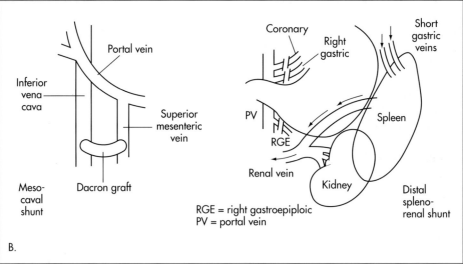

FIGURES 22.2A AND B: Portosystemic shunts. The operation aims to reduce portal pressure. Options include (A) porta-caval (end-to-side or side-to-side); (B) meso-caval (using a Dacron graft between the superior mesenteric vein and inferior vena cava) and distal splenorenal shunts (where veins feeding varices are ligated and a splenorenal vein shunt is created, preserving portal blood flow to the liver). Complications include hepatic encephalopathy (20–40%), ankle oedema, deterioration in hepatic function and shunt closure. The choice usually depends on local surgical expertise: if there is no ascites, a distal splenorectal shunt may be preferable; if ascites is present a side-to-side porta-caval shunt may be most optimal.

(Based on Sherlock S & Dooley J, Diseases of the liver and biliary system, *11th edn. Oxford: Blackwell, 2002, with permission.)*

Acute upper gastrointestinal haemorrhage in the patient with portal hypertension

History

In patients with chronic liver disease, acute gastrointestinal bleeding, especially upper gastrointestinal haemorrhage, should raise concern of a lesion consequent to portal hypertension. Oesophageal varices and portal hypertensive gastropathy are common causes.

Approximately two-thirds of cirrhotic patients develop varices and about one-third of these bleed.

Variceal haemorrhages are usually of large volume, presenting with fresh haematemesis, melaena and shock (Chapter 9). Small amounts of overt blood loss without haemodynamic changes are unlikely to be variceal in origin. Bleeding from portal hypertensive gastropathy may be slow, presenting with iron deficiency anaemia, or may be sufficient to produce overt haematemesis and melaena.

It must also be noted that peptic ulceration and other causes of upper gastrointestinal haemorrhage are also relatively common in cirrhotic patients and history should be directed to consider these conditions as well (Chapter 9).

Bleeding is a medical emergency and history should be directed to the assessment of the amount of blood loss and the probable underlying cause.

Examination

Assessment of the physical signs of blood volume loss is vital (Chapter 9). Signs of chronic liver disease (Table 22.1) support the possibility of cirrhosis and variceal bleeding. Splenomegaly suggests portal hypertension. In acute-on-chronic liver disease, the liver may be palpable and tender. The cirrhotic liver is likely to be small. Blood in the gastrointestinal tract can precipitate encephalopathy in cirrhotic patients. This should be sought and documented. There should be a search for signs of other complications of chronic liver disease including ascites and sepsis.

The chest should be carefully examined for evidence of aspiration, especially in alcoholic patients.

Investigations

Basic haematological investigations and INR are required as with any gastrointestinal haemorrhage (Chapter 9). When chronic liver disease is present, particular attention is paid to the factors of the Child-Pugh score (above). Electrolyte disturbances are not uncommon. Renal function must be checked (see hepatorenal syndrome). The source of the upper gastrointestinal haemorrhage is demonstrated by upper gastrointestinal endoscopy as soon as is practical.

Management

Significant upper gastrointestinal haemorrhage requires urgent resuscitation. Once this is achieved, endoscopy can be used to confirm and often control the source of bleeding. Acute variceal bleeding is usually controlled endoscopically by banding acutely. The long-acting somatostatin analogue, octreotide, provides an effective pharmacological means of managing acute variceal haemorrhage. This agent is often used to complement endoscopic therapy or to achieve control of blood loss while endoscopy is being arranged. A bolus dose of 50 μg is given intravenously, followed by an infusion of 50 μg/h for 24–48 hours. When endoscopic therapy is unavailable or not possible, balloon tamponade applied at the cardio-oesophageal junction can be used to control bleeding from oesophageal varices for up to 24 hours. Gastric varices respond to endoscopic glue injection.

Transjugular intrahepatic portosystemic shunting (TIPS) or surgical portosystemic shunting may be considered to control variceal bleeding when endoscopic therapy fails. TIPS involves the introduction of expandable metal stents between the portal and hepatic venous system, within the liver, placed under radiological control.

In cirrhotic patients, an acute surgical shunt has a high mortality. The risk is directly related to the Child-Pugh score. Apart from portosystemic shunting, acute surgical alternatives include transection of the oesophagus.

Liver transplantation should be considered in suitable patients with cirrhosis in the long term. When liver cell function is well preserved (as in non-cirrhotic portal hypertension), portosystemic shunting may be a viable alternative (Figure 22.2). The long-term value of the shunting procedures is questionable and careful case selection is essential.

Varices may occur anywhere in the gastrointestinal tract. Bleeding from these lesions may also be managed endoscopically if they are accessible, but surgical treatment could be required.

Prognosis

The prognosis of cirrhotic patients with an acute variceal haemorrhage is determined by their hepatic reserve. Three episodes of major variceal bleeding during a single admission is usually fatal. Once the acute haemorrhage is controlled, serial banding is performed until the oesophageal varices are obliterated. Recurrence of the varices is not unusual. Non-selective beta-adrenergic blockers, such as propranolol, may be used to reduce the chance of bleeding from oesophageal varices. A dose sufficient to reduce resting heart rate by 20–25% is effective in reducing rebleeding rates by 40%.

Prophylaxis

Not all varices bleed. However, endoscopically screening cirrhotic patients for varices has been recommended, so that primary prophylactic therapy can be instituted. Smaller varices do not necessarily require intervention. However, the larger the varices, the greater the chance of bleeding. The prophylactic use of non-selective beta-adrenergic blockers, such as propranolol, has also been shown to reduce the risk of an initial or subsequent haemorrhage, especially in those with medium to large varices or more severe portal hypertension. Endoscopic band ligation reduces the risk of variceal haemorrhage and mortality versus no intervention. Data comparing banding with beta-blocker therapy remain conflicting. Currently, for primary prophylaxis, beta-blocker therapy (e.g., propranolol) is considered first choice.

ASCITES IN THE CIRRHOTIC PATIENT

The accumulation of fluid in the peritoneal cavity is a common feature of decompensating chronic liver disease (Figure 22.3). Ascites occurs in 50% of previously compensated cirrhotic patients over a 10-year period. This complication marks a poor prognosis with a two-year survival of 50%.